Youth Gambling

Edited by Jeffrey Derevensky, Daniel T. L. Shek, Joav Merrick

Health, Medicine and Human Development

Edited by

Joav Merrick

Health is a key component of human development, growth, and quality of life. The *Health, Medicine and Human Development* book series aims to provide a public forum for book publications from a multidisciplinary group of researchers, practitioners, and clinicians for an international professional forum interested in the broad spectrum of health, medicine, and human development. We welcome research on a wide variety of substantive areas that will promote and impact healthy human development, including prevention, intervention, and care among people in vulnerable conditions.

GEOR-BK
$178.90

Youth Gambling

The Hidden Addiction

Edited by
Jeffrey Derevensky, Daniel T. L. Shek, Joav Merrick

DE GRUYTER

Editors
Jeffrey Derevensky
International Centre for Youth Gambling Problems and High-Risk Behaviors
McGill University
Montreal, Canada
jeffrey.derevensky@mcgill.ca

Daniel T.L. Shek
Department of Applied Social Sciences
The Hong Kong Polytechnic University
Hunghom, Hong Kong
daniel.shek@polyu.edu.hk

Joav Merrick
Ministry of Social Affairs
Health Services—Division for Intellectual and Developmental Disabilities
Jerusalem, Israel
jmerrick@zahav.net.il

ISBN 978-3-11-025520-1
e-ISBN 978-3-11-025569-0

Library of Congress Cataloging-in-Publication Data

Youth gambling : the hidden addiction / edited by Jeffrey Derevensky, Daniel T.L. Shek, and Joav Merrick.
    p. ; cm. — (Health, medicine and human development)
    Includes bibliographical references and index.
    ISBN 978-3-11-025520-1 (alk. paper)
    1. Youth—Gambling.   2. Teenage gamblers—Psychology.   3. Compulsive gambling—Treatment.   4. Adolescent psychology.   I. Derevensky, Jeffrey L.   II. Shek, Daniel T. L.   III. Merrick, Joav, 1950-   IV. Series: Health, medicine, and human development.
    [DNLM: 1. Gambling—psychology.   2. Gambling—therapy.   3. Adolescent.   4. Risk Factors. WM 190.5.I6]
    RJ506.O25Y68 2011
    616.85'84100835—dc23   2011021905

Bibliographic information published by the Deutsche Nationalbibliothek
The Deutsche Nationalbibliothek lists this publication in the Deutsche Nationalbibliografie; detailed bibliographic data are available in the Internet at http://dnb.d-nb.de.

Typesetting: Apex CoVantage
Printing: Hubert & Co. GmbH & Co. KG, Göttingen
Cover image: iStockphoto/Thinkstock

⊗ Printed on acid-free paper
Printed in Germany
www.degruyter.com

Contents

CORRELATES, RISK, AND PROTECTIVE FACTORS ASSOCIATED WITH YOUTH GAMBLING

4 Youth problem gambling: Our current knowledge of risk and protective factors

TREATING YOUTH PROBLEM GAMBLERS

PREVENTION INITIATIVES

Foreword

Out of the shadows but still hidden

*"Good judgment comes from experience, and often experience
comes from bad judgment"* (Rita Mae Brown)

Since I first got involved with the treatment and study of intemperate gambling almost 40 years ago, a fledgling field has emerged, with all of the attendant cottage industry features well known to more mature areas of interest. During the early years, my colleagues, friends, and the public alike had little interest in gambling-related research. There was little interest in the treatment of pathological gambling, in part, because the public thought that gamblers were responsible for their suffering. After all, they did not have to gamble. Now, intemperate gambling and gambling disorders are starting to appear on the public health and public policy radar screen. Gambling proprietors must take notice and include responsible gambling programs as part of their industry at every level. The volume of scientific and scholarly research has increased exponentially (1,2). Gambling specific treatment programs are emerging, and existing programs that focus on alcohol and other drug addiction are beginning to integrate gambling focused clinical activities into their assessment and treatment protocols.

What happened?

During the late 20th century, there was a paradigm shift. Instead of viewing gambling as an individually motivated and potentially harmful decision, the public began to recognize that exposure and access to gambling had expanded and touched the experience of most people in developed nations. The dramatic expansion of gambling raised public awareness. New gamblers suffered at a higher rate compared to more experienced gamblers, and younger gamblers evidenced more gambling-related problems compared to their more senior gambling counterparts. At about the same time, a new public health perspective was being promulgated (3-7); this view emerged on the heels of the first epidemiological studies that focused on gambling (8-9). The confluence of these events led to a new vantage point. Observers could now consider population trends as well as the risks and protective factors that might be associated with various population segments. Finally, with the various preliminary pieces in place, new research began to focus the public's attention on youth gambling (10-23). This body of work surprised many observers who did not expect that so many young people were involved with gambling activities, excessively involved with gambling activities for money and, as a result, suffered gambling–related problems. For many young people these problems were similar to their adult counterparts; for others, these problems were uniquely associated with their experience as a young person. These studies and events ignited interest and coalesced gambling proponents and opponents alike to prevent youth from illegal and underage gambling, that is, age-restricted forms of gambling. This clarion call echoed around the world and efforts began to develop primary, secondary and tertiary prevention programs – with most of the emphasis going toward primary prevention programs. For example, DiClemente, Story, and Murray (24) offered perspective about how young people begin gambling and the path that they take to stop excessive gambling; newer research reveals, to the surprise of some, that young people were more resilient than expected and could adapt successfully to the presence of gambling in their environment (25,26).

Stimulated by this new and growing interest, the field of gambling studies was bifurcating (2). Stakeholders were beginning to distinguish the study of gambling from the study of gambling-related addiction. This circumstance led to perplexity and controversy as interested parties began to enter into a sometimes confusing debate about gambling when the discussion should have been about gambling disorders. Complicating this situation even more, the stakeholders had to sort out the potential differences that might be associated with 1) preventing youth from adult gambling, 2) the need for adolescent specific assessment strategies (20), and 3) clinical issues that were central to the treatment of adolescents but less important for adults (27). Clinical researchers are still identifying the important differences between youth and adult gambling prevention, assessment and treatment.

"Youth comes but once in a lifetime" (Henry Wadsworth Longfellow)

It is essential that public health workers develop primary and secondary prevention programs that can help young people avoid or limit addiction. The evidence is very clear that adolescence is a developmental period susceptible to a variety of expressions of addiction – and intemperate gambling is no exception. Further, when young people develop these problems, they are likely to struggle with them longer and suffer more, and often different, adverse consequences than their adult counterparts who develop the same kinds of problems later in life. Effective primary prevention diminishes the need for adult treatment later. Obviously, avoiding problems also holds important social and economic benefits for the community and the individual. To develop optimally targeted prevention programs, however, we must know something about the young people who are most at risk for developing gambling–related problems. Other than knowing that the typical age-related perils of youth (e.g., impulsivity, risk-taking, peer pressure) are associated with a period of increased vulnerability, it is very difficult to determine with confidence and scientific certainty who is specifically at-risk for developing addiction, in general, and intemperate gambling problems in particular.

Identifying the distinguishable features of disordered gamblers is a thorny diagnostic problem of considerable importance; it also is a prevention problem of extraordinary significance. If we cannot identify the unique features of those who suffer with gambling disorders, how can we effectively diagnose them or target programs to prevent these behaviors. This set of identification and classification difficulties falls within the domain of taxometrics.

"Youth is a quality, not a matter of circumstances" (Frank Lloyd Wright)

Taxometrics is a statistical procedure for determining whether there is a relationship among gambling characteristics (e.g., extent of gambling, intensity of gambling, type of gambling, etc.) that permit observers to identify a distinct group (i.e., taxon) of gamblers (i.e., disordered gamblers) from the broad group of recreational gamblers. Ever since the Diagnostic and Statistical Manual of Mental Disorders (DSM) first included pathological gambling as a diagnostic classification (28), interested stakeholders have presumed that identifying excessive gamblers was a straightforward task – just apply the diagnostic criteria. Unfortunately, not all of the current DSM criteria (29) distinguish pathological gamblers from their recreational gambling counterparts (30), making early identification, screening and diagnosis a difficult and complicated task.

The title of the present book "Youth gambling: The hidden addiction", reflects an identification problem that prevention and treatment efforts must solve. More specifically, once gambling disorders entered the diagnostic nosology, observers began to assume that people with this disorder evidenced different characteristics compared to those without this disorder. Observers assumed that they could distinguish disordered gamblers from recreational gamblers because these patterns of gambling were qualitatively and, therefore, perceptibly different. New research, however, raises important questions about this matter. For example, Braverman and Shaffer conducted the first taxometric study of Internet sports gamblers (31). This research failed to identify a unique taxon or group of heavy gamblers (as defined by total amount wagered, total number of bets, average bet size, duration of betting, frequency of betting, number of bets per day, total amount lost, and percent lost), who were characteristically different from other gamblers. Absent qualitative differences, it is likely that, similar to many other patterns of behavior, gamblers reside on a continuum. They engage in the same behaviors as recreational gamblers, but just participate in these behaviors more (e.g., frequently, intensely, financially). Consequently, it is difficult for lay and professional observers to determine with precision who is and who is not struggling with a gambling disorder. Where do we draw the line along these dimensions?

This classification problem is particularly magnified for youth, in part, because they have been gambling for less time compared to their adult counterparts. Without the qualitative features to guide an identification process, prevention efforts become even more difficult than usual. It is difficult for public health programs to target high risk and vulnerable population segments. Like other expressions of addiction (32,33), pathological gambling reflects multifactorial etiology (e.g., genetic, psychological, and social influences). This circumstance increases the already difficult task of identifying gambling disorders or those who are at risk for developing such problems. Consequently, there is a tendency to view this disorder as "hidden." However, it is more than hidden, it is often invisible, because gambling-related addiction lacks distinguishing features. Complicating matters even more for young people is that many of the characteristics of adolescence (e.g., impulsivity and risk-taking) are indistinguishable from the very attributes that clinicians might associate with a gambling-related disorder. The qualities of youth often camouflage the features of a gambling disorder. Taken together, whether hidden, invisible, or camouflaged, it is very difficult to identify young people who have gambling-related disorders or are particularly vulnerable to the development of such a disorder.

The difficulties associated with discriminating youth gambling problems are many; however, I am sanguine that these problems can be solved. It is likely that we can develop the skills necessary to identify youth gambling disorders. I am confident that we can develop the prevention and treatment programs that young people need and deserve. However, to do so, we must begin to look in the right places. It is likely that clinicians and scientists will have to look in places other than the usual ones to find answer to these vexing problems. We need more prospective incidence studies and fewer prevalence studies; we need more studies targeting risk and resilience; we need to better understand the relationship of gambling to the characteristics of developmental psychopathology; we need to better understand what gambling does for young people instead of what it does to them; most of all, we need to examine our assumptions that have limited our ability to see youth gambling problems and kept them hidden.

"Youth gambling: The hidden addiction" represents an important step along the path toward a better understanding of young people and their gambling. This volume is an essential component of our efforts to advance knowledge, address the important issues associated with youth gambling, and to facilitate the development and implementation of new youth oriented prevention and treatment efforts. Derevensky, Shek, and Merrick deserve our collective thanks for assembling a distinguished group of contributors.

Howard J Shaffer, PhD
Division on Addictions, The Cambridge Health Alliance,
Harvard Medical School,
   101 StationLanding, Medford, MA 02155
   United States.
   E-mail: howard_shaffer@hms.harvard.edu

References

1. Eber GB, Shaffer HJ. Trends in bio-behavioral gambling studies research: Quantifying citations. J Gambl Stud 2000;16(4):461-7.
2. Shaffer HJ, Stanton MV, Nelson SE. Trends in gambling studies research: Quantifying, categorizing, and describing citations. J Gambl Stud 2006;22(4):427-42.
3. Korn DA, Shaffer HJ. Gambling and the health of the public: Adopting a public health perspective. J Gambl Stud 1999;15(4):289-365.
4. Korn DA, Skinner HA. Gambling expansion in Canada: An emerging public health issue. CPHA Health Digest 2000;XXIV:10.
5. Shaffer HJ. A public health perspective on gambling: The four principles. AGA Responsible Gaming Lecture Series 2003;2(1):1-27.
6. Shaffer HJ, Kidman R. Gambling and the public health. In: Grant JE, Potenza MN, eds. Pathological gambling: A clinical guide to treatment. Washington, DC: American Psychiatric Publishing, 2004:3-23.
7. Shaffer HJ, Korn DA. Gambling and related mental disorders: A public health analysis. In: Fielding JE, Brownson RC, Starfield B, eds. Ann Rev Public Health 2002;23:171-212.
8. Kallick-Kaufmann M. The micro and macro dimensions of gambling in the United States. J Soc Issues 1979;35(3):7-26.
9. Volberg RA. The prevalence and demographics of pathological gamblers: Implications for public health. Am J Public Health 1994;84:237-41.
10. Derevensky JL, Gupta R. Prevalence estimates of adolescent gambling: A comparison of the SOGS-RA, DSM-IV-J, and the GA 20 Questions. J Gambl Stud 2000;16(2-3):227-51.
11. Fisher S. Measuring pathological gambling in children: The case of fruit machines in the U.K. J Gambl Stud 1992;8(3):263-85.
12. Govoni R, Rupcich N, Frisch G. Gambling behavior of adolescent gamblers. J Gambl Stud 1996;12(3):305-17.

13. Gupta R, Derevensky JL. Adolescents with gambling problems: From research to treatment. J Gambl Stud 2000;16(2-3):315-42.
14. Jacobs DF. Illegal and undocumented: A review of teenage gambling and the plight of children of problem gamblers in America. In: Shaffer HJ, Stein S, Gambino B, Cummings TN, eds. Compulsive gambling: Theory, research and practice. Lexington, MA: Lexington Books, 1989:249-92.
15. Kearney CA, Roblek T, Thurman J, Turnbough PD. Casino gambling in private school and adjudicated youngsters: A survey of practices and related variables. J Gambl Stud 1996;12(3):319-27.
16. Lesieur HR, Heineman M. Pathological gambling among youthful multiple substance abusers in a therapeutic community. Br J Addict 1988;83(7):765-71.
17. Saunders CS. Straight talk about teenage gambling. New York: Facts on File, 1999.
18. Shaffer HJ, George EM, Cummings T. North American think tank on youth gambling issues: A blueprint for responsible public policy in the management of compulsive gambling. Boston, MA: Harvard Medical School, 1995.
19. Shaffer HJ, Hall MN, Vander Bilt J. Estimating the prevalence of disordered gambling behavior in the United States and Canada: A research synthesis. Am J Public Health 1999;89:1369-76.
20. Shaffer HJ, Hall MN, Vander Bilt J, George E, eds. Youth, gambling and society: Futures at stake. Reno, NV: University of Nevada Press, 2003.
21. Stinchfield R. Gambling and correlates of gambling among Minnesota public school students. J Gambl Stud 2000;16(2-3):153-73.
22. Winters KC, Stinchfield RD, Kim LG. Monitoring adolescent gambling in Minnesota. J Gambl Stud 1995;11(2):165-83.
23. Zitzow D. Comparative study of problematic gambling behaviors between American Indian and non-Indian adolescents within and near a northern plains reservation. Am Indian Alaskan Native Ment Health Res 1996;7(2):14-26.
24. DiClemente CC, Story M, Murray K. On a roll: The process of initiation and cessation of problem gambling among adolescents. J Gambl Studies 2000;16(2-3):289-313.
25. Stinchfield R. Gambling among Minnesota public school students from 1992 to 2007: Declines in youth gambling. Psychol Addict Behav 2011;25(1):108-17.
26. Winters KC, Stinchfield RD, Botzet A, Slutske WS. Pathways of youth gambling problem severity. Psychol Addict Behav 2005;19:104-7.
27. Petry NM. Pathological gambling: etiology, comorbidity, and treatment, 1st ed. Washington, DC: American Psychological Association, 2005.
28. American Psychiatric Association. DSM-III: Diagnostic and statistical manual of mental disorders, 3rd ed. Washington, DC: American Psychiatric Association, 1980.
29. American Psychiatric Association. Diagnostic and statistical manual of mental disorders, text revision, 4th ed. Washington, DC: American Psychiatric Association, 2000.
30. Gebauer L, LaBrie RA, Shaffer HJ. Optimizing DSM IV classification accuracy: A brief biosocial screen for detecting current gambling disorders among gamblers in the general household population. Can J Psychiatry 2010;55(2):82-90.
31. Braverman J, Labrie RA, Shaffer HJ. A taxometric analysis of actual Internet sports gambling behavior. Psychol Assessment 2011;23(1):234-44.
32. Shaffer HJ, LaPlante DA, LaBrie RA, Kidman RC, Donato AN, Stanton MV. Toward a syndrome model of addiction: Multiple expressions, common etiology. Harvard Rev Psychiatry 2004;12(6):367-74.
33. Shaffer HJ, LaPlante DA, Nelson SE, eds. The APA addiction syndrome handbook. Washington, DC: American Psychological Association Press, in press.

Author index

Paul Delfabbro, PhD
University of Adelaide
Adelaide, Australia
Chapter 3

Jeffrey L. Derevensky, PhD
International Centre for Youth Gambling
Problems and High-Risk Behaviors
McGill University
3724 McTavish Street
Quebec H3A 1Y2, Montreal
Canada
jeffrey.derevensky@mcgill.ca
Chapters 1, 2, 4, 5, 8, 10, 13, 16

Sally Gainsbury, PhD
Centre for Gambling Education
and Research
Southern Cross University
PO Box 157
NSW 2480, Lismore
Australia
sally.gainsbury@scu.edu.au
Chapter 11

Jon E. Grant, MD, JD MPH
Department of Psychiatry
University of Minnesota
Medical School
2450 Riverside Avenue
Minneapolis, MN 55454
United States
grant045@umn.edu
Chapter 12

Mark D. Griffiths, PhD
Department of Social Sciences
Nottingham Trent University
Burton Street
NG1 4BU Nottingham
United Kingdom
mark.griffiths@ntu.ac.uk
Chapters 3, 8

Rina Gupta, PhD
International Centre for Youth Gambling
Problems and High-Risk Behaviors
McGill University
3724 McTavish Street
Quebec H3A 1Y2, Montreal
Canada
rina.gupta@mcgill.ca
Chapters 2, 3, 4, 5, 10, 13, 16

Cecilia M. S. Ma, PhD
Department of Applied Social Sciences
The Hong Kong Polytechnic University
Hunghom, Hong Kong
Chapter 6

Joav Merrick, MD
Ministry of Social Affairs
Health Services
Division for Intellectual and
Developmental Disabilities
PO Box 1260
IL-91012 Jerusalem
Israel
jmerrick@zahav.net.il
Chapter 1

Daniel T. Ólason, DPhil
University of Iceland
Reykjavik, Iceland
Chapter 3

Jonathan Parke, PhD
University of Salford
United Kingdom
Chapter 8

Marc N. Potenza, MD, PhD
Departments of Psychiatry, Child Study,
and Neurobiology
Yale University School of Medicine
New Haven, Connecticut
United States
Chapter 12

N. Will Shead, PhD
Department of Psychology
Mount Saint Vincent University
166 Bedford Highway
Nova Scotia B3M 2J6, Halifax
Canada
will.shead@msvu.ca
Chapter 4

Daniel T. L. Shek, PhD
Department of Applied Social Sciences
The Hong Kong Polytechnic University
Hunghom, Hong Kong
daniel.shek@polyu.edu.hk
Chapters 1, 6, 7, 14

Randy Stinchfield, PhD
Department of Psychiatry
University of Minnesota Medical School
689 Fairmount Avenue
Saint Paul, MN 55105
United States
stinc001@umn.edu
Chapter 9

Rachel C. F. Sun, PhD
Faculty of Education
The University of Hong Kong
Hong Kong
Chapters 7, 14

Caroline Temcheff, PhD
International Centre for Youth Gambling
Problems and High-Risk Behaviors
McGill University
3724 McTavish Street
Quebec H3A 1Y2, Montreal
Canada
Chapter 10

Rachel A. Volberg, PhD
Gemini Research Ltd
PO Box 1390
Northampton, MA 01061
United States
rvolberg@geminiresearch.com
Chapter 3

Introduction

1 Adolescent gambling

Jeffrey L. Derevensky, Daniel T. L. Shek, and Joav Merrick

The landscape of gambling during the past two decades has changed dramatically. Las Vegas, Reno, and Atlantic City in the United States were once thought to be the gambling capitals of the world, but they have been overshadowed by Macau, with Singapore's two international resort casinos about to surpass Las Vegas revenues. Multinational operators continue to expand their land-based casino operations at an unprecedented rate. Governments throughout the world now view gambling as a socially acceptable form of entertainment and an excellent source of revenue. More traditional forms of gambling are being challenged by Internet and remote gambling providers.

Gambling revenues now far exceed those generated from traditional forms of entertainment – movies, the record industry, and video games combined. With the expansion of gambling has come greater accessibility, convenience, availability, and diversity of games. Whether one is purchasing a lottery ticket or scratch card, or playing traditional casino games, one can now wager via the Internet from the luxury of one's home, office, or school. You can now wager on political outcomes, winners of reality television shows, and whether your favorite Hollywood star will get arrested. Traditional sports wagering, betting on the outcome of a single or multiple games, has been replaced by proposition bets. Historically, wagering on sports meant only whether a specific team covered the point spread. Today's sports wagering can be made on not only who won or lost, but also on who was leading after a certain period of time, which player scored the most points, who is the game's most valuable player, the duration of the national anthem, how many times the star player's girlfriend is shown on camera, and the color of the star player's girlfriend's blouse, just to name a few. Individuals can virtually wager on anything via Internet gambling sites. In North America you can wager on the number of hot dogs to be eaten in a given time at the Nathan's hot dog eating contest or the number of letters in the winning word in the Scripps National Spelling Bee contest for children.

The widespread proliferation of gambling opportunities is indicative of gambling's increasing social acceptance, its popularity, and normalization. Governments throughout the world have embraced gambling as a way of providing employment, economic development, increased tourism, and improved revenues. Both the industry and general public tend to treat gambling as a form of *gaming,* which serves the functions of relaxation and social gathering. Nevertheless, similar to gambling advertisements, the downside of gambling, the social costs, has rarely been discussed, or has been dismissed as a minimal deterrent to gambling's benefits.

Whether engaged in wagering on games of personal skill, playing poker among friends, purchasing a lottery ticket, playing electronic gambling machines, sports wagering or participation in casino-type games, gambling's popularity among the young is on the rise. The new "role models" for many teens and young adults are the world champion poker players. It is not unusual for a teen to respond to the question "What would you like to do when you get older?" with "become a professional gambler." The last two multimillion-dollar winners of the World Series of Poker in Las Vegas were both under 25 years of age and college dropouts. The growing popularity of poker, in particular Texas Hold'em, is evident in the growing number of entrants into poker tournaments and its widespread television coverage.

Not surprisingly, prevalence studies continue to show gambling's popularity among adolescents as well as adults. Like their adult counterparts, the vast majority of youth who gamble do so in a responsible manner, setting and adhering to both money and time limits. Youth typically report gambling for excitement, entertainment, to social-ize, and to tempt their luck without many negative repercussions. Few experience significant adverse consequences. Yet, for a small but identifiable population, gambling is excessive and individuals suffer a host of concomitant short-term and long-term negative consequences. For these individuals, gambling problems and the nega-tive consequences associated with excessive gambling pervade most aspects of their life – employment/school (job loss, absenteeism, poor performance, early school drop-outs), interpersonal (neglect of family, peers, disrupted relationships), personal issues (stress, anxiety, depression, suicide ideation and/or attempts, poor mental and physi-cal health), finances (increased debt, loss of possessions), and legal problems (theft, delinquency, incarceration).

Prevalence research conducted over the past three decades clearly indicates that the rates of problem gambling among adolescents and young adults are typically greater than those among older adults. Although a dramatic rise in overall prevalence rates has not been observed, it is important to note that the general population has risen, thus the actual number of individuals suffering from gambling-related problems has increased. As well, we now understand that certain types of gambling may in fact be more problematic for high-risk individuals. There is speculation that electronic forms of gambling – that is, Internet and mobile wagering – may be particularly problematic for youth. Some recent research suggests that in addition to gambling for its entertainment value and to make money, a growing number of adolescents and young adults are reporting gambling on the Internet as a way of relieving boredom.

The rise and proliferation of gambling/gaming has not been without concomitant problems. The World Health Organization and the American Psychiatric Association have identified pathological gambling as a distinct psychiatric disorder, but there is a common misconception that pathological gambling is relegated only to adults, and not adolescents. Youth may be at greater risk given their belief that they can stop at any time, their perceived invulnerability, and their increased risk-taking tendencies. Adolescence, as a developmental period, is often fraught with a number of potentially risky behaviors including alcohol and substance use and abuse, eating disorders, unprotected and in-creased sexual activity, etc. As such, the focus on youth is important for several reasons. Healthy childhood development increases the likelihood that these individuals will grow into well-adjusted adults. Impeding healthy development will likely have not only a short-term impact but a long-term negative impact on an individual's psychological and emotional development.

Youth gambling represents an important public policy and health issue. Our growing knowledge and current understanding of youth gambling behaviors have only begun to be realized. The nature of adolescent gambling in Asian contexts is also a mystery for scientists because of the lack of research in this area. Though the chapters in this book provide insight into our current knowledge concerning the prevalence, risk, and protective factors associated with problem gambling, assessment issues, and prevention and treatment initiatives, much work remains to be done. Our advances during the past two decades in this field have been numerous and the authors in this book remain at the forefront of their field. Yet, technological advances, expanded venues, and the lack of youth and parental awareness concerning gambling-related problems necessitate increasing our understanding of this complex behavior.

Our enhanced understanding of the trajectory of gambling behaviors, ways to screen youth, and programs to help prevent potential gambling-related problems from emerging will ultimately minimize the numbers of youth and adults with this disorder. It is hoped that governments and the industry will work with the research and clinical community to establish coherent and responsible prevention, treatment, and social policies. More research will be needed to address the multiplicity of issues surrounding expanded gambling and to speed the development of *best practices* for prevention and treatment of problem gambling.

The current generation of youth will spend their entire lives with gambling easily accessible, readily available, and state-owned and/or regulated. We have made significant progress in our conceptualization and understanding of this problem, but more collaborative work is needed to help shape our policies. How to help adolescents acquire psychosocial competencies and to promote healthy family behavior that enables them to resist the temptation of pathological gambling are important tasks for policymakers, professionals, parents, young people, and the public to consider. Our governments will need to provide responsible social policies and regulations to protect this vulnerable population; a generation of children will depend on it.

Acknowledgements

Dr. Derevensky would like to thank the Quebec Population Health Research Network for its support in the development of several chapters.

2 Understanding the etiology of youth gambling problems

Rina Gupta and Jeffrey L. Derevensky

The complete picture of the etiology of problem gambling remains unclear at the present time, primarily due to the lack of large-scale longitudinal studies. Though a number of longitudinal studies have been conducted, they have used limited numbers of individuals in selected populations. Nonetheless, a significant body of cross-sectional research has identified individual, community, societal, and relationship factors associated with the development and maintenance of problem gambling. Some theories have been postulated both to explain the etiology of problem gambling and to identify subtypes of problem gamblers. This chapter will provide a systemic review of the current literature pertaining to how and why problem gambling develops among youth.

2.1 Introduction

The issue of youth gambling has been studied since the 1990s. During this period the prevalence studies clearly revealed that children and adolescents viewed gambling as socially acceptable, found it entertaining, and participated in various legalized and nonlegalized activities (1–3). Not only was it discovered that youth were gambling on a regular basis, but that they were doing so at rates comparable to adults, with problem gambling rates higher than those of adults (4, 5). This realization resulted in a number of empirical investigations designed to better understand why young people were more vulnerable than adults with respect to developing gambling problems, and to identify which youth are most at risk. Much of the research within this book has been devoted to better understanding some of the risk and protective factors associated with youth gambling problems. Though the research into these questions is still ongoing, a rich amount of information currently exists. There are few etiological models of addiction in general and of pathological gambling (both for adults and adolescents) in particular. Despite the paucity of theoretical paradigms to explain problem gambling, there is ample evidence to suggest that the etiology of gambling disorders is complex and multifactorial (6). A general consensus is that the risks associated with problem gambling result from an intricate relationship between one's biology, psychology, life experiences, and environmental factors. As such, a brief review in these areas will shed light on the overall etiology of problem gambling based on our knowledge to date.

2.2 Biology

Age of onset appears to have an important impact on the etiology of gambling problems. Recently, Jimenez-Murcia and colleagues (7) provided an in-depth examination of the relationship between age of onset and severity of gambling problems, and found that earlier onset of gambling was associated with increased severity of gambling problems, whereas older age of onset was associated with higher levels of psychopathology such as depressive, paranoid, and psychotic symptoms. Earlier research had previously established that people experiencing gambling problems were more likely to have started gambling at young ages, even prior to adolescence. Based on retrospective data, from samples of adult problem gamblers (8–10), the mean age of onset of gambling activity was found to be 13 years, with 37% reporting starting gambling before 10 years of age, and 49% between 11 and 19 years. Studies not of a retrospective nature have also concluded that children frequently begin gambling at the primary-school level (3, 11).

Historically, gambling has been a male-dominated activity, with significantly more males engaging in gambling activities than females (12–15). More recently, however, likely due to increased offers of various types of gambling and also to more relaxed societal attitudes toward gambling, women have been found to be just as likely to gamble as males (16). Although rates of pathological gambling remain higher among males, it is now being argued that women are also quite vulnerable and that each gender carries its own set of unique risk factors (17) and therefore should be examined individually. A telescoping effect for gender has been found such that males start gambling at younger ages whereas females tend to start gambling later in life but progress toward gambling problems at a faster pace (18–20). Differences between male and female adolescent gamblers have also been found such that males tend to gamble to satisfy their need for risk taking and sensation seeking, whereas females tend to turn toward excessive gambling as a means of escape from depression or stressful circumstances (4). It is also important to note that despite gender differences, commonalities also exist, such that poor coping skills and life stressors represent salient risk factors for both males and females (4, 17), and that excessive gambling involvement, in itself, may represent a form of maladaptive coping. Furthermore, an examination of 2,889 twin pairs ages 32 to 43 years concluded that genetic traits are as important in our understanding of the etiology of problem gambling for women as they are for men, and that specific genes resulting in greater susceptibility for problem gambling likely overlap considerably for men and women (21).

Despite the ongoing controversy over its categorization, pathological gambling is currently classified as a disorder of impulse control (22–30). In fact, impulsivity traits present early in life have been linked to the onset of problem gambling (7, 31). There is also evidence of a high comorbidity rate of substance use and abuse among problem gamblers. It is believed that impulsive tendencies are partially responsible for these co-occurring disorders (32–34).

2.3 Individual factors

It is widely recognized that addictive activities can serve as temporary escapes from life stressors and daily problems (35). As previously mentioned, research studies have demonstrated that young problem gamblers have poor coping skills, and tend to resort to gambling as a way to cope with difficulties (4, 36, 37). In addition, adult problem gambling has been linked to multiple mental health disorders, including personality disorders, paranoia, depression, anxiety, chronic understimulation, and criminal activity (38–42).

Personality characteristics have also been examined among adolescent problem gamblers. Using discriminant analysis, Gupta and her colleagues found that traits of sensation-seeking, high levels of disinhibition, boredom susceptibility, cheerfulness and excitability, as well as low levels of conformity and self-discipline, were found to be strongly associated with the prediction of problem gambling severity (43). Similar results were obtained with undergraduate students from two Canadian universities, whereby negative affect and disinhibited traits were found to be risk factors for the development of gambling problems (44). Such findings lend support to the premise that certain types of individuals, especially those who are impulsive and have difficulty with self-discipline and the inhibiting of behavioral responses, are likely more susceptible than others to developing gambling problems. These findings are in line with recent research that documents the presence of a serotonergic dysfunction (a neurotransmitter that plays an important role in impulse control) among pathological gamblers (45).

2.4 Life experiences

Adolescent gambling frequency has been found to be related to parental gambling behaviors and problems, low levels of parental monitoring, and higher levels of inadequate disciplinary practices (46–48). In contrast, positive parenting practices can serve as a protective mechanism, with higher levels of parental attachment, supervision, and monitoring resulting in lower overall levels of adolescent gambling (46, 49, 50).

Childhood maltreatment has been found to be a significant risk factor in the development of gambling problems. Responses were collected in a study of 1,324 adolescents and young adults, age 17–22 years, who completed self-report measures on gambling behaviors, gambling severity, and childhood maltreatment (physical and verbal abuse as well as neglect). Problem gamblers reported higher levels of childhood maltreatment in comparison to non-gamblers and social gamblers (51). These results highlight the importance of the interrelationship between multiple types of childhood abuse and gambling severity.

Life experiences that trigger social stress and anxiety tend to place young people (52) and adults (53) at greater risk for the development of gambling problems. It is not only the fact that one experiences major life stressors and daily hassles that renders a person vulnerable; how an individual interprets this stressor is also a major determinant (54, 55).

In contrast to the risk factors, school connectedness was found to be a protective factor that serves as a buffer against the development of gambling problems in youth (56). It is plausible that a lack of connectedness with one's school or community could similarly represent a risk factor in the etiology of problem gambling, although no study has directly assessed this relationship.

A combination of contributing factors, in contrast to a single contributing factor, appears to explain one's vulnerability to gambling problems. A discriminant function analysis using demographic, individual, family, and peer factors as potential discriminators, indicated that pathological gamblers reported the highest level of peer and parent gambling, susceptibility to peer pressure, conduct problems, binge drinking, suicide attempts, and drug use (57).

2.5 Environmental factors

There is little doubt that there is a growing proliferation of gambling opportunities and venues internationally. Gambling availability and accessibility are two factors that have been suggested as links to increases in levels of gambling participation (58). Today's culture involving a high presence of gambling opportunity and exposure (i.e., poker) surely factors into the popularity of gambling among children and adolescents, accounting for the increasing number of individuals reporting having gambled, and very likely in the etiology of gambling problems at all age levels. It is important to note that our current conceptualization of problem gambling suggests it is a progressive disorder. Pathological or problem gambling does not result from single-trial learning, but rather from repeated access, exposure, and engagement. With the ever increasing availability and accessibility of gambling, especially in the context of Internet and mobile gambling, this remains of significant concern.

Societal attitudes toward the proliferation of legalized gambling tend to be quite accepting, with a general consensus that communities benefit from direct revenues, employment and tourism, that there is little inherent harm in the activity, and that gambling or gaming is an enjoyable form of entertainment in which individuals can exercise free will and freedom of choice (59–61). A study examining attitudes of community leaders in seven different U.S. communities being introduced to local casinos highlights the acceptance of gambling within our communities. The vast majority of leaders provided support for the presence of legalized gambling, believing the casinos enhance the quality of life in a community and have a positive effect on the economy (62). Of greater concern is the fact that parental attitudes toward gambling reflect a lack of awareness that gambling participation could result in a behavioral addiction. Parents are often responsible for introducing their young children to gambling activities, view it as a harmless activity, and condone their children's gambling (63). In a recent national Canadian study examining 13 potentially risky behaviors among adolescents (e.g., drug and alcohol use, unprotected sex, bullying, eating disorders, etc.), gambling was viewed as the least potentially problematic behavior by parents (48).

Not only is there a prominent presence of legalized gambling in most communities (frequently through lottery sales in convenience stores), but there is also a significant amount of gambling advertisements to which people of all ages are exposed. Not surprisingly, a relationship between exposure to gambling advertisements and gambling participation has been demonstrated among adolescents. Results from focus groups conducted with youth concluded that adolescents perceive messages about gambling as a fun activity that is exciting/entertaining and that facilitates the attainment of wealth as well as happiness. These factors likely increase their probability of engaging in future gambling activities despite the fact that the advertisements were not specifically designed to target youth (64).

2.6 Theoretical frameworks

Several divergent theoretical approaches have attempted to explain problem and pathological gambling, including addiction, psychodynamic, biological/genetic, neurobiological, learning, cognitive-behavioral, and sociological theories (65, 66). Conceptually, most of these models perceive pathological gambling either as a categorical or a spectrum disorder. Though many of these models share common elements, they each assume that the interaction of significant bio-psycho-social variables in the etiological process may be accounted for by one set of fundamental principles, presuming that disordered gamblers are essentially a relatively homogeneous population. The corollary is that theoretically driven treatments are applied universally to all individuals with gambling problems irrespective of gender, ethnicity, type of gambling developmental history, or neurobiology, although some attention has more recently been given to the type of gambling activity (e.g., machine player, poker player, sports gambler, etc.) preferred.

Having a theoretical framework within which all the contributing factors can be understood in terms of their salience and contribution to the development of problem gambling, as well as understanding problem gambling subtypes, is necessary to the advancement of our understanding of the etiology of problem gambling.

Currently, there are a limited number of theoretical models explaining addiction in general and pathological gambling in particular. In describing adult pathological gambling, Shaffer (6, 67) has suggested a syndrome model of addiction where shared neurobiological, psychological, and social risk factors and their interactions influence the development and maintenance of the different manifestations associated with an addictive behavior. He contends that an addiction develops into specific manifestations as a result of exposure to and positive subjective experiences associated with the addictive behavior. Once the expression(s) of the addiction syndrome emerge(s), the manifestations of the syndrome simultaneously reflect both the object of the addiction (for pathological gambling it would result in the debt associated with excessive gambling) and more general characteristics associated with the addictive behavior (e.g., tolerance, withdrawal, habituation). Two predominant overarching etiological theories exist by which the development of problem gambling is conceptualized for adolescents: the *general theory of addiction* (68) and the *pathways model* (69, 70). The pathways model is more complex and elucidates different etiologies that result in gambling subtypes, whereas the general theory of addiction more generally accounts for the development of addictive behaviors and does not postulate the idea of varying typologies.

2.6.1 General theory of addictions

Jacobs (68) defines an addiction as a "dependent state acquired over time by a predisposed person in an attempt to relieve a chronic stress condition." In this definition, only certain individuals can fall victim to an addiction, and the chosen addiction provides relief from a stressed state.

Jacobs postulates several basic premises that constitute one's overall addiction risk. First, he contends that two sets of interdependent, predisposing factors must be present for an individual to be at risk for developing and maintaining an addictive behavior, the first being an abnormal physiological resting state that is chronically either excessively excited or hypotensive, and the second reflecting a psychological makeup characterized by feelings of inferiority, rejection, inadequacy, and/or guilt stemming from childhood, and low self-esteem. Accordingly, "both sets of predisposing factors must coexist and exercise their respective effects before an individual will maintain an addictive pattern of behavior *in a conducive environment*" (71).

A physiological condition of being either chronically hyper- or hypo-aroused is believed to be stress-inducing. Individuals suffering from either of these extreme arousal levels are subsequently motivated to seek activities or substances that correct their resting state, with the goal of obtaining a more comfortable homeostatic state. It remains plausible that a person with a hypotensive physiological arousal level may find relief in a stimulating and exciting activity such as gambling, temporarily eliminating their boredom and possible depression. It follows that such individuals would likely have a greater propensity for risk taking and sensation seeking than the norm. In contrast, a person with a hypertensive arousal state would likely find more relief in alcohol or marijuana – two substances known for their depressant effects. In both these examples, gambling and substances serve to regulate and "normalize" one's physiological resting states.

According to Jacobs' theoretical framework, an addictive preoccupation, such as gambling, enables the individual to find escape from painful realities and further fosters the sense of being a highly successful and admired individual who, at the time of indulgence, feels invulnerable. Dissociative states are common to all forms of addiction and permit the individual to escape into denial and bliss from psychological distress. This "altered state of identity" is believed to be the common goal of all addictive patterns of behavior. It remains extremely rewarding, reinforcing, and is believed to play an instrumental role in the maintenance of the addiction. More specifically, Jacobs views addictive behaviors as a method of self-treatment, considering they permit escape from, and momentarily correct, a chronic stress condition.

Jacobs further postulated that a conducive environment is a necessary prerequisite and must accompany the coexisting predisposing factors in the development of an addictive behavior pattern. It is likely that the individual will by chance happen upon an activity (such as gambling, overeating, or drug consumption) that eventually serves to regulate his or her abnormal physiological resting state and alleviate psychological distress. This "chance triggering event" must present the individual with sufficient intensity and novelty in order to motivate them to actively pursue a similar activity in the future.

The *general theory of addiction* was empirically tested and supported with an adolescent population (4). Gender differences were noted, such that males and females varied in their needs to modulate their physiological resting states or escape emotional distress. This theoretical framework is very useful in understanding the etiology of addiction, but lacks specificity that would allow a deeper understanding of contributing factors and possibly subtypes of problem gamblers.

2.6.2 Pathways model

Blaszczynski and Nower (69, 70) have hypothesized a conceptual *pathways model* that identifies three primary subgroups/clusters of gamblers: *behaviorally conditioned*, *emotionally vulnerable*, and *biologically based impulsive* pathological gamblers. All three groups have common exposure to related ecological factors (e.g., availability, accessibility, and acceptability), cognitive processes and distortions, and contingencies of reinforcement. However, according to the proposed model, predisposing emotional stressors and affective disturbances for some individuals and biological impulsivity for others represent significant additive risk factors. The differential pathways model has significant implications for both the assessment and treatment of adult and adolescent

pathological gamblers. Originally formulated for better understanding of adult pathological gamblers (69), it was subsequently modified to explain adolescent pathological
gamblers (70).

Based on the research literature, the *pathways model* proposes three subtypes of gamblers who display similar problem gambling features resulting from distinctly different
etiological factors. The three gambling pathways put forward are distinguishable from
each other in their presence (and/or absence) of specific pre-morbid psychopathological and biological vulnerabilities. This theory takes into consideration most of the biological, psychological, and environmental factors previously mentioned. The following
is a description of the three pathways by which it is hypothesized someone can become
addicted to gambling.

Pathway 1: Behaviorally conditioned problem gamblers

Pathway 1 gamblers are normal and psychologically healthy by most accounts, and
are distinguished by the absence of specific pre-morbid features of psychopathology.
They fluctuate between regular/heavy and excessive gambling largely as a result of
the effects of conditioning (i.e., an early big win), distorted cognitions surrounding the
probability of winning, as well as a disregard for the notion of erroneous cognitions
(e.g., independence of events), and/or a series of bad judgments/poor decision–making,
rather than from impaired control. *Pathway 1* gamblers initially gamble primarily for
entertainment, enjoyment, and socialization, facilitated by easy access and availability.
Problem gambling–related symptoms, such as a preoccupation with gambling, chasing losses, substance dependence, depressive symptomatology, and state anxiety, are
conceptualized as the consequence, not the cause, of patterns of excessive gambling
behavior.

Pathway 2: Emotionally vulnerable problem gamblers

Pathway 2 gamblers share ecological determinants, conditioning processes, and cognitive schemas of erroneous misbeliefs similar to Pathway 1 individuals. However, these
individuals are quite different, as they also present with anxiety and/or depression, a
history of poor coping under adverse conditions, and ineffective problem-solving skills,
problematic family background experiences, and major traumatic life events. Together,
these factors contribute to an emotionally vulnerable individual whose participation
in gambling is motivated by a desire to modulate affective states and/or meet specific psychological needs. As in Jacobs' (68) theory, gambling and pre-morbid drug
abuse are used to relieve aversive psychological states by providing escape or arousal.
Psychological dysfunction in these gamblers results in more resistance to change and
necessitates differential treatment addressing underlying vulnerabilities as well as
excessive gambling and drug abusing behaviors.

Pathway 3: Biologically vulnerable problem gamblers

Pathway 3 gamblers also possess psychosocial and biologically based vulnerabilities
similar to Pathway 2 gamblers, but are primarily distinguished by features of impulsivity,
antisocial personality traits and behaviors, and attention deficits, manifesting in severe
multiple maladaptive behaviors. Specifically, impulsivity directly affects the gambler's

general level of psychosocial functioning. Clinically, these impulsive gamblers exhibit a wide array of behavioral and mental health problems independent of their gambling (72–74). Excessive alcohol and multiple drug experimentation, poor interpersonal relationships, nongambling-related criminality, and a family history of antisocial behavior and alcohol problems are typically characteristic of *Pathway 3* individuals. These gamblers are reported to be less motivated to seek treatment, have poor treatment compliance rates, and generally respond poorly to any form of intervention.

Though prevalent in the gambling literature, and frequently referred to for close to a decade, the *pathways model* has not been widely empirically validated. A number of studies have found some evidence suggesting the validity of the pathways model subtypes for adults. For example, a cluster analysis conducted on responses from 110 males in treatment for pathological gambling yielded three distinct gambler subtypes; the first cluster reported little or no psychopathology, the second cluster reported anxiety and depression, and the third cluster was similar to the second cluster, with added impulsivity (40). More recently, the *pathways model* was tested empirically with an adolescent population, also with the use of cluster analyses, and the findings were highly supportive of the three subtypes hypothesized, differentiated by factors of emotional and experiential factors, impulsivity, conditioning, and other psychopathology. Gupta and her colleagues (75) did note some findings that were different from what is hypothesized in the pathways model, such that impulsivity did not play a very defining role in differentiating Pathway 2 from Pathway 3, nor did the presence of ADHD differentiate Pathway 3. However, consistent with the pathways model, Pathway 3 individuals were primarily defined by antisocial tendencies. Overall, the pathways model was found to be a very useful theoretical framework in describing the etiology of gambling problems among youth.

In summary, our understanding of the etiology of problem gambling is still immature, yet several meaningful contributing interacting factors have been identified. Undoubtedly, it is a complex interaction of biological, psychological, environmental, and societal factors that lays the path toward gambling problems. As accessibility and availability increase, as new opportunities and games become readily available to our youth, a better understanding of etiological factors remains imperative. Though there are individual factors that place a person at heightened risk, societies bear a responsibility in the prevalence of problem gambling. Laws and regulatory bodies designed to monitor and limit gambling offer and expansion, as well as other preventative measures (education of parents, prevention messages to youth and vulnerable groups) are necessary to safeguard individuals. Future research is fundamental to our ongoing understanding of how problem gambling develops, and is required for the development of more effective, empirically based prevention and treatment approaches.

References

1. Fisher S. Adolescent slot machine dependency and delinquency: Questions on a question of methodology. J Gambl Stud 1995;11:303–10.
2. Griffiths M, Sutherland I. Adolescent gambling and drug use. J Community Appl Soc Psychol 1998;8:423–7.
3. Gupta R, Derevensky J. The relationship between gambling and video-game playing behavior in children and adolescents. J Gambl Stud 1996;12:375–94.

4. Gupta R, Derevensky J. An empirical examination of Jacobs' General Theory of Addictions: Do adolescent gamblers fit the theory? J Gambl Stud 1998;14:17–49.
5. Shaffer HJ, Hall MN. Estimating the prevalence of adolescent gambling disorders: A quantitative synthesis and guide toward standard gambling nomenclature. J Gambl Stud 1996;12:193–214.
6. Shaffer HJ, Martin R. Disordered gambling: Etiology, trajectory, and clinical considerations. Annu Rev Clin Psychol 2011;7:483–510.
7. Jimenez-Murcia S, Alvarez-Moya E, Stinchfield R, et al. Age of onset in pathological gambling: Clinical, therapeutic, and personality correlates. J Gambl Stud 2010;26:235–48.
8. Dell LJ, Ruzicka MF, Palisi AT. Personality and other factors associated with the gambling addiction. Int J Addict 1981;16:149–6.
9. Productivity Commission. Australia's Gambling Industries: Australian Government;.1999: Report No. 10.
10. Wynne H, Smith G, Jacobs DF. Adolescent Gambling and Problem Gambling in Alberta. Prepared for the Alberta Alcohol and Drug Abuse Commission, Edmonton;.1996.
11. Ladouceur R. The prevalence of pathological gambling in Canada. J Gambl Stud 1996;12(2):129–42.
12. Ellenbogen S, Derevensky J, Gupta R. Gender differences among adolescents with gambling related problems. J Gambl Stud 2007;23:133–43.
13. Hraba J, Lee G. Gender, gambling, and problem gambling. J Gambl Stud 1996;12:83–101.
14. Lindgren HE, Youngs GAJ, McDonald TD, Klenow DJ, Schriner EC. The impact of gender on gambling attitudes and behavior. J Gambl Behav 1987;3:155–67.
15. Wolfgang AK. Gambling as a function of gender and sensation seeking. J Gambl Behav 1988;4:71–7.
16. Welte J, Barnes G, Wieczorek W, Tidwell M, Parker J. Gambling participation in the U.S. Results from a national survey. J Gambl Stud 2002;18(4):313–37.
17. Afifi TO, Cox BJ, Martens PJ, Sareen J, Enns MW. Demographic and social variables associated with problem gambling among men and women in Canada. Psychiatry Res 2010;178:395–400.
18. Grant JE, Kim SW. Gender differences in pathological gamblers seeking medication treatment. Compr Psych 2002;43(1):56–62.
19. Ladd GT, Petry NM. Gender differences among pathological gamblers seeking treatment. Exp Clin Psychopharmacol 2002;10:302–9.
20. Ibanez A, Blanco C, deCastro IP, Fernández-Piqueras J, Siez-Ruiz J. Genetics of pathological gambling. J Gambl Stud 2003;19(1):11–22.
21. Slutske WS, Zhu G, Meier MH, Martin NG. Genetic and environmental influences on disordered gambling in men and women. Arch Gen Psychiatry 2010;67(6):624–30.
22. Monopolis SJ, Dion JR. Disorders of impulse control: Explosive disorders. Pathological gambling, pyromania and kleptomania. In: Curran WJ, McGarry AL, Shah SA, eds. Forensic Psychiatry and Psychology: Perspectives and Standards for Interdisciplinary Practice. Philadelphia, PA: FA Davis; 1986.
23. Petry N. Substance abuse, pathological gambling, and impulsiveness. Drug Alcohol Depend 2001;63(1):29–38.
24. Nower L, Derevensky J, Gupta R. The relationship of impulsivity, sensation seeking, coping and substance use in youth gamblers. Psychol Addict Behav 2004;18:49–55.
25. Steel Z, Blaszczynski AP. Impulsivity, personality disorders and pathological gambling activity. Addiction 1998;69:81–9.
26. McDaniel S, Zuckerman M. The relationship of impulsive sensation seeking and gender to interest and participation in gambling activities. Pers Individ Differ 2003;35(6):1385–400.
27. Blaszczynski AP, Wilson A, McConaghy N. Sensation seeking and pathological gambling. Addiction 1986;81(1):113–7.
28. Nower L, Blaszczynski A. Impulsivity and pathological gambling: A descriptive model. IGS 2006;6(1):61–75.

29. Chambers R, Potenza M. Neurodevelopment, impulsivity, and adolescent gambling. J Gambl Stud 2003;19(1):53–84.
30. American Psychiatric Association. Diagnostic and Statistical Manual of Mental Disorders: DSM-1V-TR (4th Edition). Washington, DC: APA; 2000.
31. Pagani L, Derevensky J, Japel C. Predicting gambling behavior in sixth grade from kindergarten impulsivity: A tale of developmental continuity. Arch Pediatr Adolesc Med 2009;163(3):238–43.
32. Cunningham-Williams R, Cottler L, Compton W, Spitznagel E, Ben-Abdallah A. Problem gambling and comorbid psychiatric and substance use disorders among drug users recruited from drug treatment and community. J Gambl Stud 2000;16:347–76.
33. Maccallum F, Blaszczynski A. Pathological gambling and comorbid substance use. Aust NZ J Psychiatry 2002;36(3):411–5.
34. Petry N, Stinson FS, Grant BF. Comorbidity of DSM-IV pathological gambling and other psychiatric disorders: Results from the national epidemiologic survey on alcohol and related conditions. J Clin Psychiatry 2005;66(5):564–74.
35. Jacobs DF. Evidence for a common dissociative-like reaction among addicts. J Gambl Behav 1988;4(1):27–37.
36. Gupta R, Derevensky J, Marget N. Coping strategies employed by adolescents with gambling problems. Child Adolesc Ment Health 2004;9(3):115–20.
37. Turner NE, Macdonald J, Bartoshuk M, et al. Adolescent gambling behavior, attitudes, and gambling problems. IJMA 2008;6:223–37.
38. McCormick RA. Pathological gambling: A parsimonious need state model. J Gambl Behav 1987;3(257–263).
39. Blaszczynski AP, McConaghy N, Frankova A. Boredom proneness in pathological gambling. Psychol Rep 1990;67:35–42.
40. Gonzalez-Ibanez A, Aymani MN, Jimenez S, Domenech JM, Granero R, Lourido-Ferreira MR. The subtyping of pathological gambling: A comprehensive review. Psychol Rep 2003;93:707–16.
41. Graham JR, Lowenfeld BH. Personality dimensions of the pathological gambler. J Gambl Behav 1986;2:58–66.
42. Desai RA, Potenza MN. Gender differences in the association between gambling problems and psychiatric disorders. Soc Psychiatry Psychiatr Epidemiol 2008;43(3):173–83.
43. Gupta R, Derevensky JL, Ellenbogen S. Personality characteristics and risk-taking tendencies among adolescent gamblers. Can J Behav Sci 2006;3:201–13.
44. MacLaren V, Best L, Dixon M, Harrigan K. Problem gambling and the five factor model in university students. Pers Individ Differ 2011;50(3):335–8.
45. Pallanti S, Bernardi S, Allen A, Hollander E. Serotonin function in pathological gambling: Blunted growth hormone response to sumatriptan. J Psychopharmacol 2010;24(12):1802–9.
46. Vachon J, Vitaro F, Wanner B, Tremblay RE. Adolescent gambling: Relationships with parent gambling and parenting practices. Psychol Addict Behav 2004;18(4):398–401.
47. Felsher J, Derevensky J, Gupta R. Parental influences and social modeling of youth lottery participation. J Community Appl Soc Psychol 2003;13:361–77.
48. Campbell C, Derevensky J, Meerkamper E, Cutajar J. Parents' perceptions of adolescent gambling: A Canadian national study. JGI in press.
49. Magoon ME, Ingersoll GM. Parental modeling, attachment, and supervision as moderators of adolescent gambling. J Gambl Stud 2006;22(1):1–22.
50. Griffiths M. The role of parents in the development of gambling behaviour in adolescents. Educ Health 2010;28:51–4.
51. Felsher J, Derevensky J, Gupta R. Young adults with gambling problems: The impact of childhood maltreatment. IJMA 2010;8:545–56.
52. Ste-Marie C, Gupta R, Derevensky J. Anxiety and social stress related to adolescent gambling behavior. IGS 2002;2(1):123–41.

53. Coman GJ, Burrows GD, Evans BJ. Stress and anxiety in the onset of problem gambling: Implications for treatment. Stress Med 1997;13:235–44.
54. Taber JI, McCormick RA, Ramirez LF. The prevalence and impact of major life stressors among pathological gamblers. Int J Addict 1987;22:71–9.
55. Bergevin T, Derevensky J, Gupta R, Kaufman F. Adolescent gambling: Understanding the role of stress and coping. J Gambl Stud 2006;22(2):195–208.
56. Dickson L, Derevensky J, Gupta R. Youth gambling problems: An examination of risk and protective factors. IGS 2008;8(1):25–47.
57. Langhinrichsen-Rohling J, Rohde P, Seeley JR, et al. Individual, family, and peer correlates of adolescent gambling. J Gambl Stud 2004;20:23–46.
58. Jacques C, Ladouceur R, Ferland F. The impact of availability on gambling: A longitudinal study. Can J Psychiatry 2000(45):810–5.
59. Abbott DA, Cramer SL. Gambling attitudes and participation: A midwestern survey. J Gambl Stud 1993;9:247–63.
60. Derevensky J, Dickson L, Gupta R, Hardoon K. Adolescent attitudes toward gambling. Brazilian J Cognitive Psychology 2008;4:17–28.
61. Azmier J, Smith G. The Scope of Gambling in Canada: An Interprovincial Roadmap of Gambling and Its Impacts. Calgary, AB: Canada West Foundation; 1998.
62. Giacopassi D, Nichols M, Stitt BG. Attitudes of community leaders in new casino jurisdictions regarding casino gambling's effects on crime and quality of life. J Gambl Stud 1999;15:123–47.
63. Ladouceur R, Jacques C, Ferland F, Giroux I. Parents' attitudes and knowledge regarding gambling among youths. J Gambl Stud 1998;14:83–90.
64. Derevensky J, Sklar A, Gupta R, Messerlian C. An empirical study examining the impact of gambling advertisements on adolescent gambling attitudes and behaviors. IJMA 2010;8:21–34.
65. Gupta R, Derevensky JL. A treatment approach for adolescents with gambling problems. In: Derevensky JL, Gupta R, eds. Gambling Problems in Youth: Theoretical and Applied Perspectives. New York: Kluwer Acad/Plenum; 2004: p. 165–88.
66. Petry N. Pathological Gambling. Etiology, Co-morbidity and Treatment. Washington DC: American Psychological Association; 2005.
67. Shaffer HJ, LaPlante DA, LaBrie RA, Kidman R, Donato A, Stanton M. Toward a syndrome model of addiction: multiple expressions, common etiology. Harv Rev Psychiatry 2004;12:367–74.
68. Jacobs DF. A general theory of addictions: A new theoretical model. J Gambl Behav 1986(2):15–31.
69. Blaszczynski AP, Nower L. A pathways model of problem and pathological gambling. Addiction 2002;97:487–99.
70. Nower L, Blaszczynski A. A pathways approach to treating youth gamblers. In: Derevensky JL, Gupta R, eds. Gambling Problems in Youth: Theoretical and Applied Perspectives. New York: Kluwer Acad/Plenum; 2004: 189–209.
71. Jacobs DF. A general theory of the addictions: Rationale for and evidence supporting a new approach for understanding and treating addictive behaviors. In: Shaffer HJ, Stein SA, Gambino B, Cummings TN, eds. Compulsive Gambling: Theory, Research, and Practice. Lexington, MA: Lexington; 1989: 35–64.
72. Blaszczynski AP, Steel Z, McConaghy N. Impulsivity in pathological gambling: The antisocial impulsivist. Addiction 1997;92(1):75–87.
73. Rugle L, Melamed L. Neuropsychological assessment of attention problems in pathological gamblers. J Nerv Ment Dis 1993;181:107–12.
74. Vitaro F, Arseneault L, Tremblay R. Impulsivity predicts problem gambling in low SES adolescent males. Addiction 1999;94(4):565–75.
75. Gupta R, Nower L, Derevensky J, Blaszczynski AP. Problem Gambling in Adolescents: An Examination of the Pathways Model. Ontario: Report prepared for the Ontario Problem Gambling Research Centre; 2009.

Prevalence of youth gambling and problem gambling

3 An international perspective on youth gambling prevalence studies

Rachel A. Volberg, Rina Gupta, Mark D. Griffiths, Daniel T. Ólason, and Paul Delfabbro

In the wake of rapid expansion of legal gambling internationally, studies of adolescent gambling involvement and problem gambling prevalence have been carried out in numerous jurisdictions. This chapter reviews adolescent gambling prevalence studies carried out in North America, Europe, and Oceania. Based on this review, work is clearly needed to assess the impact of survey methods on identified prevalence rates and to improve the measurement of problem gambling among adolescents. From a substantive perspective, several clear demographic and behavioral characteristics are associated with gambling involvement and problem gambling among youth. However, early assumptions about youth gambling and problem gambling must give way to more nuanced understandings of how these phenomena change in response to changes in the social and cultural environment. We have traveled some distance down the road toward understanding the determinants as well as the distribution of youth gambling and problem gambling, but there is still a long way to go.

3.1 Introduction

Few people regard gambling as a serious issue for adolescents, although many researchers have noted that an entire generation has now grown up in an era when lottery and casino gambling is widely available and heavily advertised (1–4). Concern among researchers and clinicians who treat people with gambling problems is that increased availability and decreased stigma has led to increases in adolescent gambling as well as the prevalence and severity of gambling problems among adolescents and young adults.

There are many other reasons to be concerned about adolescent gambling. Research among adults has shown that individuals with severe gambling-related difficulties begin gambling much earlier than those without gambling problems (5, 6). Another reason for concern is that adolescents tend to begin gambling before they begin experimenting with tobacco, alcohol, drugs, and/or sexual behavior (7–9). A third, related concern is that gambling often co-occurs with other risky behaviors and mental health problems and, if unaddressed, could affect adolescents' success in overcoming other difficulties in their lives (10–12). Finally, although access to most legal forms of gambling is age-restricted, the evidence suggests that large numbers of high school and underage college students are able to gamble in casinos and buy lottery tickets (13, 14).

The impact on adolescents of the widespread availability, heavy advertising, and sanctioning of multiple forms of legal gambling is an increasing concern in the fields of public health and addictions. Nevertheless, a significant lack of consensus remains around the question of what constitutes problem gambling among adolescents and how to measure the disorder. Although well-accepted methods for identifying pathological gambling in the adult population have emerged (15), there are good reasons for caution in applying such methods to adolescents. The psychiatric criteria for identifying pathological gambling among adults were developed based on adult life experiences, and younger individuals have not yet had time to develop the same depth of experience. Another concern is that the psychiatric criteria for pathological gambling have never been clinically tested among adolescents, and little information has emerged about their validity in this subgroup of the population.

The few instruments developed to measure adolescent problem gambling are primarily derived from instruments developed to assess adults. The majority of adolescent studies have used either an adaptation for adolescents of the widely used South Oaks Gambling Screen (SOGS-RA) (16) or an adaptation of the adult psychiatric criteria for pathological gambling (DSM-IV-J and DSM-IV-MR-J) (17, 18). In a study comparing these two screens and one other measure of problem gambling (Gamblers Anonymous 20 Questions), Derevensky and Gupta (19) found substantial agreement among all three instruments, although the DSM-IV-J yielded a lower prevalence estimate than either the SOGS-RA or the GA 20 Questions. The three measures identified between 3.4% and 5.8% of participants in the study as probable pathological gamblers. However, only 1.1% of the participants in the study classified themselves as such (20).

Despite uncertainty about precisely what adolescent problem gambling screens measure, work has been carried out to identify the patterns of gambling and problem gambling among adolescents in many jurisdictions. Given the amount of research that has been done, there is value in taking a comparative look at what these studies can tell us about youth gambling and problem gambling from an international perspective. In this chapter, we review the methods and results of adolescent prevalence surveys that have been carried out in North America (the United States and Canada), Europe and the Nordic countries, and Oceania (Australia and New Zealand). We conclude by reviewing some of the consistent findings across these studies and drawing some important lessons for the future. A synopsis of the key features of all of these surveys is provided in ▶Tab. 3.1.

3.2 United States of America

The development of adolescent gambling prevalence research in the United States spans three distinct periods. The early period (1984 to 1989) coincided with the growth of state-run lotteries. The middle period (1990 to 1999) coincided with a rapid expansion of casino gambling in the wake of the passage of the Indian Gaming Regulatory Act of 1988. The past decade (2000 to 2009) saw changes in strategies for collecting data about adolescent gambling and problem gambling, increased analytic sophistication, and growing interest in the links between adolescent gambling and other risky behaviors.

3.2.1 Early period (1984–1989)

In an early review of adolescent prevalence surveys, Jacobs (21) identified six studies that were completed before 1990 (22–27). Carried out in California, Connecticut, New Jersey, and Virginia, all the studies were conducted in high schools using self-completed

Tab. 3.1: Summary of adolescent prevalence surveys carried out internationally

Location	Author	Year Data Collected	Sample Size and Ages	Method	Measure	Gambling Participation (past year)	Problem/ Pathological Gambling
UNITED STATES							
Early Period (1984–1989)							
California	Jacobs et al.	1985	843 14–18	Classroom	GA 20 Questions	20	4
California	Jacobs et al.	1987	257 14–18	Classroom	GA 20 Questions	45	4
Connecticut	Steinberg	1988	573 14–18	Classroom	SOGS	60	5
New Jersey	Lesieur and Klein	1984	892 16–18	Classroom	PGSI	86	5.7
Virginia	Kuley and Jacobs	1987	212 14–18	Classroom	GA 20 Questions	40	Not reported
Virginia	Kuley and Jacobs	1989	147	Classroom	GA 20 Questions	58	Not reported
Middle Period (1990–1999)							
Georgia	Volberg	1996	1,007 13–17	Telephone	SOGS-RA MFM	52	2.8
New York	Volberg	1997	1,103 13–17	Telephone	SOGS-RA MFM	75	2.4
Oregon	Volberg	1998	997 13–17	Telephone	SOGS-RA	66	1.4
Texas	Wallisch	1992	924 14–17	Telephone	SOGS-RA MFM	66	5.0
Texas	Wallisch	1995	3,079 14–17	Telephone	SOGS-RA MFM	67	2.3
Washington	Volberg	1993	1,045 13–17	Telephone	SOGS-RA MFM	70	0.9

(Continued)

Tab. 3.1: Summary of adolescent prevalence surveys carried out internationally (Continued)

Location	Author	Year Data Collected	Sample Size and Ages	Method	Measure	Gambling Participation (past year)	Problem/ Pathological Gambling
Washington	Volberg and Moore	1999	1,000 13–17	Telephone	SOGS-RA MFM	65	0.9
Louisiana	Westphal, Rush and Stevens	1998	11,736 6th–12th grades	Classroom	SOGS-RA	86	5.8
Vermont	Proimos et al.	1995	16,948 8th–12th graders	Classroom	Single item	53	7.0
Minnesota	Winters, Stinchfield and Fulkerson	1992	75,806 9th and 12th graders	Classroom	2-item screen	M9=83 F9=60 / M12=86 F12=63	2.4 0.7 / 2.6 0.6
Minnesota	Winters, Stinchfield and Kim	1995	73,897 9th and 12th graders	Classroom	2-item screen	M9=77 F9=50 / M12=82 F12=59	2.3 0.5 / 2.9 0.4
Minnesota	Stinchfield	1998	78,564 9th and 12th graders	Classroom	2-item screen	M9=70 F9=38 / M12=81 F12=54	2.3 0.5 / 2.9 0.6
Recent Period (2000–2009)							
Nevada	Volberg	2002	1,004 13–17	Telephone	SOGS-RA DSM-IV-MR-J	66	1.9
New York	Rainone and Gallati	2006	5,844	Classroom	DSM-IV-MR-J	72	3.0
Oregon	Volberg, Hedberg and Moore	2007	1,555 12–17	Telephone	SOGS-RA DSM-IV-MR-J	46	1.3
National	Welte et al.	2005–2007	2,274 14–21	Telephone	SOGS-RA DIS	67	1.3

Notes:

MFM = Multi-Factor Method for scoring the SOGS-RA; PGSI = Pathological Gambling Signs Index

CANADA

Early Investigations (1988–1995)

Location	Author	Year	N / Age	Mode	Instrument		Prevalence
Alberta	Wynne Resources	1995	972 12–17	Telephone	SOGS-R	67	7.9
Windsor, Ontario	Govoni et al.	1994	935 14–19	Classroom	SOGS-RA	90	8.1
Ontario	Insight Canada Research	1994	400 12–19	Not reported	SOGS-R	65	4
Quebec City, Quebec	Ladouceur and Mireault	1988	1,612 14–19	Classroom	PGSI	65	3.6
Nova Scotia	Omnifacts Research	1993	300 13–17	Not reported	SOGS	60	3

Recent Period (1998–2009)

Location	Author	Year	N / Age	Mode	Instrument		Prevalence
Canada	Huang and Boyer	2002	5,666 15–24	Face-to-face	CPGI	61	2.2
British Columbia	Gregg	2001/2	454 15–19	Classroom	SOGS-RA	90	5
Alberta	AADAC	2002	3,394 Grades 7–12	Classroom	SOGS-RA	41	3.8
Alberta	AADAC	2005	3,915 Grades 7–12	Classroom	SOGS-RA	63	3.6
Saskatchewan	Dickinson and Schissel	2003	1,884 15–18	Classroom	Not assessed	81	Not reported
Manitoba	Wiebe	1999	1,000 12–17	Telephone	SOGS-RA	78	3
Manitoba	Lemaire	2002/2003	410 15–20	Telephone	SOGS-RA	78	3
Manitoba	Mackay, Patton, and Broszeit	2004	6,673 Grades 7–12	Classroom	DSM-IV-MR-J	35	2.3
Ontario	Adlaf et al.	2005	7,726 Grades 7–12	Classroom	SOGS-RA6	33	4.5

(Continued)

Tab. 3.1: Summary of adolescent prevalence surveys carried out internationally (*Continued*)

Location	Author	Year Data Collected	Sample Size and Ages	Method	Measure	Gambling Participation (past year)	Problem/ Pathological Gambling
Quebec	Martin, Gupta, and Derevensky	2006	4,571 Grades 7–11	Classroom	DSM-IV-J	*French 35 Other 42 Total 36	French 2 Other 4 Total 2
Atlantic Provinces	Poulin	1998	13,549 Grades 7–12	Classroom	SOGS-RA	70	2.2

Notes: *French = French mother tongue, Other = Mother tongue other than French.

EUROPE

Belgium	Kinable	2006	38,357 12–18	Classroom	Not assessed	40 (lifetime)	Not reported
Estonia	Laansoo	2006	2,005 15–74	Telephone	SOGS	75 (lifetime)	3.4 (lifetime)*
Germany***	Hurrelmann et al.	2003	5,000 13–19	Not reported	DSM-IV-MR-J	62	3
Great Britain	Fisher and Balding	1996	3,724 12–15	Classroom	DSM-IV-J	15 (7 day lottery)	Not reported
Great Britain	Fisher	1997	9,774 12–15	Classroom	DSM-IV-MR-J	19 (7 day fruit machines)	5.6
Great Britain	Ashworth and Doyle	1999	9,529 12–15	Classroom	DSM-IV-MR-J	75	5.4
Great Britain	Ashworth et al.	2000	11,581 12–15	Classroom	DSM-IV-MR-J	70	4.9
Great Britain	MORI/IGRU	2006	8,017 12–15	Classroom	DSM-IV-MR-J	54	3.5
Great Britain	Ipsos MORI	2009	8,598 12–15	Classroom	DSM-IV-MR-J	21 (7 day all activities)	2.0**
Italy***	Capitanucci et al.	2006	579 13–20	Classroom	SOGS-RA	Not reported	6

Country	Author	Year	Sample (n / age)	Method	Instrument		
Lithuania***	Skokauskas et al.	2007	835 9–16	Classroom	DSM-IV-MR-J SOGS-RA	83 (lifetime)	4 5
Romania***	Lupu et al.	2002	500 14–19	Classroom	GA-20	82 (lifetime)	7 (lifetime)
Slovakia***	Kotrc	2006	1,142	Classroom	Not assessed	27.5 (lifetime)	Not assessed
Spain***	Becona et al.	2001	11–16	Classroom	DSM-IV-J SOGS-RA	Not reported	0.8 4.6

Notes:

* Problem gambling prevalence for adolescents and adults combined.

** Scoring requirement that all screener questions be answered was dropped in 2009.

*** Used regional (not national) samples.

NORDIC COUNTRIES

Country	Author	Year	Sample (n / age)	Method	Instrument		
Denmark	Sörensen et al.	2007	3,814 12–17	Telephone	Five item NODS	51 (lifetime)	0.8
Finland	Ilkas and Aho	2006	5,000 12–17	Telephone	SOGS-RA	52	2.3
Iceland*	Ólason et al.	2003	750 16–18	Classroom	DSM-IV-MR-J SOGS-RA	Not reported	2.0 2.7
Iceland*	Ólason et al	2004	3,511 13–15	Classroom	DSM-IV-MR-J SOGS-RA	70	1.9 2.8
Iceland*	Baldursdottir et al.	2005	1,513 16–18	Classroom	DSM-IV-MR-J	62	3.0
Iceland*	Kristjansdottir	2007	1,537 13–18	Classroom	DSM-IV-MR-J	57	2.2
Norway	Johansson and Götestam	1999	3,237 12–18	Telephone Postal	10-item DSM-IV	82	1.8
Norway	Rossow and Hansen	2002	13,000 13–19	Classroom	Lie/Bet + Chasing	78	3.2

(Continued)

Tab. 3.1: Summary of adolescent prevalence surveys carried out internationally (*Continued*)

Location	Author	Year Data Collected	Sample Size and Ages	Method	Measure	Gambling Participation (past year)	Problem/ Pathological Gambling
Norway	Rossow and Molde	2004	20,703 13–19	Classroom	SOGS-RA	74	2.5
Sweden	Rönnberg et al.	1997	1,000 15–17	Telephone Postal	SOGS-R	76	0.9

Notes:
* *Used regional (not national) samples.*

AUSTRALIA and NEW ZEALAND

Location	Author	Year Data Collected	Sample Size and Ages	Method	Measure	Gambling Participation (past year)	Problem/ Pathological Gambling
Australian Capital Territory	Delfabbro, Lahn and Grabosky	2003	926	Classroom	DSM-IV-J	70	4.4
South Australia	Delfabbro and Thrupp	2000–2001	505	Classroom	DSM-IV-J	62	3.5
South Australia	S. A. Dept for Families and Communities	2005	605	Telephone	DSM-IV-J	43	1.0
South Australia	Lambos et al.	2007	2,669	Classroom	DSM-IV-J	56	2.4
Victoria	Moore and Ohtsuka	1997	1,017 14–25	Classroom	10-item SOGS	75 (lifetime)	3.1
Victoria	Moore and Ohtsuka	1998	796 13–17	Classroom	10-item SOGS	89 (lifetime)	3.8
Victoria	Jackson	1997	2,788 13	Classroom	Not assessed	41	Not assessed
New Zealand	Sullivan	2001	547	Classroom	DSM-IV-J	65	13.0
New Zealand	Rossen	2008	2,005	Classroom	DSM-IV-MR-J	68	3.8

questionnaires. The students participating in these studies were probably not representative of their schools or of adolescents in their states because as Jacobs noted, "none of these independent unsponsored investigators had the resources to employ formal stratified sampling procedures" (21:433). Sample sizes were relatively small, ranging from 147 to 892, and different instruments were used in each study. In California and Virginia, separate surveys were carried out before and after state lotteries were introduced. In the wake of the introduction of lotteries, Jacobs (21) reported that past-year gambling participation among high school students rose from 20% to 45% in California and from 40% to 58% in Virginia.

In a subsequent analysis that included these six studies along with nine additional surveys carried out between 1989 and 1999, Jacobs (1:120) concluded that the rise in the median level of gambling participation from 45% before 1990 to 66% "leaves little doubt that juvenile gambling throughout the US has increased significantly." Jacobs (1:134) further concluded that "the dominant long term trend has been a progressive increase in the amount of serious gambling-related problems reported by juveniles in the US." This view is in contrast to the conclusion reached by other researchers (3, 28, 29) that rates of youth gambling and problem gambling tend to be quite stable over time.

3.2.2 Middle period (1990–1999)

In the United States, the decade from 1990 to 1999 saw rapid growth in the number and quality of adolescent gambling prevalence surveys. Although some states funded only one such survey during the decade, several states funded two or more surveys.

Single surveys

During the 1990s, single school-based or telephone surveys were completed in several states, including Georgia, Louisiana, New York, and Vermont. The reasons for funding these studies varied. In Georgia, there was concern about the impact of a new state lottery on adolescent gambling and, in New York, concern about the impact of a new lottery game, five-minute keno. In Louisiana, the State Health Department desired information on which to base a youth gambling prevention program.

In 1995, Vermont was the first state to add a gambling module to the Youth Risk Behavior Survey (YRBS) conducted annually by the Centers for Disease Control and Prevention (30). The survey was administered to 8th to 12th grade students (n = 21,297) in public and private schools across the state. Two questions related to gambling were included in the survey, one assessing past-year gambling participation and the other assessing problems caused by gambling. Apart from gambling, the risk behaviors assessed in this survey included drug and alcohol use, seatbelt use, violence, and sexual activity. Among the 16,948 students who answered both gambling questions, problem gamblers reported significantly more risky behaviors than gamblers, and gamblers reported significantly more risky behaviors than nongamblers. The Vermont researchers recommended that gambling be included as a regular part of health assessments of adolescents and used to identify youth at risk of developing other risk behaviors.

In 1996, the Georgia Department of Human Resources funded an adolescent prevalence survey (31). Telephone interviews with a sample of 1,007 Georgia adolescents aged 13 to 17 used the SOGS-RA to assess problem gambling. A modified scoring method was used to classify respondents in this survey as nonproblem, at-risk, and problem gamblers. Based on this multi-factor method (also used in surveys in Texas and Washington State), 2.8% of the Georgia adolescents surveyed were classified as problem gamblers. Logistic regression analysis showed that male adolescents with high weekly incomes but low self-esteem were more likely to be classified as problem gamblers than were other adolescents in the study. A similar adolescent survey was carried out in 1997 in New York State (32). The sample in New York included 1,103 adolescents aged 13 to 17 years and the SOGS-RA was used to assess problem gambling. Based on the multi-factor method, 2.4% of the adolescent respondents were classified as problem gamblers.

In 1998, Westphal and colleagues (33) conducted a large school-based prevalence survey in Louisiana. The study included a random sample of 11,736 students in grades 6 through 12 attending both public and private schools throughout the state. One third (34%) of the final sample was African American. Based on the SOGS-RA, 5.8% of students were classified as problem gamblers. The researchers noted that the age of onset for gambling participation was significantly younger than for smoking tobacco and use of marijuana and alcohol.

Repeat cross-sectional surveys

In the 1990s, several states funded multiple adolescent prevalence surveys (e.g., Oregon, Texas, and Washington State). In all these states, the surveys used methods very similar to those employed in the surveys in Georgia and New York. The major difference across these states was the interval between the baseline and replication surveys. In Texas, the gap was 3 years (34, 35); in Washington State, the gap was 6 years (36, 37); and in Oregon, the gap was 9 years (38, 39).

In Texas, Wallisch (34, 35) found that whereas lifetime gambling participation among adolescents aged 14 to 17 years increased in the wake of the introduction of a state lottery, past-year gambling participation remained stable. The prevalence of problem gambling, assessed using the SOGS-RA, declined from 5.0% in 1992 to 2.3% in 1995. In Washington State, Volberg and Moore (37) found that past-year gambling participation declined slightly from 70% to 65%, whereas the prevalence of problem gambling, using the SOGS-RA, was unchanged at 0.9%.

In Oregon, Volberg et al. (39) found a significant decline in gambling participation among adolescents over a 9-year period, from 66% in 1998 to 46% in 2007, with no change in the prevalence of problem gambling. The researchers hypothesized that the substantial drop, particularly in age-restricted gambling activities, could be due to several factors, including sampling error, lifelong exposure to gambling, changes in attitudes toward youth gambling, and extensive efforts undertaken by the state of Oregon to educate youth, parents, and teachers about the risks of adolescent gambling.

In Minnesota, the presence of a well-established research center on adolescent risk behavior combined with the introduction of a state lottery to support an extensive program of research into adolescent gambling in the 1990s. In 1990, Winters, Stinchfield, and Fulkerson (40) conducted a telephone survey of 702 Minnesota youth aged 15 to 18 years to obtain a baseline measure of youth gambling before the introduction of the state lottery. One year later, 532 participants from the baseline survey (76%) were re-interviewed by telephone (41). Although no statistically significant changes were found in regular participation in specific gambling activities, a shift from informal private games to legal gambling activities over the 1-year interval was observed. This report was the first instance of a prospective study of gambling behavior.

A series of three school-based prevalence surveys was subsequently carried out in Minnesota in 1992, 1995, and 1998 (29, 42). In each year, two items (feeling bad about gambling and wanting to stop gambling) were added to the Minnesota Student Survey, a self-administered questionnaire that inquires about multiple behavioral domains and is administered every 3 years to nearly all 9th and 12th graders in Minnesota. Between 1995 and 1998, the researchers found that although fewer youth gambled, the proportion of youth who gambled frequently increased. The researchers also found that the proportion of youth self-reporting gambling problems based on these two items remained relatively stable between 1992 and 1998.

Native American youth

In the 1990s, Class III (casino) gambling on Native American reservations expanded rapidly. In the wake of this development, two small prevalence studies were carried out among Native American adolescents (43, 44). One of these two school-based surveys was carried out on a Northern Plains reservation ($n = 227$ students, ages 12–19) and the other was completed on a Great Lakes reservation ($n = 185$ students, ages 12–19). The two surveys used identical methods, and the results focused on comparisons of American Indian and non-Indian adolescents living on or near the reservations. The self-administered questionnaire included a combination of SOGS, GA 20 Questions, and DSM-III-R items.

Both studies found that the majority of Native American youth gambled and that Native American youth started gambling at an earlier age than non-Indian youth. Zitzow (44) reported that 5.6% of the non-Native American youth scored as "pathological gamblers" compared with 9.6% of Native American youth. Peacock et al. (43) did not report on the proportion of youth in their sample that scored as problem or pathological gamblers. However, these researchers concluded that Native American youth were at greater risk for developing gambling problems because of extremely high rates of loss of important people in their lives and the widespread belief that money would solve their problems.

Interestingly, in considering the impact of the introduction of casino gambling in Indian country, Zitzow concluded that "the recent introduction of a large stakes casino within this reservation community may not be the most significant event in promoting gambling . . . The most significant events appear to have already occurred within the last 15 years due to the onset of bingo, pulltabs, state-supported scratch tabs, and the state lottery" (44: 25).

3.2.3 Present period (2000–2009)

Since 2000, the number of surveys designed specifically to measure adolescent gambling prevalence has declined in the United States. Instead, researchers are finding new ways to obtain information about adolescent gambling and are focusing more on risk and protective factors associated with problem gambling.

Adding gambling modules to other surveys of youth

Ten years ago, the National Gambling Impact Study Commission (45) recommended add-ing gambling components to existing research panels. Although this recommendation was never implemented at the national level, several states (e.g., Arizona, Louisiana, New York) added gambling modules to existing surveys of youth (46–48). Unfortunately, only the New York survey included any questions about gambling-related problems.

Because the focus of these surveys is on risk and protective factors for a range of behaviors, all include large samples of students. Adding questions that assess past-year involvement in a range of gambling activities enables an examination of gambling in-volvement in relation to gender and age, as well as in relation to other risk behaviors, such as alcohol and substance use, anti-social behavior, and school performance. One interesting finding from the surveys in Arizona and Louisiana is that, in contrast to many other adolescent gambling prevalence studies, older youth in these states were less likely than younger youth to say that they gambled.

Another advantage to adding gambling modules to youth risk behavior surveys is that changes in gambling participation can be tracked over time. In Arizona, where gambling questions were asked in 2006 and 2008, significant increases in gambling participation were identified among 8th, 10th, and 12th graders (46). In New York, where gambling questions were included in the 1998 and 2006 annual School Survey of the Office of Alcoholism and Substance Abuse Services, students were 15% more likely to have played card games for money and 43% more likely to have played lottery games in 2006 compared with 1998 (48). The 2006 survey in New York was the only one that included a problem gambling screen; notably, 28% of the students in New York who were deemed to be in need of chemical dependence treatment services had experienced gambling problems in the past year.

The national picture

As part of the national Gambling Impact and Behavior Study, Gerstein et al. (49) completed a survey of 534 youths aged 16 to 17 via a randomized telephone survey of U.S. households. Youth were interviewed with the same questionnaire used in an accompanying adult survey and screened for gambling problems using the NODS, a screen derived from the DSM-IV criteria for pathological gambling and designed spe-cifically for telephone survey administration. The most striking finding relates to the different pattern of youth gambling compared with adults. Adolescent gambling was predominantly composed of private betting on games of skill, particularly card games. Over one-quarter of youths (28%) compared with just 11% of adults had bet on such games in the past year. The other most prominent youth games were betting in sports pools and buying lottery tickets. Another interesting finding was that the prevalence of at-risk, problem, and pathological gambling among the adolescent respondents was substantially lower than among adults, if the same cutpoints were used.

Between 2005 and 2007, a nationally representative survey of youth gambling and problem gambling was carried out with funding from the National Institutes of Health (4, 10). Telephone interviews were completed with 2,274 youths and young adults aged 14 to 21 years in all 50 states and the District of Columbia. The data were weighted to adjust for household size and to match the gender, age, and race distributions of the U.S. Census. The primary measure of problem gambling was the SOGS-RA, although the researchers also included a 13-item module from the Diagnostic Interview Schedule that was used to assess pathological gambling in an earlier adult survey (50). The study found that 68% of the youth and young adult respondents had gambled in the past year. Males were much more likely than females to gamble regularly, as were older adolescents. African Americans were less likely than youth of other races to have gambled in the past year but, if they gambled, they were more likely to do so regularly. As with the earlier national survey, this study found that rates of problem and pathological gambling were lower than those in the adult sample assessed by the same research team and with the same questionnaire. A separate analysis of the data found a close relationship between the mean number of gambling activities engaged in by youth and problem gambling (51). After controlling for involvement in other games, the researchers found that card games, games of skill, and gambling at casinos were the activities most closely associated with an increased risk of gambling-related problems among adolescents and young adults.

Since 2002, the Adolescent Risk Communication Institute (created by the Annenberg Foundation) has funded an annual telephone survey of youth aged 14 to 22 years. The sample size was 900 in each year except for 2004 and 2008. Respondents are asked questions about a range of risky activities, including frequency of engaging in specific gambling activities in an "average" month. Respondents who have engaged in one or more activities in an average month are asked four questions about difficulties related to their gambling that assess the DSM-IV criteria of preoccupation, tolerance, loss of control, and withdrawal. In 2008, the Institute reported that monthly rates of card playing, particularly on the Internet, had spiked in 2005 and 2006 in the wake of a "card playing (poker) fad" and had since declined and stabilized. The researchers reported that sports betting increased among male youth in 2008 but that the long-term trend in overall weekly gambling since 2002 had been downward for both male and female youth (52).

3.3 Canada

Although there have been numerous studies of adolescent gambling in Canada, relatively few prevalence surveys have been completed. Most studies consist of convenience samples, assessing adolescents within the school system, and usually include only youth living close to major city centers. Nonetheless, such studies have proved useful in understanding gambling patterns, preferences, and trends, as well as a sense of the proportion of youth in Canada who experience gambling-related problems.

3.3.1 Early investigations (1988–1995)

Early surveys of adolescents, completed in Nova Scotia in 1993, in Ontario in 1994, and in Alberta in 1996, included the adult SOGS rather than a problem gambling screen specifically designed for adolescents (53–55). Wynne Resources reports that the Alberta youth survey was carried out by telephone, but the modality used in the Nova Scotia and Ontario adolescent surveys is unclear. Two early surveys in Quebec City and Windsor, Ontario, were classroom-based but included different problem gambling screens. The Quebec City survey was based on the "pathological gambling signs index" used in another early youth survey in New Jersey (26, 56). The Windsor survey used the

SOGS-RA to assess the extent of problem gambling (57). Both past-year gambling and the rate of pathological gambling were lower in Quebec City than in New Jersey; the Windsor survey found higher rates of both past-year gambling and problem gambling than reported in other provinces.

Across the board, these early investigations found that Canadian youth participated in a multitude of gambling activities, usually self-organized forms of wagering (e.g., card games for money, betting on games of skill including video games), although lottery products were also popular among adolescents (7).

3.3.2 Recent period (1999–2009)

The national survey

The Canada-wide mental health survey (Canadian Community Health Survey: Mental Health and Well-Being 1.2) is the largest nationally representative data set assessing gambling participation and problem gambling prevalence among individuals aged 15 years and older. The youth data consist of a subset of 5,666 Canadian residents aged 15 to 24 years. Respondents were interviewed face-to-face, and the Canadian Problem Gambling Index (CPGI) was used to measure gambling and problem gambling. Although minor regional differences were seen, overall 61% of youth reported gambling in the previous year, 56% ranked as nonproblem gamblers, 3.5% scored as being at slight risk for gambling problems, and 2.2% ranked as being moderately at risk for and/or meeting the criteria for problem gambling. Those at greatest risk were young, male, and living in the Prairie region (58).

The rates of problem gambling identified among adolescents in the national prevalence survey in Canada were substantially lower than rates identified in provincial prevalence surveys conducted in roughly the same period. This finding is particularly true for British Columbia and the Prairie provinces of Alberta, Saskatchewan, and Manitoba. Also noteworthy is that the national survey included individuals to age 24 years who were interviewed in person, whereas provincial surveys have focused primarily on those under the age of 18 or 19 years and have been completed in classrooms or by telephone. Accordingly, differences between the provincial surveys and the national survey must be interpreted with caution.

British Columbia

Aside from the national prevalence study, little research on adolescent gambling has been carried out in British Columbia. One small study, conducted in Langley in 2001–2002 among 454 students aged 15 to 19 years, included the SOGS-RA. Ninety percent of the participants in this study reported gambling in the previous year and five percent met the narrow criteria for serious gambling-related problems (59).

The Prairie provinces

Based on recent studies in all three provinces (Alberta, Saskatchewan, and Manitoba), the rates of adolescent gambling participation appear lower in Alberta than in the other two provinces. In 2002 and 2005, the Alberta Youth Experience Survey, completed with students in grades 7 through 12 (60, 61), included questions about gambling participation and problem gambling. In 2002, 41% of the students reported gambling in the past year. The most popular gambling activities included scratch tabs (31%), playing cards for money (23%), and betting on sports events (21%). Alberta adolescents held favorable attitudes toward gambling and perceived it as a socially acceptable activity. Based on the SOGS-RA, 3.8% of Alberta students were considered problem gamblers, of which the majority were male, in high school, Aboriginal, and from larger cities. Three years later, a repeat survey found that past-year gambling participation had increased to 63%, with scratch tabs replaced by card playing as the most frequent activity (41%). The prevalence of problem gambling based on the SOGS-RA remained almost unchanged at 3.6%; but the prevalence of at-risk gambling rose from 5.7% to 8.8% (61).

A study commissioned by Saskatchewan Health in 2003 included a sample of 1,884 students aged 15 to 18 years (62). The majority of youth (81%) reported gambling with scratch tickets, games of skill, and self-organized poker games among the most popular activities. Although problem gambling was not assessed, the authors concluded that Saskatchewan youth were actively involved in gambling, and that gambling represented a significant proportion of their monthly expenditures.

The Addictions Foundation of Manitoba conducted a prevalence study of youth in 1999. One thousand youth, aged 12 to 17 years, were interviewed by telephone and administered the SOGS-RA. The majority of the adolescents (78%) reported gambling in the previous year, with the most popular activities being the purchase of raffle tickets, playing cards for money, and betting on dice or games of skill. Based on the SOGS-RA, 8% of these adolescents were at-risk gamblers and 3% were problem gamblers (63). Three years later, a follow-up study was completed with 410 individuals from the 1999 cohort, now aged 15 to 20 years (64). Looking only at the 32% of the sample still under 18 years of age, the study found that the overall rate of gambling participation had not changed. However, respondents were more likely to participate in legal, age-restricted forms of gambling, such as casinos and VLTs, and less likely to gamble in home or school settings. The at-risk and problem gambling rates decreased slightly from 1999, but the authors concluded that these changes were not statistically significant.

In 2004, a study conducted in Manitoba schools included 6,673 students aged 12–18 years from across the province. The sample included more rural schools than in previous surveys in Manitoba and was more representative of the youth population of Manitoba. Using the DSM-IV-MR-J the results differed significantly from previous adolescent surveys in Manitoba, with only 35% of the students reporting having gambled in the previous 12 months. However, the rate of problem gambling (2.3%) is very similar to rates previously reported in Manitoba (65). These results suggest that youth in rural areas are less likely than urban youth to gamble.

Ontario

The Centre for Addiction and Mental Health's Ontario Student Drug Use Survey (OSDUS) is the longest ongoing school survey of adolescents in Canada, having been conducted every two years since 1977. Beginning in 1999, the OSDUS included questions about gambling and gambling problems in these surveys, which encompass students in grades 7 to 12 (ages 12–18 years). Although the full SOGS-RA was used until 2003, the 12-item screen was reduced to 6 items in the 2005 survey. In 2005, 33% of the students acknowledged playing cards for money in the past year, 18% purchased lottery tickets, and 17% bet money in sports pools. The least prevalent activity was casino gambling (1%), followed by Internet gambling (2%). Among all the students, 6% were identified as heavy gamblers and 4.5% were classified as problem gamblers. Developmentally, heavy gambling rates were found to vary significantly by grade, peaking in grade 12 at 8.5%. Although the researchers identified a sharp decrease in the rate of problem gambling between 1999 and 2003 (from 6.2% to 3.5%), between 2003 and 2005 they found a slight increase in problem gambling prevalence (from 3.5% to 4.5%), a change that was not statistically significant (66, 67).

Quebec

Quebec is a unique province with known meaningful cultural differences between Francophones (French-speaking), Anglophones (English-speaking), and Allophones (neither English-speaking nor French-speaking). Whereas Quebec's population is predominantly Francophone, significant numbers of Anglophones and Allophones live around the major city centers, primarily Montreal. Problem gambling rates in Quebec have been shown to vary according to these cultural differences. In 2006, a province-wide, representative sample of 4,571 students in grades 7 to 11 was surveyed using the DSM-IV-J to assess problem gambling (68). The results showed that 36% of high-school students had gambled in the past 12 months, with participation rates being higher among Allophone students (42% vs. 35%). Thirty percent of students were classified as occasional gamblers and 6% were classified as habitual gamblers (i.e., gambling at least once per week). The rate of habitual gambling was higher among Anglophone and Allophone students compared to Francophone youth (9% vs. 5%). The most popular forms of gambling among Quebec high-school students included card games (21%), instant lotteries (17%), games of skill (14%), and private sports gambling (13%). Approximately 4% of these high school students were at-risk gamblers and 2% were problem gamblers. The prevalence of problem gambling was twice as high among students who spoke a language other than French at home (Anglophones/Allophones) compared with Francophones (4% vs. 2%) (68).

The Atlantic provinces

In 1998, a survey was conducted across all four Atlantic provinces: Nova Scotia, New Brunswick, Newfoundland and Labrador, and Prince Edward Island. A total of 13,549 students from grades 7 through 12 in the public school systems completed a questionnaire that included the SOGS-RA. Overall, 70% of the students reported gambling in the previous year; the most popular gambling activities were scratch tabs (60%), playing cards for money (35%), and betting on sports (30%). The prevalence of at-risk gambling among these adolescents was 3.8% and the prevalence of problem gambling was 2.2%. The prevalence of problem gambling did not vary on the basis of age (69).

3.4 Europe

Recent reviews of gambling participation across many European countries suggest that research into adolescent gambling is comparatively rare in this part of the world. In this section, research conducted in the Baltic and Balkan countries, Germany and Belgium, the Latin European countries of Italy and Spain, and Great Britain is reviewed. This is followed by a review of research conducted in the Nordic countries of Denmark, Finland, Iceland, Norway, and Sweden.

3.4.1 Baltic and Balkan states

Central and Eastern European countries in which some adolescent gambling research has been completed include Estonia, Lithuania, Romania, and Slovakia. In Estonia, two prevalence surveys have been carried out among residents aged 15 to 74 years (70, 71). The 2004 survey included 1,000 respondents and the 2006 effort surveyed 2,005 respondents. The SOGS was translated into Estonian and used to assess problem and pathological gambling in both studies (72). In comparing the results of the two surveys, Laansoo and Niit (73) observed that younger respondents in these surveys were more likely to gamble and more likely to be classified as probable pathological gamblers.

A youth gambling study was recently completed in Kaunas, Lithuania's second largest city (74). The sample comprised 835 randomly selected adolescents between the ages of 9 and 16 years from all of the Kaunas secondary schools (47% male, 53% female). Two problem gambling screens, the SOGS-RA and the DSM-IV-MR-J, were translated into Lithuanian (75, 76). The results showed that males were significantly more likely than females to be both occasional and regular gamblers. Based on the DSM-IV-MR-J, 4% of the study participants were identified as pathological gamblers. Compared with other gamblers, the pathological gamblers in this study were significantly more likely to gamble on slot machines (51% vs. 8%), cards (17% vs. 7%), and Short Message Service (SMS) gambling (27% vs. 9%). Being male, having cognitive distortions regarding gambling, having parents who gambled, having parents who gambled to excess, using alcohol regularly, and smoking regularly all contributed independently to pathological gambling status.

As in Lithuania, some research on adolescent gambling has been conducted in Romania (77). Lupu, Onaca, and Lupu (78) examined the prevalence of problem gambling using the GA 20 Questions in three Romanian counties. Based on a sample of 500 high-school students (57% female and 43% male) between the ages of 14 and 19, the games most frequently played by Romanian teenagers were football pools (56%), poker (35%), and bingo (32%). Two-thirds of the sample (64%) gambled frequently and 82% indicated that they gambled in groups. The mean age at which these Romanian youth began gambling was 14 years. Among the 7% of participants identified as problem gamblers, 82% were male. Analysis showed that 18% of the problem gamblers had fathers who were alcoholics and 12% had fathers who were problem gamblers. No significant differences were found between problem and nonproblem gamblers in relation to family income or social status.

In a separate study, Lupu and colleagues (79) examined the risk factors for problem gambling among 231 Romanian adolescents aged 14 to 18 years. Using the GA 20 Questions, the researchers categorized the participants into three groups based on their level of gambling and problem gambling severity. Among these youth, 54% endorsed between two and six of the GA 20 Questions and another 12% endorsed seven or more items. Risk factors for the most severe problem group included parental divorce, serious physical illness in a family member, death of a family member, family break-up, psychological illness in a family member, sexual abuse, and being in a severe accident. Based on the data, Lupu et al. (79) identified two distinct types of adolescent problem gambler:

- adolescents from unfavorable family and social environments who were dealing with stress and trauma (e.g., neglect, physical and/or sexual abuse); and
- adolescents from favorable family and social environments, where parents neglected the child because of work involvement.

Among the first group, gambling was a coping mechanism to deal with chronic stress; among the second group, gambling was a way to spend time and/or attract a parent's attention.

Finally, a recent overview by Zivny and Okruhlica (80) made reference to a study that examined the comorbidity of gambling and psychoactive substance use in primary and secondary schools in Slovakia (81). In this survey of 1,142 primary and secondary students, 12% of primary school children reported they had gambled occasionally and 1.5% admitted gambling regularly. Among secondary school children, 15.5% gambled occasionally whereas 1.6% played regularly.

3.4.2 Germany and Belgium

The only study examining the prevalence of adolescent problem gambling in Germany was carried out by Hurrelmann, Schmidt, and Kähnert (82). Comprising 5,000 youth aged 13 to 19 years from the Federal State of North Rhine-Westphalia, the results showed that 62% of the respondents had gambled for money in the past year. Scratch cards (36%) and private card games for money (29%) were the most popular activities. Other popular activities included state-run sports betting (18%), amusement-with-prizes machines (17%), private games of skill (17%), and private dice games (15%). The prevalence rate of problem gambling using the DSM-IV-MR-J was 3% among all participants. However, boys were five times more likely than girls to be problem gamblers. Problem gamblers reported significantly more stressful life events than nonproblem gamblers, consumed psychoactive substances more frequently, and were dissatisfied with their life situation. The researchers concluded that these adolescent problem gamblers lacked coping skills for handling day-to-day demands.

The only study of adolescent gambling in Belgium was part of a larger study of youth risk habits (83). This survey of 38,357 youth aged 12 to 18 examined participation in four gambling activities (slot machines, lotteries, card games, and betting). Results showed that 40% of these adolescents had gambled on one or more of the four activities in their lifetime, reflecting a decrease from 53% in 2001 and 42% in 2005.

3.4.3 Latin Europe

Very little research has been done on adolescent gambling in any of the Latin European countries. In Italy, Capitanucci, Biganzoli, and Smaniotto (84) examined youth gambling in a student sample from a technical college in Northern Italy (520 males and 59 females; aged between 13 and 20 years). A translated version of the SOGS-RA used to assess problem gambling found that the most popular form of gambling among these Italian youth was sports betting (14% of the respondents bet on sports once a week or more often), and 6% of the respondents were classified as problem or pathological gamblers. Pathological gambling was strongly correlated with being male, gambling out of habit or for relaxation, and believing chance games to be skilful (e.g., erroneous cognitions). A separate study by Baiocco, Couyoumdjian, Langellotti, and Del Miglio (85) examined aspects of pathological gambling among adolescents living in Rome. The sample comprised 300 adolescents (118 boys, 182 girls; aged between 14 and 20 years). The results showed that Roman adolescents preferred games of skill to games of chance or card games, with just over 2% of the sample being classified as problem gamblers. These adolescent problem gamblers had greater difficulties in terms of school performance and discipline, higher scores on impulsiveness, aggressiveness, and resentment toward their parents, and higher rates of parental gambling.

In contrast to other Latin European countries, substantial research has been done on problem gambling in Spain. A number of studies have been carried out with adolescent gamblers, although most have been on small local samples (e.g., 86–90). Two extensive studies have been completed among primary and secondary school children in Galicia (89). In the first study, the DSM-IV-J and the SOGS-RA were used to assess problem gambling among children aged 11 to 16 years. The researchers found that 0.8% of their respondents scored as severe problem gamblers on the DSM-IV-J, whereas 4.6% of their respondents scored as problem gamblers on the SOGS-RA. In a separate study of youth aged 14 to 21 years, Becoña, Miguez, and Vazques (89) found that 4.6% scored as problem gamblers based on the SOGS-RA. Finally, in a study with a large sample of university students from Madrid (aged 17 to 35 years), Viloria (91) found 4.5% scored as probable pathological gamblers and 6.6% scored as problem gamblers based on the SOGS.

3.4.4 Great Britain

More research into adolescent gambling has been completed in Britain than in any other European country. This is likely due to the widespread availability and accessibility of fruit (slot) machines in Britain. Early large-scale studies carried out by local councils and voluntary organizations in the United Kingdom (UK) did not investigate problem gambling. However, these studies did show that the majority of British children gambled occasionally and nearly 20% gambled weekly (92). In the wake of the introduction of a National Lottery, a study of 4,516 adolescents aged between 11 and 16 years found that 24% of respondents reported gambling on the lottery or buying scratch cards once a week or more (93). In the same period, a school-based study of approximately 1,000 adolescents aged 11 to 15 years found that 6% of respondents met the DSM-IV-J criteria for problem gambling (94), and another small-scale study of 204 boys aged 11 to 16 years found 5% who met these criteria (95).

National youth prevalence surveys in Britain were conducted in 1996, 1997, 1999, 2000, 2006, and 2009 under the aegis of the Office of the National Lottery (later the National Lottery Commission) (96–101). The 1996 survey included 7,200 pupils aged 12 to 15 drawn from 48 schools around the country. The survey found that 15% of a representative subsample of 3,724 pupils had spent their own money on the National Lottery in the preceding week, with the majority of these purchases (60%) made legally by a parent. Past-week lottery purchases were significantly associated with being male and having a higher level of spending money (96). The most recent wave of this ongoing youth-tracking study found that slot machines were the most popular form of commercial gambling among adolescents, with 9% of the sample of 8,598 adolescent participants having played these machines in the past week (down from 17% in 2006) (101). A review of over 30 British studies of youth gambling (102) indicated that

- At least two-thirds of adolescents have ever played slot machines;
- One-third of adolescents have played slot machines in the last month;
- Up to 20% of adolescents are regular slot machine players (playing at least once a week) (9% in the latest 2009 national prevalence survey); and
- Up to 6% of adolescents are probable pathological gamblers and/or have severe gambling-related difficulties (2% in 2009, down from 3.5% in 2006, 4.9% in 2000, and 5.4% in 1999).

In some areas of Britain (e.g., Scotland), adolescent problem gambling prevalence rates two to four times higher than those identified in the adult British population have been reported (103).

Research in the UK has found that very few female adolescents have gambling problems on slot machines. A strong correlation between adolescent gambling and parental gambling (94,104) suggests that adults may to some extent foster adolescent gambling in Britain. Other factors that have been linked with adolescent problem gambling in Britain include working class youth culture, delinquency, alcohol and substance abuse, poor school performance, theft, and truancy (e.g., 93, 105, 106).

3.4.5 Nordic countries

All of the Nordic countries have conducted one or more epidemiologic studies of adult gambling and problem gambling in the past 5 years. Research on adolescent gambling is less extensive and differs widely between countries (107, 108).

Denmark

A prevalence survey of adolescent gambling in Denmark was recently completed, with a sample of 5,096 adolescents aged 12 to 17 years randomly selected from the national register (109, 110). A total of 3,814 youth participated in the study (representing 75% of the drawn sample), with results showing that 51% of youth had gambled at least once and 7.2% had gambled in the past month. Boys were more likely to gamble than girls and older adolescents (16 to 17) were more likely to gamble than younger adolescents. The most popular gambling activities among Danish youth were scratch tickets, slot machines, and Lotto.

Problem gambling was assessed using a modified version of the NODS. A total of 7.5% of the adolescents endorsed one or more of the abbreviated five-item NODS, with 0.8% endorsing three or more items. Boys were more likely to have gambling problems than girls and prevalence was higher in the oldest age group (16 to 17 years) than in the younger age groups. Further analysis suggested that problematic gamblers played mostly scratch tickets, slot machines, and poker (110).

Finland

Only one study of adolescent gambling has been carried out in Finland (111). This study included a random sample of 5,000 adolescents aged 12 to 17 years selected from the personal register and interviewed by telephone (112). The results showed that 52% of the adolescents had gambled in the past year and 18% in the past week. Gambling was more common among boys than girls and among adolescents aged 15 to

17 years compared with younger age groups. The most popular gambling activity was slot machines, followed by scratch cards and the Lotto (111, 112). A Finnish version of the SOGS-RA was administered to adolescents who gambled at least twice a month. Overall, 2.3% of Finnish adolescents were classified as problem gamblers. Boys were three times more likely than girls to score as problem gamblers. Further analysis showed that adolescent problem gamblers were most likely to gamble on slot machines, scratch cards, Internet poker, and sports betting (111).

Iceland

In Iceland, four school surveys have been carried out in the capital of Reykjavik or in surrounding towns. The first survey, completed in 2003, included 750 students aged 16 to 18 years from 12 upper secondary and comprehensive schools in the greater Reykjavik area and Akureyri. Some differences were found in problem gambling rates between the two instruments used; the DSM-IV-MR-J identified 2.0% of the sample as problem gamblers (score 4+) with another 3.2% at risk for gambling problems. Based on the SOGS-RA, 2.7% were classified as problem gamblers and 4.4% were classified as at risk (113).

In 2004, a larger study was completed with 3,511 students aged 13 to 15 in Reykjavik (114). The results showed that about 70% of the participants had gambled in the past 12 months and 8% gambled weekly. Using the DSM-IV-MR-J, 1.9% of the students were classified as problem gamblers and another 3.7% were deemed at risk for gambling problems. Based on the SOGS-RA, 2.8% were classified as problem gamblers and 4.1% were classified as at-risk.

Two more recent studies on adolescent gambling and problem gambling in the greater Reykjavik area found similar results. In 2007, a sample consisting of 1,513 students aged 16 to 18 was surveyed (115). In this study, 62% acknowledged gambling in the past year, with 11% gambling on a weekly basis. Using the DSM-IV-MR-J, the study found that 3.0% scored as problem gamblers and 3.8% as at-risk gamblers. Also in 2007, a study was conducted in Hafnarfjörður, a neighboring town to Reykjavik. From the total population aged 13 to 18 years in Hafnarfjörður, 1,537 participated in the study (a response rate of 81%). The results showed that 57% of the adolescents had gambled in the preceding year and 8% gambled weekly. Based on the DSM-IV-MR-J, 2.2% were classified as problem gamblers with another 2.7% classified as at-risk gamblers (116). In all four Icelandic studies, boys were more likely to gamble than girls and were more likely to be classified as having gambling problems.

In all these studies, potential risk factors of problem gambling were systematically evaluated. In general, problem gambling among adolescents in Iceland is strongly related to illicit drug taking and alcohol abuse, cognitive distortions, emotional and conduct problems, attention deficit hyperactivity disorder, poor attendance at school, and poorer grades. Gambling on slot machines, poker, and on the Internet are the favorite gambling activities among problem gamblers (107, 113–116).

Norway

Three adolescent prevalence studies have been completed in Norway since 1999. The first Norwegian study of youth aged 12 to 18 years included both telephone interviews and a postal survey. The telephone survey was based on a representative sample of

10,000 telephone numbers drawn from households likely to include adolescents. The sample for the postal survey was based on 3,000 participants aged 12 to 18 years drawn from the Norwegian central register (117, 118). The overall response rate for the study was 45%. Gambling participation rates were high, with about 82% of the participants having gambled in the past 12 months and 25% having gambled weekly. Boys were more likely to gamble than girls. Problem gambling was assessed using a 10-item version of the DSM-IV that was administered only to those who gambled weekly or more often. The study found that 1.8% of the total sample scored as potential pathological gamblers (answering yes to at least five criteria), and an additional 3.5% were denoted as "at risk" gamblers (three or four DSM-IV criteria). Boys were four times more likely than girls to be classified as potential pathological gamblers. One interesting finding was that the prevalence of potential pathological gambling was two times higher among the adolescents interviewed by telephone compared with those who answered the postal survey (117).

The second and third Norwegian studies share a number of similarities (119, 120). Both studies were school-based surveys of students aged 13 to 19 years. The second study was conducted in 2002 and included about 13,000 adolescents from 72 schools, with a response rate of 92% (119). The third study was carried out in 2004 and included all primary and secondary schools in Norway. A total of 20,703 Norwegian adolescents participated in the study, resulting in a response rate of 80% (120). Past-year gambling participation declined slightly from 78% in 2002 to 74% in 2004, and weekly gambling declined from 14% in 2002 to 11% in 2004. In both studies, boys gambled more than girls, and scratch cards and slot machines were the most popular activities.

In 2002, problem gambling was estimated using the two-item Lie/Bet screen (121) and an additional item assessing chasing behavior. Respondents were classified as problem gamblers if they endorsed all three items. The rate of problem gambling was 3.2% using this approach. If problem gambling was defined as endorsing the two Lie/Bet questions, the prevalence rate increased to 6%. Regardless of the scoring method, boys were much more likely than girls to be classified as problem gamblers (119). In 2004, problem gambling was estimated using both the Lie/Bet screen and the SOGS-RA (120). Problem gambling prevalence based on the Lie/Bet (lifetime) was 3.5%, whereas problem gambling prevalence based on the SOGS-RA was 2.5%. Based on the SOGS-RA, an additional 6% of the respondents were classified as at-risk gamblers. Again, boys were more likely than girls to be classified with gambling problems, regardless of the screen used.

Further analysis, comparing the classification rates between instruments, suggested only moderate congruence between the two problem-gambling screens, but this result may be due to the different time frames of the instruments, with Lie/Bet estimating lifetime prevalence and SOGS-RA 12-month prevalence (120). It is interesting that problem gambling prevalence based on the Lie/Bet screen was considerably lower in 2004 (3.5%) than in 2002 (6.0%).

Sweden

Studies of gambling and problem gambling among Swedish adolescents are scarce, and no recent studies of adolescent gambling appear to have been done. In 1997, however, a large-scale epidemiologic study on gambling and problem gambling was conducted that included a sample of 9,917 individuals aged 15 to 74 randomly selected from the Swedish personal register (122, 123). The survey included an over-sample of 1,000 adolescents aged 15 to 17 years. Specific analysis of youth showed that 76% had gambled in the past year and 16% gambled weekly or more often. Youth were most likely to have gambled on fast lottery games, slot machines, and local lottery games. Using a Swedish translation of the SOGS-R (124), this study found 0.9% of the Swedish youth sample to be probable pathological gamblers (≥ 5) with another 4.2% scoring as problem gamblers (scores 3–4) (122). Two years after the original survey, follow-up interviews were completed with 93 adolescents from the study. Based on the SOGS-R, two-thirds of the adolescents who were classified as problem gamblers in 1997 scored as nonproblem gamblers in the follow-up. Among those youth classified as probable pathological gamblers in 1997, about half were classified as problem gamblers two years later. However, several youth classified as problem gamblers in 1997 were classified as probable pathological gamblers in 1999 (125). As in other longitudinal studies, these findings support the notion that problem gambling is a highly transitional state among adolescents and young adults (126, 127).

3.5 Australia and New Zealand

In both Australia and New Zealand, empirical evidence derived from large-scale population surveys has consistently shown that the highest rates of problem gambling tend to be observed in the 18 to 24 age range and particularly among males (e.g., 128–135). The results from these studies suggest that gambling may often have its origins in adolescence so that problems observed during early adulthood reflect patterns of involvement that extend back several years.

3.5.1 Survey studies in Australia and New Zealand

Although most adolescent gambling studies in Australia and New Zealand have been undertaken with very similar purposes, there have been some differences in the methodologies employed. Some studies have been entirely confined to individuals under the age of 18 years, whereas others have included young adults. The data have been collected from both school-based surveys and through telephone interviews. The studies have also differed in terms of the measures used to capture the frequency of gambling, as well as the prevalence of problem and pathological gambling.

The first major study of youth gambling in Australia was undertaken by Moore and Ohtsuka (136, 137) in the State of Victoria. Over 1,000 school and university students aged 14 to 25 completed a questionnaire about their gambling habits, gambling attitudes, the role of family and social influences, and a modified 10-item version of the original SOGS (138). The researchers found that 3.1% scored in the pathological range, and regular gambling was found to be associated with having more positive attitudes toward gambling and having friends and family members who approved of gambling. A similar study involving 769 individuals from Melbourne under the age of 18 found that 3.8% of students scored in the pathological range (139). Other relevant Victorian research conducted during this period was undertaken in 1997, although the full results were not published until quite recently (140). In this study, 2,788 secondary school students aged 13 were asked if they had participated in the last year in five gambling activities. Problem gambling was not assessed, although a distinction was made between students who had gambled at all in the past year and those who had gambled on three or more activities. Overall, 41% of the students had gambled in the past year and 8% had gambled on three or more activities. Multivariate analyses indicated that significant independent predictors of greater involvement in gambling for males were drinking, marijuana use, and antisocial behavior. For females, greater involvement in gambling was predicted by dissatisfaction with peer relationships and low perceived rewards at school.

Since the late 1990s, five studies to examine the prevalence of gambling and pathological gambling among youth using instruments validated for use in this population have been carried out in Australia and New Zealand (135, 141–145). Although not all of these studies were entirely confined to under-aged populations (some of Rossen's New Zealand sample were aged 18 to 21), the results are unlikely to have been significantly influenced by these sampling differences. Almost all of these studies used the DSM-IV-J or DSM-IV-MR-J as developed and validated by Fisher (17, 18). All but one of the studies were based on the complete school population or a random sampling of students from classrooms in secondary level schools (high schools and colleges).

Some consistency was found in the overall participation rates across these studies (mean past-year gambling—64%). With the exception of the South Australian Department for Families and Communities telephone survey in South Australia (135), the prevalence rates for pathological gambling clustered around 3.5%. Notably, the prevalence rate obtained in the only randomized telephone survey of adolescents was significantly lower than in the other studies.

3.5.2 Variations in activity preferences and individual differences

Across these five surveys, the most popular activities among young people have tended to be scratch tickets, lotteries, card games, and betting on sports. In the two South Australian classroom surveys, approximately 40% of students gambled on scratch tickets, approximately 25% gambled on card games, and 15% to 20% gambled on sports; relatively few gambled on gaming machines (only 5% in the most recent South Australian survey). In all these studies, boys were found to gamble on a wider range of activities than girls, with the largest differences observed for card games, racing, and sports. Boys were also significantly more likely than girls to be classified as pathological gamblers (e.g., 7.8% vs. 2.7% in South Australia; 3.5% vs. 1.2% in the ACT) (141, 143). Pathological gambling rates have also been found to be higher in specific ethnic groups. For example, the two largest classroom studies in Australia found that indigenous students were much more likely than non-indigenous students to be classified as pathological gamblers (28% vs. 4.1% in the ACT; 9% vs. 2.2% in South Australia). In New Zealand, Pacific Island students were 11.5 times more likely than other students to be pathological gamblers (144).

Another consistent finding has been the strong link between gambling and other risk-taking behavior, as well as various measures of psychosocial adjustment. For example, in the ACT study (146), three-quarters of pathological gamblers reported drinking alcohol on a weekly basis as compared with only 50% of the rest of the sample. Cigarette-smoking rates among pathological gamblers were four times higher than among nonproblem gamblers, marijuana rates were six times higher, and hard drug involvement was 10 to 20 times higher, depending on the type of drug. The ACT study also showed that young pathological gamblers scored poorly on measures of self-esteem, negative mood, and general health, and had poorer family adjustment. Similar findings were reported by Rossen (144) in New Zealand. Young pathological gamblers in that country were more likely to have been suspended from school, to feel alienated, and to report having poorer attachments to their parents.

3.5.3 Links between adolescent and adult gambling

Australian research has also provided insight into the association between adolescent gambling and gambling during early adulthood. A South Australian study conducted by Delfabbro, Winefield, and Anderson (147) investigated the gambling habits of 578 young people who were tracked for 4 years from mid-adolescence (age 15 years) into adulthood (18–19 years). Each year, the same participants were administered standardized measures of gambling participation. The results showed that, although mid-adolescent gambling was positively associated with later gambling as adults, there was considerable individual variability in gambling patterns from one year to the next. Only one in four young people who gambled at the age of 15 years continued gambling yearly, and it was rare to find young people whose participation in specific activities was consistent from one year to the next. Using logistic regression models, participation data obtained from young people closer to the time they left school were more predictive of adult gambling patterns than those obtained at a younger age. The findings highlighted the importance of using longitudinal analyses to study the stability of gambling patterns over time.

3.6 Conclusions

Several conclusions can be drawn from this extended review of adolescent prevalence studies. First, from a methodological perspective, this review has shown that school-based surveys and telephone surveys are the primary modalities used in adolescent prevalence surveys. In Australia, the one survey conducted by telephone obtained a significantly lower prevalence rate than in the classroom studies. Similarly in the United States, surveys conducted by telephone obtained somewhat lower prevalence rates than those conducted in classrooms. In Canada, the prevalence rates obtained in classroom and telephone surveys were generally higher than the prevalence rate obtained (using a different problem gambling screen) using face-to-face interviews. In Norway, problem gambling prevalence was two times higher among adolescents interviewed by telephone compared with those who answered a postal survey. Clearly, work is needed to assess the impact of survey modality on identified prevalence rates among adolescents, as has recently been done among adults (148).

Another important methodological trend is that the sample sizes for adolescent surveys have increased over time. Early stand-alone adolescent gambling surveys tended to include samples of only a few hundred participants, as in the period 1984 to 1989 in the United States, in the mid-1990s in Canada, and in recent studies in the Balkan and Baltic countries. In cases in which gambling modules are added to larger health surveys of adolescents, the sample sizes can be extremely large, as in Louisiana and Minnesota in the United States and the national survey in Canada. These studies, along with surveys in Britain, the Nordic countries, and Australia and New Zealand, have been valuable in documenting the links between gambling and other risk behaviors (e.g., drug and alcohol use, seatbelt use, poor school performance, conduct problems, truancy, delinquency, violence, and sexual activity). However, except in cases such as Britain, where the focus of the program of research is primarily on gambling, a significant limitation in large school-based studies is the trade-off between the size and focus of the overall study and the number of gambling items that can be added. An important direction for future research will be assessing the relationship between reduced sets of gambling items and their full-length versions.

A particular concern with regard to measurement is that the problem gambling instruments most widely used with adolescents are derived from adult problem gambling screens and may not be suited to assessing gambling-related problems in younger people. Questions have been raised regarding the validity of both the SOGS-RA and DSM-IV-MR-J (e.g., 19, 149–155). However, pending a better-validated problem gambling instrument for adolescents (a recent report details the performance of one candidate, the Canadian Adolescent Gambling Inventory [CAGI]) (156), these two instruments are likely to continue to be viewed as the best approximations for the measurement of problem gambling among adolescents. Their use is probably preferable to the use of either full-length or shortened versions of adult instruments.

From a substantive perspective, some generalizations can be made with regard to the demographic characteristics of adolescent gamblers and problem gamblers. Across the board, boys are more likely to gamble than girls and more likely to experience problems. Although many of these differences in gambling behavior may be due to social influences in relation to gender, one recent study of adolescent twins found that, though genetic factors explained most of the variance in gambling and problem gambling among male twins, shared environment explained more of the variance among female twins (157). This is clearly an area where further research is needed.

Other important factors in shaping adolescent gambling behavior relate to ethnicity and culture. There is good evidence across multiple jurisdictions that although ethnic and indigenous youth are less likely than other youth to gamble, the former are more likely to gamble regularly when they do gamble and to experience problems (e.g., Native American and African American youth in North America, non-Francophone youth in Quebec, indigenous youth in Australia, and Pacific Island youth in New Zealand). There are other clear demographic patterns. For example, the most popular youth gambling activities tend to be private, peer-related activities, such as card games and betting on sports. Older youth are more likely to engage in accessible forms of age-restricted gambling, such as lotteries. However, studies that have compared gambling patterns of youth with those of adults in the same jurisdiction found that older youth tend to migrate toward age-restricted gambling activities, such as casino gambling, only as they near the age when they would be legally able to participate. Other common demographic characteristics are that youth problem gamblers are more likely to start gambling at a younger age and to have parents who gamble.

From a theoretical perspective, this review suggests that early assumptions about youth gambling and problem gambling must give way to a more nuanced understanding of how these behaviors change in response to changes in the social and cultural environment. For example, it has been widely assumed that gambling participation among youth in jurisdictions where legal gambling is widespread will be higher than in jurisdictions where legal gambling is restricted. It has also been widely assumed that large numbers of underage youth will be able to participate in age-restricted gambling activities when these become available. Finally, it has been widely assumed that problem gambling prevalence rates will be much higher among youth in jurisdictions where legal gambling is broadly available compared with youth in jurisdictions where legal gambling is both less visible and less available. However, as a recent study of youth in Nevada (158) as well as several of the surveys reviewed here have shown, rates of gambling participation can be substantially lower among youth in mature gambling jurisdictions; access by underage youth to some (but not all) age-restricted forms of gambling can be very low; and problem gambling prevalence rates can be significantly lower among adolescents in such jurisdictions compared with others where gambling is less available.

An emerging concern is the recent explosion of Internet and mobile gambling, although, as yet, little research has been done looking at these phenomena (159, 160). Since its inception in 1996, online gambling has become one of the most popular Internet activities and though base rates are still low, gambling via the Internet has increased (161). Strong links between online gambling and nongambling fantasy games, role-playing games, board games, and card games are an additional cause for concern as youth migrate from free gaming sites to online gambling sites. The most recent survey of adolescents in Oregon found that gambling for free on the Internet is now the most popular gambling activity among adolescents, although only a few of these youth have gambled on the Internet using money (39).

Perhaps most significantly, this review underscores the value of conducting repeated studies of adolescent gambling within jurisdictions to improve our understanding of how youth gambling patterns change over time and in relation to lifelong exposure, changes in attitudes toward youth gambling, and efforts at prevention. Repeat studies in Minnesota, Oregon, Washington state, and Manitoba in North America as well as in Belgium, Britain, and Norway in Europe, clearly demonstrate that since the early 1990s, adolescent gambling participation has remained stable or has decreased substantially in those jurisdictions. Similarly, repeat studies in North America and in Europe have shown that since the early 1990s, adolescent problem gambling prevalence rates have remained stable or decreased. More frequent surveys have the added value of helping to monitor trends in adolescent participation in specific activities. For example, in the wake of extensive media coverage of professional poker tournaments in the first half of the decade, in 2005 and 2006 the ARCI surveys documented a spike in card playing among youth and young adults. After 2006, the ARCI surveys showed that the monthly rate of card playing declined and then stabilized. Subsequently, the surveys showed that following the "poker" spike, sports betting increased and card playing declined (52).

A recent systematic review of research on adolescent gambling includes several recommendations that echo the conclusions reached here (162). The reviewers argue that more work is needed to develop and validate survey instruments intended specifically to assess adolescent gambling. They call for greater attention to racial and ethnic differences in the study of adolescent gambling. Finally, in relation to comborbidity, they highlight the importance of looking beyond alcohol and drugs to focus on violence, delinquency, and sexual activity as important correlates of adolescent gambling. Other recent reviews urge greater attention to family influences and the impact of advertising on adolescent gambling behavior (163, 164).

Beyond the cross-sectional research reviewed here, there is a growing body of prospective, longitudinal research on adolescents and young adults that yields important new findings. Longitudinal research is better suited than cross-sectional studies for identifying causal factors that contribute to changes in gambling and problem gambling status over time. Prospective longitudinal studies of adolescent gambling also yield vital information about how gambling and problem gambling status can change at the individual level as well as in the aggregate.

As noted above, the earliest longitudinal study of adolescent gambling was carried out in Minnesota (41). This study and more recent studies completed in Europe, North America, and Australia have all pointed to the highly transitional nature of gambling and problem gambling among youth. Several studies of adolescents who have been followed into young adulthood have found stronger relationships between past-year gambling or problem gambling and the same behavior in proximal rather than distal years (147, 165). Other studies have found links between gambling and personality disorders, most specifically impulsivity (165, 166). Still other longitudinal studies have found that different groups of adolescent gamblers are characterized by different trajectories toward problem gambling. In an update to their earlier study of adolescents in Minnesota, Winters and colleagues (167) found that at-risk gambling and problem gambling in young adulthood were associated with different independent predictors. In a study of Canadian boys, Vitaro and colleagues (168) identified three groups with significantly different gambling careers and found that impulse control deficits, low inhibition, and high risk-taking both preceded the development of gambling problems and differentiated the boys who developed problems from those who did not.

Although we have learned a great deal over the last 25 years, research on adolescent gambling and problem gambling to date has been largely descriptive. As this review has shown, we have traveled some distance down the road toward a better understanding of the determinants as well as the distribution of youth gambling and problem gambling, but there is still a long way to go.

Acknowledgements

This chapter is updated, revised, and adapted from Volberg RA, Gupta R, Griffiths MD, Ólason DT, Delfabbro P. An international perspective on youth gambling prevalence studies. Int J Adolesc Med Health 2010;22:3–38.

References

1. Jacobs DF. Juvenile gambling in North America: An analysis of long-term trends and future prospects. J Gambl Stud 2000;16(2/3):119–52.
2. Shaffer HJ, Hall MN. Estimating prevalence of adolescent gambling disorders: A quantitative synthesis and guide toward standard gambling nomenclature. J Gambl Stud 1996;12: 193–214.
3. Stinchfield R, Winters KC. Gambling and problem gambling among youths. Ann Am Acad Political Soc Sci 1998; 556:172–85.

4. Welte JW, Barnes GM, Tidwell MC, Hoffman JH. The prevalence of problem gambling among U.S. adolescents and young adults: Results from a national survey. J Gambl Stud 2008;24(2):119–33.

5. Burge AN, Pietrzak RH, Petry NM. Pre/early adolescent onset of gambling and psychosocial problems in treatment-seeking pathological gamblers. J Gambl Stud 2006;22(3):263–74.

6. Kessler RC, Hwang I, LaBrie RA, et al. DSM-IV pathological gambling in the National Comorbidity Survey Replication. Psychol Med 2008;38:1351–60.

7. Gupta R, Derevensky JL. Adolescent gambling behavior: A prevalence study and examination of the correlates associated with problem gambling. J Gambl Stud 1998;14(4):319–45.

8. Jacobs DF. Illegal and undocumented: A review of teenage gambling and the plight of children of problem gamblers in America. In: Shaffer HJ, Stein SA, Gambino B, Cummings TN, eds. Compulsive Gambling: Theory, Research, and Practice. Lexington, MA: Lexington Books; 1989: 249–92.

9. Westphal JR, Rush B, Stevens L, Johnson LJ. Pathological gambling among Louisiana students: Grades six through twelve. Paper presented at the Am Psychiatr Assoc Ann Meet, Toronto, 1998.

10. Barnes GM, Welte JW, Hoffman JH, Dintcheff BA. Shared predictors of youthful gambling, substance use and delinquency. Psychol Addict Behav 2005;19:165–74.

11. Vitaro F, Brendgen M, Ladouceur R, Tremblay RE. Gambling, delinquency, and drug use during adolescence: Mutual influences and common risk factors. J Gambl Stud 2001;17(3):171–90.

12. Winters KC, Anderson N. Gambling involvement and drug use among adolescents. J Gambl Stud 2000;16(2–3):175–98.

13. Arcuri AF, Lester D, Smith FO. Shaping adolescent gambling behavior. Adolescence 1985;20:935–8.

14. Felsher JR, Derevensky JL, Gupta R. Lottery playing amongst youth: Implications for prevention and social policy. J Gambl Stud 2004;20(2):127–54.

15. Abbott MW, Volberg RA. The measurement of adult problem and pathological gambling. Int Gambl Stud 2006;6(2):175–200.

16. Winters KC, Stinchfield R, Fulkerson J. Toward the development of an adolescent gambling problem severity scale. J Gambl Stud 1993;9:63–84.

17. Fisher SE. Measuring pathological gambling in children: The case of fruit machines in the UK. J Gambl Stud 1992;8:263–85.

18. Fisher SE. Developing the DSM-IV-MR-J criteria to identify adolescent problem gambling in non-clinical populations. J Gambl Stud 2000;16(2/3):253–73.

19. Derevensky JL, Gupta R. Prevalence estimates of adolescent gambling: A comparison of the SOGS-RA, DSM-IV-J, and the GA 20 Questions. J Gambl Stud 2000;16(2/3):227–51.

20. Hardoon KK, Derevensky JL, Gupta R. Empirical measures vs. perceived gambling severity among youth. Addict Behav 2003;28(5):933–46.

21. Jacobs DF. A review of teenage gambling in the US. In: Eadington WR, Cornelius JA, eds. Gambling Behavior and Problem Gambling. Reno, NV: Institute for the Study of Gambling and Commercial Gaming; 1993: 431–41.

22. Jacobs DF, Marston AR, Singer RD. Study of gambling and other health-threatening behaviors among high school students. Loma Linda, CA: Jerry L. Pettis Memorial Veterans Hospital; 1985.

23. Jacobs DF, Marston AR, Singer RD. A post-lottery study of gambling behaviors among high school students. Loma Linda, CA: Jeffrey L. Pettis Memorial Veterans Hospital; 1987.

24. Kuley N, Jacobs DF. A pre-lottery benchmark study of teenage gambling in Virginia. Loma Linda, CA: Loma Linda University, Department of Psychiatry; 1987.

25. Kuley N, Jacobs DF. A post-lottery impact study of effects on teenage gambling behaviors. Loma Linda, CA: Loma Linda University, Department of Psychiatry; 1989.

26. Lesieur HR, Klein R. Pathological gambling among high school students. Addict Behav 1987;12:129–35.

27. Steinberg M. Gambling behavior among high school students in Connecticut. Paper presented at the Third National Conference on Gambling, New London, CT, 1988.
28. Shaffer HJ, LaBrie R, LaPlante DA, Nelson S, Stanton M. The road less travelled: Moving from distribution to determinants in the study of gambling epidemiology. Can J Psychiatry 2004;49:504–16.
29. Stinchfield R. A comparison of gambling among Minnesota public school students in 1992, 1995 and 1998. J Gambl Stud 2001;17(4):273–96.
30. Proimos J, DuRant RH, Dwyer Pierce J, Goodman E. Gambling and other risk behaviors among 8th to 12th grade students. Pediatrics 1998;102(2):e23.
31. Volberg RA. Gambling and problem gambling among adolescents in Georgia. Atlanta, GA: Georgia Department of Human Resources; 1996.
32. Volberg RA. Gambling and problem gambling among adolescents in New York. Albany, NY: New York State Council on Problem Gambling; 1998.
33. Westphal JR, Rush JA, Stevens L, Johnson LJ. Gambling behavior of Louisiana students in grades 6 through 12. Psychiatr Serv 2000;51(1):96–9.
34. Wallisch L. Gambling in Texas: The 1992 Texas survey of adolescent gambling behavior. Austin, TX: Texas Commission on Alcohol and Drug Abuse; 1993.
35. Wallisch L. Gambling in Texas: The 1995 Texas survey of adolescent gambling behavior. Austin, TX: Texas Commission on Alcohol and Drug Abuse; 1995.
36. Volberg RA. Gambling and problem gambling among adolescents in Washington State. Olympia, WA: Washington State Lottery; 1993.
37. Volberg RA, Moore WL. Gambling and problem gambling among Washington State adolescents: A replication study, 1993 to 1999. Olympia, WA: Washington State Lottery; 1999.
38. Carlson MJ, Moore TL. Adolescent gambling in Oregon. Salem, OR: Oregon Gambling Addiction Treatment Foundation; 1998.
39. Volberg RA, Hedberg EC, Moore TL. Oregon youth and their parents: Gambling and problem gambling prevalence and attitudes. Salem, OR: Oregon Department of Human Services; 2008.
40. Winters KC, Stinchfield R, Fulkerson J. Patterns and characteristics of adolescent gambling. J Gambl Stud 1993;9(4):371–86.
41. Winters KC, Stinchfield R, Kim LG. Monitoring adolescent gambling in Minnesota. J Gambl Stud 1995;11(2):165–83.
42. Stinchfield R, Cassuto N, Winters KC, Lassiter W. Prevalence of gambling among Minnesota public school students in 1992 and 1995. J Gambl Stud 1997;13(1):25–48.
43. Peacock P, Day A, Peacock TD. Adolescent gambling on a Great Lakes Indian reservation. J Hum Behav Soc Environ 1999;2:5–17.
44. Zitzow D. Comparative study of problematic gambling behaviors between American Indian and non-Indian adolescents within and near a Northern Plains reservation. Am Indian Alsk Native Ment Health Res 1996;7(2):14–26.
45. National Gambling Impact Study Commission. Final report. Washington, DC: National Gambling Impact Study Commission; 1999.
46. Arizona Criminal Justice Commission. 2008 Arizona Youth Survey: Shining light on Arizona youth. Phoenix, AZ: Arizona Criminal Justice Commission; 2008.
47. Esters I, Biggar R, Lacour J, Reyes M. 2008 Louisiana study on problem gambling. Lafayette, LA: Cecil. J. Picard Center for Child Development, University of Louisiana at Lafayette; 2008.
48. Rainone G, Gallati RJ. Gambling behaviors and problem gambling among adolescents in New York State: Initial findings from the 2006 OASAS school survey. New York, NY: NYS Office of Alcoholism and Substance Abuse Services; 2007.
49. Gerstein DR, Volberg RA, Harwood H, Christiansen EM, et al. Gambling impact and behavior study: Report to the National Gambling Impact Study Commission. Chicago, IL: National Opinion Research Center at the University of Chicago; 1999.

50. Welte JW, Barnes G, Wieczorek WF, Tidwell M-C, Parker J. Alcohol and gambling among U.S. adults: Prevalence, demographic patterns and comorbidity. J Stud Alcohol 2001;62(5):706–12.
51. Welte JW, Barnes GM, Tidwell M, Hoffman J. The association of form of gambling with problem gambling among American youth. Psychol Addict Behav 2009;23(1):105–12.
52. Adolescent Risk Communication Institute. Internet gambling stays low among youth ages 14 to 22 but access to gambling sites continues; sports gambling makes resurgence. Philadelphia, PA: Annenberg Public Policy Center; 2008.
53. Insight Canada Research. An exploration of the prevalence and pathological gambling behaviour among adolescents in Ontario. Report to the Canadian Foundation on Compulsive Gambling; 1994.
54. Omnifacts Research. An examination of the prevalence of gambling in Nova Scotia. Halifax: Nova Scotia Department of Health; 1993.
55. Wynne Resources. Adolescent gambling and problem gambling in Alberta. Report to the Alberta Alcohol and Drug Abuse Commission; 1996.
56. Ladouceur R, Mireault C. Gambling behaviors among high school students in the Quebec area. J Gambl Beh 1988;4(1):3–12.
57. Govoni R, Rupcich N, Frisch GR. Gambling behaviour of adolescent gamblers. J Gambl Stud 1996;12(3):305–17.
58. Huang JH, Boyer R. Epidemiology of youth gambling problems in Canada: A national prevalence study. Can J Psychiatry 2007;52(10):657–65.
59. Gregg JD. Youth gambling in British Columbia. Master's thesis. Langley: Trinity Western Univ; 2003.
60. Alberta Alcohol and Drug Abuse Commission. The Alberta youth experience survey 2002. Edmonton: Alberta Alcohol and Drug Abuse Commission; 2003.
61. Alberta Alcohol and Drug Abuse Commission. Gambling among Alberta youth: The Alberta youth experience survey 2005. Edmonton: Alberta Alcohol and Drug Abuse Commission; 2007.
62. Dickinson H, Schissel B. University of Saskatchewan survey—youth gambling in Saskatchewan: Perceptions, behaviours, and youth culture. Regina: Saskatchewan Ministry of Health; 2003.
63. Wiebe J. Manitoba youth gambling prevalence study: Summary of findings 1999. Winnipeg: Addictions Foundation of Manitoba; 1999.
64. Lemaire J. Manitoba youth gambling behaviour: Follow-up to the 1999 AFM report. Winnipeg: Addictions Foundation of Manitoba; 2004.
65. Mackay TL, Patton D, Broszeit B. Student gambling report 2005. Winnipeg: Addictions Foundation of Manitoba; 2005.
66. Adlaf EM, Ialomiteanu A. Prevalence of problem gambling in adolescents: Findings from the 1999 Ontario Student Drug Use Survey. Can J Psychiatry 2000;45(8):752–5.
67. Adlaf EM, Paglia-Boak A, Beichman JH, Wolfe D. The mental health and well-being of Ontario students 1991–2005: Detailed OSDUS findings. Toronto: Centre for Addiction and Mental Health; 2006.
68. Martin I, Gupta R, Derevensky JL. Participation aux jeux de hasard et d'argent. In: Dubé G (ed). Enquête québécoise sur le tabac, l'alcool, la drogue et le jeu chez les élèves du secondaire, 2006. Montreal: Institut de la statistique du Québec: 2007: 125–44.
69. Poulin C. Problem gambling among adolescent students in the Atlantic provinces of Canada. J Gambl Stud 2000;16(1):53–78.
70. Faktum Uuringukeskus. Elanike kokkupuuted hasart-ja õnnemängudega [Gambling prevalence in Estonia]. Tallinn; 2004.
71. Laansoo S. Patoloogiline hasart-mängimine: ulatus Eestis ning seosed käitumuslike ja isiksuslike riski-faktoritega (Pathological gambling in Estonia and the relationships with behavioral and personal risk factors). Master's thesis. Talinn: Tallinna Ülikool Eesti; 2006.

72. Laansoo S, Niit T. South Oaks Mängurisõel (South Oaks Gambling Screen). Talinn: Tallinna Ülikool Eesti; 2004.
73. Laansoo S, Niit T. Estonia. In: Meyer G, Hayer T, Griffiths MD, eds. Problem gaming in Europe: Challenges, prevention, and interventions. New York, NY: Springer; 2009.
74. Skokauskas N. Lithuania. In: Meyer G, Hayer T, Griffiths MD, eds. Problem gaming in Europe: Challenges, prevention, and interventions. New York, NY: Springer; 2009.
75. Skokauskas N, Satkeviciute R. Adolescent pathological gambling in Kaunas, Lithuania. Nord Psykiatr Tidsskr 2007;61(2):86–91.
76. Skokauskas N, Satkeviciute R, Burba B, Rutkauskiene I. Gambling among adolescents in Kaunas. Lithuanian Gen Pract 2005;5(9):11–15.
77. Lupu V. Romania. In: Meyer G, Hayer T, Griffiths MD, eds. Problem gaming in Europe: Challenges, prevention, and interventions. New York, NY: Springer; 2009.
78. Lupu V, Onaca E, Lupu D. The prevalence of pathological gambling in Romanian teenagers. Minerva Med 2002;93:413–8.
79. Lupu V, Boros S, Miu A, Iftene F, Geru A. Factori de risc pentru jocul patologic de noroc la adolescenţii români [Risk factors in pathological gambling in Romanian adolescents]. Revista SNPCAR 2001;4(4):33–8.
80. Zivny H, Okruhlica L. Slovakia. In: Meyer G, Hayer T, Griffiths MD, eds. Problem gaming in Europe: Challenges, prevention, and interventions. New York, NY: Springer; 2009.
81. Kotrc D. Uzívanie psychoaktívnych látok a patolokické hrácstvo na základnych a strednych skolách v obvode Kysucké Nové Mesto [Using drugs and gambling in elementary and high school in the Kysucké Nové Mesto region]. Alkoholizmus a drogové závislosti 2005;40:223–39.
82. Hurrelmann K, Schmidt L, Kähnert H. Konsum von Glücksspielen bei Kindern und Jugendlichen—Verbreitung und Prävention [Participation in gambling of children and adolescents—Prevalence and prevention]. Düsseldorf: Ministerium für Gesundheit, Soziales, Frauen und Familie des Landes Nordrhein-Westfalen; 2003.
83. Kinable H. Bevraging van Vlaamse leerlingen in het kader van een Drugbeleid Op School. Synthese-rapport schooljaar 2005–2006 [Inquiry of Flemish students within the framework of a School Drug Policy. Summary report school year 2005–2006]. Brussels: VAD; 2006.
84. Capitanucci D, Biganzoli A, Smaniotto R (eds). Reti d'azzardo [Gambling networks]. Varese: Edizioni And-In-Carta; 2006.
85. Baiocco R, Couyoumdjian A, Langellotti M, Del Miglio C. Gioco d'azzardo problematico, tratti di personalità e attaccamento in adolescenza [Problematic gambling, personality traits and adolescence attachment]. Età Evolutiva 2005;1:56–65.
86. Arbinaga F. Conductas de juego con apuestas y uso de drogas en una muestra de adolescentes de la ciudad de Huelva [Game of chance behavior and drug consumption in a sample of adolescents of the city of Huelva]. Análisis y Modificación de Conducta 1996;22:577–601.
87. Becoña E. Pathological gambling in Spanish children and adolescents: An emerging problem. Psychol Rep 1997;81:275–87.
88. Becoña E, Gestal C. El juego patológico en niños del 2º ciclo de E.G.B [Pathological gambling in children of primary school]. Psicothema 1996;8:13–23.
89. Becoña E, Míguez MC, Vázquez FL. El juego problema en los niños de Galicia [Problem gambling in the children of Galicia]. Madrid: Sociedad Española de Psicopatología Clínica, Legal y Forense; 2001.
90. Villa A, Becoña E, Vázquez FL. Juego patológico con máquinas tragaperras en una muestra de escolares de Gijón [Pathological gambling with slot machines in a sample of Gijón scholars]. Adicciones 1997;9:195–208.
91. Viloria C. El juego patológico en los estudiantes universitarios de la Comunidad de Madrid [Pathological gambling in university students of the region of Madrid]. Clínica y Salud 2003;14:43–65.
92. Abbott MW, Volberg RA, Bellringer M, Reith G. A review of research on aspects of problem gambling. London: Responsibility in Gambling Trust; 2004.

93. Griffiths MD, Sutherland I. Adolescent gambling and drug use. J Community Appl Soc Psychol 1998;8:423–7.
94. Wood RTA, Griffiths MD. The acquisition, development and maintenance of lottery and scratchcard gambling in adolescence. J Adolesc 1998;21:265–73.
95. Griffiths MD. Scratchcard gambling among adolescent males. J Gambl Stud 2000;16(1):79–91.
96. Fisher SE, Balding J. Under sixteen's find the Lottery a good gamble. Educ Health 1996;13(5):5–7.
97. Fisher SE. Gambling and problem gambling among young people in England and Wales. Plymouth: Centre for Research Into the Social Impact of Gambling, University of Plymouth; 1998.
98. Ashworth J, Doyle N. Under 16s and the National Lottery 1999. London: BMRB Social Research; 2000.
99. Ashworth J, Doyle N, Howat N. Under 16s and the National Lottery: Tracking survey July 2000. London: BMRB Social Research; 2000.
100. MORI. Under 16s and the National Lottery: Final report. London: National Lottery Commission; 2006.
101. Ipsos MORI. British survey of children, the National Lottery and gambling 2008–09: Report of a quantitative survey. London: National Lottery Commission; 2009.
102. Griffiths MD. Great Britain. In: Meyer G, Hayer T, Griffiths MD, eds. Problem gaming in Europe: Challenges, prevention, and interventions. New York, NY: Springer; 2009.
103. Moodie C, Finnigan F. Prevalence and correlates of youth gambling in Scotland. Addict Res Theory 2006;14:365–85.
104. Wood RTA, Griffiths MD. Adolescent lottery and scratchcard players: Do their attitudes influence their gambling behaviour? J Adolesc 2004;27:467–75.
105. Griffiths MD. Adolescent gambling. London: Routledge; 1995.
106. Yeoman T, Griffiths MD. Adolescent machine gambling and crime. J Adolesc 1996;19:183–8.
107. Ólason DT. Youth gambling in the Nordic countries. Sixth Nordic Conference on Gambling Studies and Policy Issues. Copenhagen; 2007.
108. Ólason DT. Gambling and problem gambling studies among Nordic adults: Are they comparable? Seventh Nordic Conference on Problem Gambling, Treatment and Prevention. Helsinki; 2009.
109. Nielsen C, Heideman J. Pengespil blandt unge: En rapport om 12–17 åriges spillevaner [Gambling among youth: A report on gambling habits among 12–17 years old]. Copenhagen: SFI—Det Nationale Forskningscenter For Velfærd; 2008.
110. Sørensen NU, Nielsen JC, Wittendorff N. Unge og Gambling: 12–17 åriges pengespiladfærd i et risiko-og trivselperspektiv [Young and gambling: 12 to 17 years old gambling habits within a risk perspective]. Copenhagen: Aarhus University, Center for Ungdomsforskning; 2008.
111. Jaakkola T. Finland. In: Meyer G, Hayer T, Griffiths MD, eds. Problem gaming in Europe: Challenges, prevention, and interventions. New York, NY: Springer; 2009.
112. Ilkas H, Aho P. Nuorten Rahapel-aaminen. 12–17 vuotiaiden nuorten rahapelaaminen ja peliongelmat—puhelinhaastattelu [Youth gambling. Youth of 12–17 years gambling and gambling problems—telephone survey]. Helsinki: Taloustutkimus Ltd.; 2006.
113. Ólason DT, Sigurdardottir KJ, Smari J. Prevalence estimates of gambling participation and problem gambling among 16–18-year old students in Iceland: A comparison of the SOGS-RA and DSM-IV-MR-J. J Gambl Stud 2006;22(1):23–39.
114. Ólason DT, Skarphedinsson GA, Jonsdottir JE, Mikaelsson M, Gretarsson SJ. Prevalence estimates of gambling and problem gambling among 13–to 15-year-old adolescents in Reykjavík: An examination of correlates of problem gambling and different accessibility to electronic gambling machines in Iceland. J Gambl Issues. 2006;18:39–56.
115. Baldursdottir K, Ólason DT, Gretarsson SJ, Davidsdottir ÁR, Sigurjonsdottir AM. Peningaspil og algengi spilavanda meðal 16 til 18 ára framhaldsskólanemenda: Mat á áhættupáttum [Gambling and problem gambling prevalence among 16 to 18 year old adolescent

in comprehensive schools: Evaluation on risk factors]. Sálfræðiritið [Icelandic J Psychol] 2008;13:27–46.

116. Kristjansdottir E. Þátttaka í peningaspilum, spilavandi og tengsl við áhættuþætti hjá 13–18 ára nemendum í Hafnarfirði [Gambling participation, problem gambling and association with risk factors among 13–18 year old students in Hafnarfjörður]. Dissertation. Reykjavik: University of Iceland; 2008.

117. Götestam KG, Johansson A. Norway. In: Meyer G, Hayer T, Griffiths MD, eds. Problem gaming in Europe: Challenges, prevention, and interventions. New York, NY: Springer; 2009.

118. Johansson A, Götestam KG. Gambling and problematic gambling with money among Norwegian youth (12–18 years). Nord Psykiatr Tidsskr 2003;57:317–21.

119. Rossow I, Hansen M. Underholdning med bismak: Ungdom og pengespill [Entertainment with a smack: Youth and gambling]. Oslo: NOVA—Norwegian Social Research; 2003.

120. Rossow I, Molde H. Chasing the criteria: Comparing SOGS-RA and the Lie/Bet screen to assess prevalence of problem gambling and 'at-risk' gambling among adolescents. J Gambl Issues 2006;18:57–71.

121. Johnson EE, Hamer R, Nora RM, Tan B, Eisenstein N, Engelhart C. The lie/bet questionnaire for screening pathological gamblers. Psychol Rep 1997;80:83–8.

122. Rönnberg S, Volberg RA, Abbott MW, et al. Gambling and problem gambling in Sweden. Stockholm: National Institute of Public Health; 1999.

123. Volberg RA, Abbott MW, Rönnberg S, Munck IM. Prevalence and risks of pathological gambling in Sweden. Acta Psychiatr Scand 2001;104(4):250–6.

124. Abbott MW, Volberg RA. The New Zealand National Survey of problem and pathological gambling. J Gambl Stud 1996;12(2):143–60.

125. Jonsson J, Rönnberg S. Sweden. In: Meyer G, Hayer T, Griffiths MD, eds. Problem gaming in Europe: Challenges, prevention, and interventions. New York, NY: Springer;, 2009.

126. Slutske WS, Jackson KM, Sher KJ. The natural history of problem gambling from age 18 to 29. J Abnorm Psychol 2003;112(2):263–74.

127. Winters KC, Stinchfield RD, Botzet A, Slutske WS. Pathways of youth gambling problem severity. Psychol Addict Behav 2005;19(1):104–7.

128. Abbott MW, Volberg RA. Frequent and problem gambling in New Zealand. Wellington: Department of Internal Affairs; 1992.

129. Dickerson M, Maddern R. The extent and impact of gambling in Tasmania with particular reference to problem gambling: A follow up to the baseline study conducted in 1994. Sydney: Australian Institute for Gambling Research; 1997.

130. McMillen J, Marshall D, Ahmed E, Wenzel M. 2003 Victorian longitudinal community attitudes survey. Melbourne: Gambling Research Panel; 2003.

131. Productivity Commission. Australia's Gambling Industries. Canberra: Aus Info; 1999.

132. Queensland Treasury. Queensland household gambling survey 2001. Brisbane: Queensland Government; 2001.

133. Queensland Treasury. Queensland household gambling survey 2003–04. Brisbane: Queensland Government; 2005.

134. Roy Morgan Research. The third study into the extent and impact of gambling in Tasmania with particular reference to problem gambling. Hobart: Department of Health and Human Services; 2001.

135. South Australia Department for Families and Communities. Gambling prevalence in South Australia. Adelaide: Government of South Australia; 2007.

136. Moore S, Ohtsuka K. Gambling activities of young Australians: Developing a model of behavior. J Gambl Stud 1997;13:201–36.

137. Moore S, Ohtsuka K. Beliefs about control over gambling among young people, and their relation to problem gambling. Psychol Addict Behav 1999;13:339–47.

138. Lesieur HR, Blume SB. The South Oaks Gambling Screen (SOGS): A new instrument for the identification of pathological gamblers. Am J Psychiatry 1987;144:1184–8.

139. Moore S, Ohtsuka K. Youth gambling in Melbourne's West: Changes between 1996 and 1998 for Anglo-European background and Asian background school-based youth. Int Gambl Stud 2001;1:87–102.

140. Jackson AC, Dowling N, Thomas SA, Bond L, Patton G. Adolescent gambling behaviour and attitudes: A prevalence study and correlates in an Australian population. Int J Ment Health Addict 2008;6(3):325–52.

141. Delfabbro PH, Lahn J, Grabosky P. Further evidence concerning the prevalence of adolescent gambling and problem gambling in Australia: A study of the ACT. Int Gambl Stud 2005;5:209–28.

142. Delfabbro PH, Thrupp L. Youth gambling in South Australia: The role of attitudes and economic socialization. J Adolesc 2003;26:313–30.

143. Lambos C, Delfabbro PH, Pulgies S, DECS. Adolescent gambling in South Australia. Adelaide: Independent Gambling Authority of South Australia; 2007.

144. Rossen F. Adolescent gambling in New Zealand: An examination of protective and risk factors. Dissertation. Auckland: University of Auckland; 2008.

145. Sullivan S. Gambling amongst New Zealand high school students. In: Blaszczynski A, ed. Proceedings of the 11th annual conference of the National Association for Gambling Studies. Sydney: National Association for Gambling Studies, 2001:345–9.

146. Delfabbro PH, Lahn J, Grabosky P. Psychosocial correlates of problem gambling among adolescents. Aust NZ J Psychiatry. 2006;40:587–95.

147. Delfabbro PH, Winefield AH, Anderson S. Once a gambler-always a gambler: Longitudinal analysis of adolescent gambling patterns. Int Gambl Stud 2009;9:151–63.

148. Williams RJ, Volberg RA. Impact of survey description, administration format, and exclusionary criteria on population prevalence rates of problem gambling. Int Gambl Stud 2009;9:101–17.

149. Derevensky JL, Gupta R. Measuring gambling problems among adolescents: Current status and future directions. Int Gambl Stud 2006;6: 201–15.

150. Derevensky JL, Gupta R, Winters KC. Prevalence rates of youth gambling problems: Are the current rates inflated? J Gambl Stud 2003;19:405–25.

151. Jacques C, Ladouceur R. DSM-IV-J Criteria: A scoring error that may be modifying the estimates of pathological gambling among youths. J Gambl Stud 2003;19:427–31.

152. Ladouceur R, Bouchard C, Rhéaume N, et al. Is the SOGS an accurate measure of pathological gambling among children, adolescents and adults? J Gambl Stud 2000;16(1):1–24.

153. Langhinrichsen-Rohling J, Rohling ML, Rohde P, Seeley JR. The SOGS-RA vs. the MAGS-7: Prevalence estimates and classification congruence. J Gambl Stud 2004;20:259–81.

154. Pelletier A, Ladouceur R, Fortin J, Ferland F. Assessment of high school students' understanding of DSM-IV-MR-J items. J Adolesc Res 2004;19:224–32.

155. Poulin C. An assessment of the validity and reliability of the SOGS-RA. J Gambl Stud 2002;18:67–93.

156. Tremblay, J., Stinchfield, R., Wiebe, J., Wynne, H. Canadian Adolescent Gambling Inventory (CAGI): Phase III final report. Toronto: Canadian Centre on Substance Abuse; 2010.

157. Beaver KM, Hoffman T, Shields RT, Vaughn MG, DeLisi M, Wright JP. Gender differences in genetic and environmental influences on gambling: Results from a sample of twins from the National Longitudinal Study of Adolescent Health. Addiction 2010;105:536–542.

158. Volberg RA. Why pay attention to adolescent gambling? In: Romer, D, ed. Reducing adolescent risk: Toward an integrated approach. Thousand Oaks, CA: Sage Publications; 2003:256–261.

159. Derevensky JL, Gupta R. Internet gambling amongst adolescents: A growing concern. Int J Ment Health Addict 2007;5(2):93–101.

160. Griffiths MD, Wood RTA. Adolescent Internet gambling: Preliminary results of a national survey. Educ Health 2007;25:23–7.

161. Wood RT, Williams RJ. Internet gambling: Past, present, and future. In: Smith G, Hodgins DC, Williams RJ, eds. Research and Measurement Issues in Gambling Studies. London: Elsevie;, 2007:491–514.
162. Blinn-Pike L, Worthy SL, Jonkman JN. Adolescent gambling: A review of an emerging field. J Adolesc Health 2010;47:223–36.
163. McComb JL, Sabiston CM. Family influences on adolescent gambling behavior: A review of the literature. J Gambl Stud 2010;26(4):503–20.
164. Derevensky JL, Sklar A, Gupta R, Messerlian C. An empirical study examining the impact of gambling advertisements on adolescent gambling attitudes and behaviors. Int J Ment Health Addiction 2010;8(1):21–34.
165. Goudriaan AE, Slutske WS, Krull JL, Sher KJ. Longitudinal patterns of gambling activities and associated risk factors in college students. Addiction 2009;104(7):1219–32.
166. Slutske WS, Caspi A, Moffitt TE, Poulton R. Personality and problem gambling: A prospective study of a birth cohort of young adults. Arch Gen Psychiatry 2005;62:769–75.
167. Winters KC, Stinchfield RD, Botzet A, Anderson N. A prospective study of youth gambling behaviors. Psychol Addict Behav 2002;16(1):3–9.
168. Vitaro F, Wanner B, Ladouceur R, Brendgen M, Tremblay RE. Trajectories of gambling during adolescence. J Gambl Stud 2004;20(1):47–69.

Correlates, risk, and protective factors associated with youth gambling

4 Youth problem gambling: Our current knowledge of risk and protective factors

N. Will Shead, Jeffrey L. Derevensky, and Rina Gupta

Risk factors for youth gambling problems are best understood within an ecological model recognizing the interwoven relationship that exists between the individual and his or her environment. Empirical studies covering individual, relationship, community, and societal factors associated with adolescent gambling problems are presented. This cumulative body of research suggests that males exposed to gambling at an earlier age are at greater risk of developing gambling problems. Individuals who report poor family cohesion, have family members or friends who gamble, and those exposed to and engaged in a wider diversity of gambling options remain at greater risk for future gambling problems. Adolescents with impulsive, high sensation-seeking personalities, and those who exhibit emotion-focused coping styles, mental health disorders, substance use, and antisocial behaviors are more likely to experience gambling problems. Many of these risk factors appear to predict a more general behavior problem syndrome. Greater emphasis and additional research into the causal risk factors that lead to gambling problems among youth will ultimately improve our prevention efforts.

4.1 Introduction

The field of gambling research has grown dramatically over the past two decades but there remains a paucity of research on some of the risk and protective factors associated with problem gamblers (1). Although considerable research has been conducted in the past two decades, a lack of consensus regarding the risk factors and their relative weight in contributing to problem gambling among youth still remains. Studying the risk factors among youth is particularly important given that severe gambling problems often originate during adolescence (2). A better understanding of the factors contributing to the acquisition and development of disordered gambling behaviors among youth will ultimately help clarify the etiology of gambling problems.

   Some strides have been made to foster a better understanding of the onset and developmental course of gambling problems, and those advances form the basis of this review. This growing body of research focuses on identification of the bio-psycho-social and environmental mechanisms underlying excessive gambling behavior among youth. As risk and protective factors that contribute to gambling problems are better elucidated, the information can be used to improve assessment, treatment, and prevention programs. With more knowledge about which youth are at the highest risk of becoming problem gamblers, these programs will be able to better target specific types of youth with the goals of stopping or minimizing gambling problems before they occur and improving the effectiveness of treatment for those who suffer from gambling problems.

Examination of the factors associated with youth gambling problems provides a more complete description of the nature of these problems, their onset, and how they are maintained. Knowledge about these risk factors is also critical for better identifying the potential warning signs associated with gambling problems. This information can be used to develop prevention initiatives geared toward youth with gambling problems. For example, public service announcements aimed at youth gambling prevention can incorporate aspects that appeal to youth who are at greatest risk of becoming heavily involved in gambling activities. Such an approach has been taken by developers of anti-drug media campaigns in designing public service announcements with high sensation value to appeal to youth who are at greater risk for substance use problems (3).

As risk factors become better understood, a complementary understanding of resiliency can be achieved. Risk factors tend to represent extremes on certain bio-psycho-social dimensions such that opposing ends of the same dimensions may represent important protective factors. For instance, if lack of family cohesion is associated with gambling problems, greater family connectedness should by its very nature lower the risk of developing a gambling problem. Thus, risk factors should help to extrapolate significant protective factors that offset their impact and increase resiliency (although empirical research will be needed to validate these findings).

In addition, raising public awareness of the factors that contribute to the development and maintenance of problem gambling among youth will ultimately bolster the advancement of services for young problem gamblers (4). The more society understands about the short- and long-term consequences of disordered gambling, the more likely it will be viewed as an important public health concern. Parents, teachers, health professionals, policymakers, and the public in general need to stay informed about risk factors and consequences in order to help youth avoid and overcome gambling problems.

This review outlines our current knowledge of the risk factors associated with child and adolescent problem gambling. Empirical studies covering several categories of risk factors are examined. These categories of risk factors are presented using an ecological model to recognize the multiple interacting contexts in which gambling problems occur. The ecological model addresses individual risk factors as well as overlapping interpersonal, community, and societal systems that create the conditions for youth to develop gambling problems (5). At an individual level, personal psychological attributes that increase the likelihood of gambling problems are examined. Interpersonal level influences address the potential of relationships with significant others such as family and friends to shape an individual's gambling behavior. Community factors, encompassing the influences of the greater environment in which the individual lives, are also presented. When considering youth gambling behavior, availability, accessibility, and marketing of gambling within a community are particularly relevant. Finally, at the societal level, the influence of broad, macro-level factors is examined. These risk factors address cultural beliefs, societal norms, and worldwide trends that can potentially lead to gambling problems among children and adolescents. The ecological model provides an appropriate framework for understanding the multitude of risk factors that contribute to youth gambling problems and the complex interactions that exist between factors nested within different ecological systems.

4.2 Demographic factors

There is widespread acceptance and strong support for the circumstance that adolescent problem gamblers are more likely to have reported gambling at a younger age (approximately 10 years of age) (6–8). Similarly, adults with gambling problems report having been introduced to gambling earlier in their childhood compared with adults who do not experience problems (9). Together, these findings suggest that youth who are exposed to gambling at an early age are at increased risk of developing problems. Delaying the onset of gambling exposure as long as possible appears to be an important protective factor, especially given the fact that, among adolescents, the transition between social gambler and problem gambler is even more rapid than with adults (10).

4.3 Gender

The cumulative body of gambling research clearly shows that gambling is more popular among males than females and males are more likely to experience problem or pathological gambling behaviors (11, 12). This gender difference has been found in adolescents as well as adults (8, 13–15). More frequent gambling among boys compared with girls has also been shown in a sample of primary school children (16). In a recent study of middle and high school students, males were found to be almost six times more likely than females to be identified as having a gambling problem and twice as likely to be classified as at-risk gamblers, endorsing a number of criteria for gambling problems but not meeting the clinical cut-off for pathological gamblers (17).

An early study by Gupta and Derevensky (7), testing Jacobs' General Theory of Addictions (18), which proposed that disordered gambling is a habitual coping response to abnormal physiological resting states, revealed that male and female adolescents may be differentially predisposed to gambling problems. Among males, high excitability and dissociation while gambling predicted categorization as problem or pathological gamblers, whereas among females, depressed mood, dissociation, and stimulant drug use were better predictors. These findings suggest that among adolescents who gamble to relieve chronic stress conditions, males and females generally differ in terms of how they experience and manifest abnormal resting states.

4.4 Racial and ethnic groups

There is mounting evidence that adult members of racial/ethnic minority groups and lower socioeconomic classes may be at a significantly greater risk of developing gambling problems (19, 20), a finding that has been replicated in adolescent studies (21, 22). In a sample of U.S. adults, gambling problems were significantly more common among minority groups, with Blacks, Hispanics, Asians, and Native Americans being 3 to 5 times more likely to experience at least some gambling problems compared with Whites when holding gender, age, and socioeconomic status (SES) constant (19). Yet, a study of adolescents showed contradictory results (13). After controlling for SES, black youth actually reported gambling less frequently than white youth. A study of youth in

Montreal, Canada (22), revealed that Allophone adolescents (neither French nor English being the primary language) had the highest rates of reported weekly gambling and experienced more gambling problems. Anglophones were the next highest, whereas Francophones seemed to experience the least problems. The paucity of cultural research and inconsistent findings suggest that these may well be one additional factor contributing to problem gambling. Further research is necessary to determine the impact on youth of racial/ethnic group, socioeconomic status, and their interaction.

4.5 Personality

Research has pointed toward the presence of dispositional attributes of problem gamblers (23–25). The suggestion is that certain personality characteristics, most of which emerge at a young age and are fairly stable over the lifespan, likely contribute to problem gambling. Examining personality traits associated with problem gambling among youth is particularly useful in terms of determining the direction of the relationship between gambling problems and personality traits.

Although most studies examining personality risk factors have focused on specific personality variables, a recent study by Gupta and her colleagues examined a wide variety of personality factors to help identify those most highly associated with gambling problems among youth (26). High school students with moderate to severe gambling-related problems obtained scores that deviated significantly from the normative means on four personality traits: excitability, conformity, self-discipline, and cheerfulness. These findings suggest that adolescents with gambling problems tend to exhibit less self-regulatory behavior (i.e., impulsivity, distractibility, over-activity, self-indulgence, difficulty conforming to group norms) while exuding the impression of being carefree, sociable, and happy. Those adolescents with the most severe gambling problems reported the highest levels of frustration, impulsivity, anxiety, impatience, and irritability. Still further, adolescents with gambling problems obtained higher scores on the Disinhibition and Boredom Susceptibility subscales of the Sensation Seeking Scale, indicating that they have higher risk-taking tendencies.

4.6 Impulsivity

It has been proposed that gambling among youth is the product of an impulsive personality type (27–30). Such lack of impulse control is the hallmark of problem gambling as currently defined. Impulsivity can be described as behavior carried out in a spontaneous or unintentional manner without thought or self-control. This definition describes many of the features of disordered gambling; accordingly, pathological gambling is currently classified as a disorder of impulse control in the *Diagnostic and Statistical Manual of Mental Disorders, Fourth Edition-Text Revision* (DSM-IV-TR) (31). Indeed, research has consistently shown that adults as well as youth with gambling problems exhibit higher scores on both self-report and behavioral measures of impulsivity (23, 25, 26).

Studies have shown that the relationship between impulsivity and problem gambling has direct implications for youth as well (29, 30, 32, 33). A study of 754 adolescent boys from low socioeconomic environments investigated the relationship between impulsivity and problem gambling severity (27). Self-reports and teacher ratings of impulsivity when the boys were 13 years old were compared with problem gambling status in later adolescence (age 17 years). Nongamblers had the lowest impulsivity scores, followed by those with few gambling problems and problem gamblers.

Vitaro and his colleagues reported findings in several studies based on a sample of young low SES boys who were assessed on various personality variables when they were 12 to 14 years old and again at age 17. Disinhibition and response modulation deficits in early adolescence predicted gambling problems at a later age (28). In addition, problem gamblers with substance use problems were more likely to have high self-reports of impulsivity and to exhibit impulsivity-related behaviors at a younger age compared with those with only gambling problems (30). Together, the findings of these prospective studies emphasize the significance of impulsivity as a personality trait among youth that is highly predictive of gambling problems at a later age. It also raises the possibility that impulsivity may be an important focal point of treatment for youth with gambling problems. For example, treatment for adolescents might aim to help individuals develop skills for delaying immediate gratification and placing more weight on the long-term consequences of their behavior.

4.7 Risk behavior

Risk-taking is an intrinsic element of gambling. Problem gamblers have been shown to take greater risks in general and on gambling tasks in particular (23). Problem gamblers have been shown to be associated with high sensation-seeking behavior (23). A study of middle school and high school students found that risk propensity was a particularly strong predictor of being at-risk or having a gambling problem, even after controlling for other predictors (17). Youth who perceive their involvement in risky activities as highly positive while not appreciating the immediate costs and negative consequences of such activities are at greater risk of developing gambling problems. In an interesting study paralleling alcohol studies, Gillespie, Derevensky and Gupta (34) showed that youth with gambling problems do perceive both the benefits and risks associated with gambling. They concluded that those with gambling problems see the risks but assume these are long-term risks and that by the time their problems are serious they will have ceased or cut back their gambling.

4.8 Coping styles

The way in which people cope with life circumstances is a function of both personality and experience. Some individuals use gambling as a form of maladaptive coping in response to problems and stresses in their daily lives (35). Problem gamblers commonly report "gambling to escape," achieved through mood modification as a means of coping with stressful life events and negative affective mood states. Accordingly, problem gamblers are hypothesized to face more life challenges and use less effective coping styles that employ avoidance or mood modification tactics rather than proactively dealing with the cause of the problem. Adolescents with gambling problems report more stress, daily hassles, and major traumatic life events (36) and have been shown to have poor general coping skills (10, 17, 32).

A pattern of more stressful life events and ineffective coping strategies among adolescent problem gamblers was demonstrated in a study that examined stress, coping, and gambling severity in a sample of 11- to 20-year-olds (37). Adolescents with gambling problems reported more negative and major life events compared with social and non-gamblers. In addition, adolescents with gambling problems used less task-focused coping and more avoidance-focused coping. Males with gambling problems reported using more emotion-focused coping strategies but there were no differences among females in terms of emotion-focused coping. A study of gambling and childhood maltreatment showed that, among adolescents and young adults, reports of maltreatment increased as gambling severity increased (36). At-risk and pathological gamblers reported more childhood maltreatment of all types (physical/verbal abuse and neglect) and acknowledged that the effects of their maltreatment had negatively impacted their daily behavior, suggesting that they may be gambling as a means to cope with psychological problems and "escape" from past experiences. In sum, youth who experience more stressful life events with a tendency to use ineffective coping strategies, particularly emotion-focused strategies among males, are at greater risk of turning to gambling as a maladaptive outlet to deal with their problems.

The existing body of research on personality variables and youth gambling problems suggests that there are qualitative differences in personality traits across adolescents with varying severity of gambling behavior. Adolescents who generally exhibit less self-regulatory behavior, higher risk-taking tendencies, and ineffective coping styles are more susceptible than others to developing gambling problems.

4.9 Mental health factors

As previously noted, some individuals engage in gambling in order to modify undesirable mood states (32, 35). For these individuals, gambling becomes a form of negative reinforcement by alleviating unwanted emotions (e.g., anxiety and depression). These finding are consistent with the pathways model of problem gambling (38) and Jacobs' general theory of addictions (18) in that certain problem gamblers engage in the activity to cope with abnormal physiological resting states. Adolescents with severe gambling problems have been shown to experience higher levels of state and trait anxiety (7, 8, 36, 39). For these adolescents, their anxiety may be diminished by gambling providing an "escape" and allowing individuals to disengage from stressful life events or problems. This hypothesis is further supported by findings that adolescent problem gamblers score higher on measures of dissociation and are more likely to report gambling in order to achieve feelings of dissociation (10).

In addition to increased anxiety levels, adolescent problem gamblers report lower self esteem and greater depressive symptomatology (7, 8, 10, 26, 36, 40). Similarly, older adolescents with serious gambling problems are at a heightened risk for suicide ideation and suicide attempts (7). For these youth, gambling may provide emotional relief from symptoms of depression by inducing positive feelings of well-being. Indeed, youth with gambling problems report that they gamble for excitement, to escape problems, and to alleviate depression (7, 36, 39). Another study reported that pathological gamblers and those at risk for gambling problems more heavily anticipated pleasure and excitement from gambling and expected to feel good about themselves as a result of gambling, compared with social and nongamblers (34).

4.10 ADHD

There has been considerable research interest in the possible association between Attention Deficit Hyperactivity Disorder (ADHD) and pathological gambling. Given that ADHD is normally diagnosed during childhood, the potential link between these two psychiatric conditions is particularly important for understanding risk factors for problem gambling among youth. Notably, existing knowledge about the progression of ADHD may provide a developmental framework for understanding risk factors for gambling problems among youth.

Several studies have reported a relationship between gambling problems and ADHD (41, 42), and more recently, a study by Hardoon, Gupta, and Derevensky (43) has shown that there are similar traits that underlie ADHD and gambling problems. Adolescent problem gamblers in high school were found to be similar to those adolescents with ADHD on several dimensions (26). Youth with gambling problems tended to score high on the excitability factor of the High School Personality Questionnaire, composed of items that query the extent to which respondents are easily distracted, frustrated, annoyed, overactive, and impulsive. These characteristics match up to the criteria for ADHD, as outlined in the DSM-IV-TR (31).

A prospective study examined a sample of children diagnosed with ADHD at two points in time – initially between the ages of 7 and 11 and later between the ages of 18 and 24 (33). At the follow-up assessment, participants were identified as either still meeting the criteria for a diagnosis of ADHD or no longer meeting the criteria. No differences were found between the participants with persistent ADHD, nonpersistent ADHD, and a group of controls in terms of gambling participation or frequency. However, those with persistent ADHD were significantly more likely to be identified as pathological gamblers when compared with those with nonpersistent ADHD or no ADHD. The findings suggest that symptoms of ADHD that persist into young adulthood are particularly important risk factors for gambling problems among youth.

4.11 Academic achievement

Among adults, a negative consequence commonly associated with gambling problems is poor work performance. Apart from absences and lateness due to gambling, the quality of work tends to suffer as individuals become preoccupied with gambling, thinking about their next gambling episode and experiencing negative emotional consequences in response to losses. Although children and adolescents are often not subject to these problems, they are nevertheless subject to poor school performance as a result of excessive gambling. Dickson et al. (17) found in a sample of adolescents that school-related problems predicted at-risk and pathological gambling, with a large proportion of pathological gamblers (43.5%) experiencing significant school problems. Likewise, the proportion of students with below average, self-perceived grades increased linearly as gambling severity increased with almost one quarter of pathological gamblers perceiving that they performed worse than other students at school compared with only 6.5% of nongamblers reporting low grades. Meanwhile, feeling welcome and integrated into the school environment was a protective factor such that lower school-connectedness was associated with adolescent problem gambling. A link between gambling problems and poor school performance has been demonstrated in several studies (8, 15, 43).

Given that the above findings are correlational in nature, it is not currently possible to determine whether school problems arise as a result of gambling problems or if problems in school tend to lead to gambling problems (e.g., resulting from an inability to concentrate on school-related tasks and/or escaping from problems and not putting in the appropriate study time). It has also been shown that a high proportion of youth with gambling problems report having a learning disability (43), suggesting that innate academic difficulties may precede gambling problems. However, the relationship is most likely reciprocal with excessive gambling activity leading to poorer performance in school which, in turn, contributes to increased gambling involvement. The extent to which one causes the other cannot be determined without prospective data that examines the sequential nature of these problems.

4.12 Substance abuse

Problem gambling is often conceptualized as a nonpharmacological behavioral "addiction" because, although one does not ingest a substance with chemically addictive properties when gambling, it shares several defining features with substance use disorders. For example, in the DSM-IV-TR (31), substance dependence and pathological gambling are both characterized by preoccupation, a need to increase the behavior to achieve the desired effect, symptoms of withdrawal, loss of important social, occupational, or recreational activities, and continuation despite knowledge of its negative consequences. Among adults, there is a high co-occurrence between substance use disorders and gambling disorders (44), which is not surprising given the striking similarities in their defining features, suggesting that common variables contribute to the development of both disorders.

Research on adolescents mirrors the finding of a significant association between substance abuse and gambling problems in adults. A number of studies have shown that adolescent problem gamblers are at increased risk for the development of multiple addictions (7, 10, 15, 19). In a sample of Minnesota youth, those with greater gambling involvement were more likely to be regular drug users (15). Similarly, among New York state adolescents, heavy drinking males were significantly more likely than nondrinkers or moderate drinkers to gamble at least weekly (13). Studies assessing alcohol, tobacco, illicit drug, and marijuana use among Minnesota youth showed them to be reliable predictors of gambling frequency (14, 45) as did a study of Washington State youth demonstrating a positive association between tobacco, alcohol, and drug use and both gambling frequency and gambling problems (46). Clearly, data on adolescent substance use and gambling indicate that these behaviors tend to co-occur in youth, suggesting that substance use should be viewed as a warning sign for co-morbid gambling problems and vice versa.

4.13 Delinquency

Despite legal prohibitions and statutes prohibiting youth gambling on regulated activities, prevalence data indicate that the majority of youth have gambled (8, 10, 14, 15) (see also Volberg and her colleagues in this volume), further suggesting that gambling is becoming perceived as a normative activity. Notwithstanding the high rates of gambling participation among youth, government restrictions tend to categorize underage gambling along with underage drinking, deeming them both adult activities that pose a significant risk to youth. Disordered gambling among youth is delinquent behavior, not only in the sense that it normally involves repeated violation of the law, but also because many of the associated problems relate to other delinquent activities to fulfill gambling intentions. In fact, when one overlaps the typical personality features of problem gambling over norms for delinquent behaviors on the High School Personality Questionnaire, the profiles look remarkably similar (26).

One of the DSM-IV-TR criteria for pathological gambling is the commission of illegal acts to finance gambling, including forgery, fraud, theft, or embezzlement (31). Adolescent research has likewise demonstrated a strong association between delinquency and gambling problems (8, 10, 15). For some youth, gambling may be an outgrowth of a more general behavior problem syndrome. Youth who have difficulty following rules and behaving in socially acceptable ways are more likely to engage in delinquent activities that include gambling (13). Antisocial tendencies among youth are characteristic of conduct disorder representing a persistent pattern of behaviors that violate age-appropriate social norms (31). A recent study showed a strong co-morbidity between conduct disorder and gambling problems, particularly among younger respondents in a sample of 14- to 21-year-olds (47). Further evidence of a relationship between youth gambling and antisocial behavior was found in an analysis of Minnesota public school students which revealed that antisocial behavior – including vandalism, physical fights, stealing, and getting thrills from dangerous activities – was the strongest predictor of gambling frequency (14). Stinchfield and his colleagues posited that frequent gambling may be part of a collection of deviant behaviors including violence, vandalism, shoplifting, and substance use. This type of young gambler fits with Blaszczynski and Nower's (38) "anti-social impulsivist" pathway of problem gambling. Youth who are prone to "acting-out" behaviors, violence, deceitfulness, and consistent violation of rules may be at risk for gambling problems.

4.14 Interpersonal relationships

Children and adolescents spend a large portion of their lives with their immediate family, with behaviors being modeled on family members who have a strong impact on the future behavior of young people. Consequently, gambling by family members contributes to the gambling behavior of youth. For example, most youth become exposed early on to gambling by their parents (43). In studying children between the ages of 9 and 14, Gupta and Derevensky (6) found a large majority (86%) of those who gambled regularly reported gambling with family members. Other studies have also reported that youth with greater gambling involvement are more likely to have parents or family members that gamble (8, 15, 21).

In another study, a sample of adolescents from middle and high school were examined to test the extent to which various protective factors increased resilience to adolescent problem gambling (17). Problem gamblers were less likely to report feeling connected to their families compared to at-risk gamblers, social gamblers, and nongamblers. Self-reported ratings of family cohesion decreased from nongamblers across each level of gambling severity group. Family cohesion remained a significant predictor when tested along with other protective factors in their ability to predict participant classification as either nonproblem gamblers (i.e., nongamblers and social gamblers) or problem gamblers (i.e., at-risk and pathological gamblers). These results support previous findings in which youth with gambling problems were more likely to report having poor family connectedness, family dysfunction, low perceived social support, and low parental supervision (8, 43, 29).

In the same study, pathological adolescent gamblers were more likely to report having family members with gambling problems compared with other adolescents, and the proportions generally decreased as severity of problems diminished (17). When tested with other risk factors to predict problem gambling status, only having a sibling with a gambling problem remained a significant predictor. Other family factors related to stressful life events were examined for their ability to differentiate between gambling severity groups but were not tested in the overall prediction models. The death of a friend or close family member and the arrest of a family member differed across groups, with pathological gamblers having generally higher rates. Parental divorce and/or remarriage of parents, moving to a new town/city, loss of a parent's job, and a close family member having a serious illness did not differentiate between gambling severity groups.

Poor caregiving can also contribute to future gambling of youth. In a study of childhood maltreatment and youth gambling, pathological gamblers reported significantly higher levels of emotional and physical neglect as children compared with at-risk, social, and nongamblers (36). Living in a non-nurturing family environment appears to be an additional risk factor for gambling problems among youth.

4.15 Peers

Friends play an important role in shaping the risky activities of young people. Before adolescents are allowed to participate in regulated forms of gambling (e.g., casinos, lotteries, machine gambling), they often begin gambling among their personal friends. When gambling becomes a regular activity among friends, it may become viewed as a normative activity that is both desirable and safe. Indeed, one study found that only 10% of students aged 13 and 14 years feared being caught for gambling by parents, suggesting that gambling is generally regarded as a socially acceptable activity among adolescents (6). As such, having friends who gamble makes gambling less likely to be perceived as a high-risk activity and adolescents may exhibit less caution when gambling in the future. In the same study (6), 75% of 9- to 14-year-olds who regularly gambled reported that they gambled with their friends and the tendency to gamble more at a friend's home and at school increased with age. Not only does having friends who gamble increase the likelihood of gambling involvement, clinical evidence suggests that adolescents who develop gambling problems tend to lose their nongambling friends as they spend more time with gambling associates (48). This pattern has the

potential to be particularly harmful given that the protective factor of positive friendships is replaced with a friendship milieu in which gambling is both socially acceptable
and the predominant extracurricular activity.

Having a friend with a gambling problem has also been found to differentiate youth
based on their gambling severity groups in that over 40% of pathological gamblers and
over one third of at-risk gamblers reported having a friend with a gambling problem as
compared with only 10% of social gamblers and 6% of nongamblers (17). In addition,
it was a significant predictor of problem gambler status over and above all other risk
and protective factors. Also of note was the finding that having friends with substance
use problems increased with problem gambling severity, suggesting that having friends
who engage in any addictive behavior, not just gambling, poses a significant risk factor. Similarly, having friends who engage in antisocial delinquent behaviors is strongly
predictive of gambling problems among youth (13, 29).

The general quality of peer relationships also appears to predict problem gambling
severity among youth. A study of Australian adolescents revealed that problem gamblers
have poorer relationships with non-friend peers in their class, despite reporting having
as many close friends as nonproblem gamblers (40). Problem gamblers indicated that
they disliked twice as many classmates as nonproblem gamblers and also reported
that significantly more classmates dislike them. Among various measures of psychological well-being, social alienation was the strongest predictor of gambling severity, with
adolescent problem gamblers being significantly more disillusioned in general. Regardless of the quality of close friendships, it appears that poor relationships with peers, in
general, are a risk factor for youth problem gambling.

4.16 Community

At a community level, an obvious risk factor for problem gambling is the widespread
availability of gambling opportunities that are accessible to youth. Though research is
currently inconclusive regarding the impact of gambling availability on the prevalence of
gambling problems, there is ample evidence to suggest that youth have been engaged in
both regulated and unregulated forms of gambling. Conventional wisdom predicts that
more gambling opportunities within communities ultimately leads to higher incidences
of gambling problems. Findings are mixed in this regard and it has been suggested that
the relationship between exposure to gambling and the prevalence of gambling-related
problems is nonlinear, varying across individuals, places, and time (49). Accordingly, it
is difficult to determine whether youth who are exposed to more gambling opportunities
in their communities are at greater risk of developing problems. However, among young
people who gamble, there is evidence suggesting that specific types of gambling activities
pose a greater risk than others (50), with poker now becoming a game of choice.

A national sample of U.S. youth between the ages of 14 and 21 years clearly suggests that youth who had experience with multiple types of gambling during the past
year were more likely to have gambling problems (50). When involvement in other
games was controlled, card playing, games of skill, and casino gambling were found
to be highly associated with increased risk of gambling problems. These data merely
examined the association between specific forms of gambling and gambling-related
problems among youth, making it difficult to determine whether exposure itself leads

to more problems or if youth with gambling problems are more likely to participate in multiple forms of gambling, which is likely the case. Nonetheless, the results suggest that certain gambling activities and overall level of gambling engagement can be useful predictors of gambling problems among youth. High gambling versatility appears to be a particularly salient risk factor for youth problem gambling (40). When youth are presented with and have access to more gambling options, they may be more likely to find a preferred form of gambling, which can increase the risk of developing a problem. This finding, coupled with research suggesting that early age of onset may be problematic, remains a concern (6–8).

4.17 Marketing

Related to the availability of gambling within communities is the way gambling is marketed toward community members. Although most jurisdictions have laws prohibiting minors from participating in regulated forms of gambling, youth are exposed to the same messages advertising gambling opportunities as adults. A broad range of marketing strategies is typically used to promote gambling opportunities to the public. Television and radio commercials, billboards and other signage, point-of-sale advertisements, sponsorship arrangements, and promotional products are examples of marketing efforts that use various forms of media to endorse gambling opportunities (51). These advertisements tend to focus on the fun, entertainment, and possibility of "winning big" with no mention of the potential consequences of gambling. Adolescents report that these advertisements portray gambling as a socially acceptable, rewarding, and enriching activity that leads to a happier lifestyle (52).

Not only do these advertisements increase the availability of gambling within communities by providing information about local gambling opportunities, they normalize gambling by portraying it as an acceptable and harmless form of entertainment. As youth are exposed to more and more gambling advertisements, they are more likely to perceive it as a normative activity within their respective communities. In addition, the central message of these advertisements, that gambling is a thrilling and worry-free activity, is more likely to be accepted and pursued by children and adolescents. Derevensky et al. (52) found that 47% of adolescent males and 38% of adolescent females reported that gambling advertisements made them want to try gambling. In addition, problem gamblers were much more likely to report "sometimes" or "often" gambling after seeing an advertisement (32%) compared with social (3%) or nongamblers (0%). Such findings have led researchers to suggest that the presence of gambling advertisements is a strong risk factor for youth gambling involvement (51). The fact that the past two winners of the World Series of Poker, Joe Cada and Jonathan Duhamel, who won millions of dollars, were both under the age of 21 and college drop-outs, provides a new type of role model for youth. In a number of focus groups with children ages 12–15, many indicated that after leaving school they wanted to be professional gamblers. Accordingly, community-level regulation of these advertisements that reduces exposure to youth and prohibits overly positive portrayals of gambling would likely reduce the normalization of gambling and lead to subsequent reductions in gambling problems among youth.

4.18 Societal influences

Beyond individual, interpersonal, and community-level factors that have an impact on youth gambling behavior, there are macro-level risk factors that reflect the wider culture and society. Throughout history, cultural norms have dictated the legality and availability of gambling opportunities. At several points in time, widespread belief that gambling was sinful led to its prohibition in many parts of the world. To this day, gambling remains outlawed in most Muslim countries and public opposition, often from religious organizations, has led to the removal of gambling machines in certain jurisdictions. However, as gambling revenues have been shown to be lucrative sources of funds for governments, charities, and businesses, gambling opportunities have expanded. Coinciding with this expansion, conservative attitudes toward gambling have typically been modified, and gambling continues to gain acceptance as a socially acceptable, even charitable, form of entertainment. Consequently, this prevailing attitude poses a serious risk for youth. Children and adolescents who identify strongly with the ideological, social, economic, and political values of a gambling-permissive society will be more likely to see it as a normative activity themselves, and thus something they may choose to pursue.

As previously noted, the availability and marketing of gambling are important determinants of youth gambling. However, differences in gambling rates across communities can also be attributed to cultural differences (53). In addition, differences between cultural groups within the same geographic region can at least partially explain variations in gambling attitudes and behaviors. Thus far, the majority of the review has consisted of Western studies. Although few non-Western studies have specifically examined risk factors for youth gambling problems, it is instructive to examine some of the cultural factors known to impact the initiation and maintenance of gambling.

Existing research suggests relatively high rates of gambling among certain cultural and ethnic groups including Jewish, Chinese, and Indigenous peoples (53). There is some evidence that racial/ethnic minority groups are at greater risk of developing gambling problems. Though these higher gambling rates may be caused to some extent by noncultural factors such as low SES, there is evidence that cultural issues also play a unique role. For example, Zitzow (54) reported that American Indian adolescents reported more gambling involvement and gambling-related problems compared with non-American Indian adolescents, which was partially attributed to cultural acceptance of magical thinking among American Indians. Thus, cultural beliefs that emphasize an external locus of control and a reliance on "fate" or "luck" may encourage more gambling among youth.

Traditional family configurations may also influence gambling behavior. For example, Raylu and Oei (53) suggested that children from Chinese families with a traditional patriarchal family system have increased exposure to and parental approval of gambling. Certain cultures also transmit general attitudes toward gambling to its members. Whereas gambling is perceived as part of the lifestyle, history, and tradition of Chinese people, it has been met with steadfast disapproval in Muslim cultures. Clearly, children growing up in a Chinese culture will be more likely to develop positive attitudes and increased exposure to gambling compared with Muslim children.

Whereas cultural issues represent important macro-level factors that influence youth gambling, global trends in gambling represent another significant consideration. Most notably, the Internet gambling industry has experienced large-scale expansion that some researchers posit will lead to higher rates of gambling and related problems among youth (55) (also see the review in this volume by Griffiths and Parke). Though the presence of more gambling venues represents a potential risk factor at a community level, the emergence of Internet-based gambling circumvents the accessibility issue and allows access to gambling to virtually anyone, virtually anywhere, and at any time in the world. The high accessibility of Internet gambling presents new societal concerns, particularly for youth who have spent their entire lives adopting and embracing this technology.

Although no empirical studies have tested the causal relationship between the availability of Internet gambling and gambling problems among youth, the results of at least two correlational studies suggest that youth who gamble via the Internet are much more likely to experience significant gambling problems (56–57). These findings are alarming given that youth continue to have increased exposure to the Internet and its evolving set of applications. The academic and extracurricular activities of youth have become well integrated into advancing technologies. As the popularity and accessibility of Internet gambling has increased, so has Internet usage and computer access among youth. These combined elements make Internet gambling a potentially high-risk form of gambling with its own set of unique risk factors worthy of increased scrutiny among researchers. In addition, much of the appeal of Internet gambling appears to be related to the game of poker, which has garnered an incredible amount of international attention as a "sport" that anyone can pursue. As global interest in poker continues to grow in the form of increased television exposure, multi-million dollar tournaments, and the creation of celebrity poker professionals, children and adolescents are more likely to seek out Internet gambling sites as an opportunity to test their own poker skills. Societal acceptance of poker as a legitimate and harmless pastime poses a risk for youth gambling.

This technology is also being brought to "smart phones." As such, mobile gambling has similarly drastically increased. This trend raises new concerns, especially among youth and young adults who continue to immerse themselves in advancing technology.

4.19 Conclusions

Myriad factors are implicated in the development of gambling problems among children and adolescents. Individual, relationship, community, and societal factors all play a role in the cause and maintenance of youth gambling problems. However, variables at each of these levels cannot be considered in isolation. Rather, all risk factors should be examined within the context of other risk factors that could potentially lead to overinvolvement with gambling. At the individual level, demographic, personality, and psychological factors influence youth's susceptibility to developing gambling problems. Relationship-level factors encompass family and friends, whereas community-level factors include availability, accessibility, and marketing within the community where the child lives. Finally, at a societal level, cultural factors and worldwide trends in gambling (i.e., Internet and mobile gambling) are considered important large-scale forces that can impact the level of risk. Although these risk factors cover a wide range of variables, it is far from being a comprehensive review of factors that are relevant to youth gambling prevention.

The current review highlights research on risk factors that, for the most part, focus on examining the negative factors associated with gambling problems among youth. However, efforts to prevent tobacco, alcohol, and drug use among youth have focused on not only decreasing risk factors but also increasing protective factors (58) and resilience (59). The success of these initiatives in preventing high-risk behaviors highlights the importance of designing youth gambling prevention efforts to enhance resiliency. Although the results of one study suggested that the absence of risk factors contributes more significantly to the prediction of gambling problems among youth than the presence of protective factors (17), yet another study demonstrated that risk and protective factors each contribute uniquely to the prediction of youth gambling problems (59). Accordingly, youth gambling research should go beyond a basic risk prevention framework to one that fosters protective factors when helping develop youth gambling prevention initiatives. One category of potentially instructive protective factors is positive development constructs. Current evidence is limited on the extent to which such constructs, including cognitive and emotional competencies, serve as protective factors for youth gambling. Parker et al. (60) found that higher emotional intelligence among youth was associated with lower scores on a problem gambling measure. Among the different components of emotional intelligence, interpersonal abilities had the highest negative correlation with problem gambling severity, suggesting that youth with better interpersonal skills are less likely to spend considerable amounts of time gambling.

However, the direction of this relationship was undetermined. Cognitive competencies and their relation to youth problem gambling have been left unexplored for the most part as well. Turner and his colleagues reported that a higher score on knowledge of randomness, self-monitoring, and coping skills among older adolescents was associated with lower scores on a problem gambling measure (61). In addition, an intervention designed to improve these competencies resulted in significant increases in understanding randomness and enhancing self-monitoring, and coping skills knowledge compared with a control group. It would seem that preliminary evidence suggests that positive development constructs warrant further investigation as potential protective factors for youth gambling problems.

Much of the research reviewed tended to examine the factors that co-occur with gambling problems among youth. That is, most existing research on risk factors provides an account of the characteristics and situational factors observed in youth who already exhibit signs of disordered gambling. Though these correlational findings are useful for secondary prevention measures, they are less helpful for primary prevention efforts aimed at preventing the onset of gambling problems and other high-risk behaviors. More prospective research is needed to establish the antecedents of problem gambling among youth. Such studies should take a longitudinal approach to determine which factors are present before gambling problems emerge. Although more costly and difficult to undertake, such research would provide valuable knowledge about how gambling problems develop in youth and the resiliency factors that can help make children more resistant to gambling problems before they are initiated to gambling activities.

Most existing research on risk factors has focused on demographic and behavioral correlates of youth gambling. Much less work has been devoted to examining the unique thoughts and attitudes that are prevalent among youth with gambling problems. These factors represent a crucial area of study given that thoughts and attitudes encompass the motivation to gamble. Current evidence suggests that children and adolescents with positive attitudes toward gambling are more likely to develop gambling problems (21). In addition, adolescent problem gamblers hold more irrational beliefs about gambling, often failing to understand the true risks associated with gambling and believing that they have more control over gambling outcomes than chance dictates (62, 63). Future research on risk factors should closely examine the thoughts and attitudes that contribute to gambling problems among youth. By revealing how gambling-related thoughts and attitudes develop, such studies will ultimately impact prevention efforts that aim to counter these beliefs before they become more firmly entrenched.

Another area of inquiry that warrants further exploration is technological forms of gambling (e.g., mobile and Internet gambling) and their potentially unique set of risk factors. The daily lives of children and adolescents are becoming increasingly immersed in technology, particularly the Internet, bringing into question the extent to which Internet usage poses a major risk factor for youth gambling. With the rapid expansion of Internet gambling and governmental acceptance and licensing of such sites over the past 10 years, these concerns have become a reality. Qualitative data suggests that young people are the fastest growing segment of Internet gamblers (64). Yet, the risk factors associated with Internet gambling among youth remain largely unexplored. Video game playing, an activity that has become more technologically advanced and interactive, may also be related to problem gambling among youth. One study found that adolescents in grades 7 to 11 who experienced gambling problems were more likely to spend excessive amounts of time playing video games compared with nonproblem and social gamblers (65). Future studies should investigate the risk factors that have emerged with advancing technology, such as video games and Internet gambling.

It is noteworthy that many of the risk and protective factors associated with problem gambling are predictive of multiple other problem behaviors, including substance abuse, conduct and oppositional disorders, and delinquency, suggesting that gambling may be part of a larger constellation of high-risk behaviors that has its roots in common underlying factors. Studies on risk factors for gambling problems, delinquency, and substance use among youth suggest that all three high-risk behaviors are well predicted by a common set of risk factors, supporting the notion of a general problem behavior syndrome (13, 29, 40, 66). Prevention efforts will benefit most from research that focuses on identifying risk factors that contribute to this general problem behavior syndrome, which will ultimately have a positive impact on the overall development of youth (17, 59).

Improving youth gambling prevention efforts will require the active involvement of parents to consider their own children's level of risk and to develop open and honest communication with their children about gambling. But before parents can engage in frank discussions about gambling with their children they need to become aware of the seriousness of gambling as an issue among teens. Unfortunately, research suggests that parents are in much need of further education about youth gambling. Parents tend to underestimate the probability that their own children have gambled or have a gambling problem (67), and gambling remains very low (in fact, the lowest concern among 13 potential adolescent risk behaviors) on their priority list of teen concerns (68). It is hoped that prevention can begin with a better understanding of the risk factors for gambling problems among youth. New directions in research and the application of corresponding findings to prevention efforts will help achieve the overall goal of minimizing or reducing problems associated with gambling among youth.

Gambling behavior among youth reflects an ongoing trend in society that could be best understood within an ecological model recognizing the inter-woven relationship that exists between the individual and the environment. Though the prevalence rates for adolescent gambling problems have not dramatically increased during the past decade in spite of increased acceptance, availability, and accessibility, it is important to note that the general overall population has increased (e.g., the U.S. population has increased by 9.7% in the past decade). As a result, the total number of individuals, adolescents and adults, with gambling problems has increased. The mosaic and constellation of factors that place some youth at risk for gambling problems will be ultimately impacted by our social and public health policies. Establishing more empirically driven prevention programs will likely help in both the short-term and long-term. Educators, legislators, and parents would be wise to address this growing issue.

References

1. Johansson A, Grant JE, Kim SW, Odlaug BL, Gotestam, KG. Risk factors for problematic gambling: a critical literature review. J Gambl Stud 2009;25(1):67–92.
2. Griffiths MD. The acquisition, development, and maintenance of fruit machine gambling in adolescents. J Gambl Stud 1990;6(3):193–204.
3. Stephenson MT, Morgan SE, Lorch EP, Palmgreen P, Donohew L, Hoyle RH. Predictors of exposure from an anti-marijuana media campaign: Outcome research assessing sensation seeking targeting. Health Commun 2002;14(1):23–43.
4. Volberg RA, Dickerson MG, Ladouceur R, Abbott MW. Prevalence studies and the development of services for problem gamblers and their families. J Gambl Stud 1996;12(2):215–31.
5. Bronfenbrenner U. The ecology of human development: Experiments by nature and design. Cambridge, MA: Harvard Univ Press; 1979.
6. Gupta R, Derevensky, JL. Familial and social influences on juvenile gambling. J Gambl Stud 1997;13(3):179–92.
7. Gupta R, Derevensky, JL. An empirical examination of Jacobs' General Theory of Addictions: Do adolescent gamblers fit the theory? J Gambl Stud 1998;14(1):17–49.
8. Wynne H, Smith G, Jacobs D. Adolescent gambling and problem gambling in Alberta. Alberta Alcohol and Drug Abuse Commission; 1996.
9. Productivity Commission, Australia. Australia's gambling industries. Australian Government. Report number: 10; 1999.
10. Gupta R., Derevensky, JL. Adolescent gambling behavior: A prevalence study and examination of the correlates associated with problem gambling. J Gambl Stud 1998;14(4):319–45.
11. Volberg RA. The prevalence and demographics of pathological gamblers: Implications for public health. Am J Health Promot 1994;84 (2):237–41.
12. Welte JB, Barnes GM, Wieczorek WF, Tidwell MC, Parker J. Gambling participation in the U.S. – Results from a national survey. J Gambl Stud 2002;18(4):313–37.
13. Barnes GM, Welte JW, Hoffman JH, Dintcheff BA. Gambling and alcohol use among youth: Influences of demographic, socialization, and individual factors. Addict Behav 1999; 24(6):749–67.
14. Stinchfield R, Cassuto N, Winters K, Latimer W. Prevalence of gambling among Minnesota public school students in 1992 and 1995. J Gambl Stud 1997;13(1):24–48.
15. Winters KC, Stinchfield R, Fulkerson J. Patterns and characteristics of adolescent gambling. J Gambl Stud 1993;9(4):371–86.
16. Ladouceur R, Dubé D, Bujold A. Gambling among primary school students. J Gambl Stud 1994;10(4):363–70.

17. Dickson LM, Derevensky JL, Gupta R. Youth gambling problems: Examining risk and protective factors. Int Gambl Stud 2008;8(1):25–47.
18. Jacobs DF. A general theory of addictions: A new theoretical model. J Gambl Stud 1986;2(1):15–31.
19. Welte JB, Barnes GM, Wieczorek WF, Tidwell MC, Parker J. Alcohol and gambling pathology among U.S. Adults: Prevalence, demographic patterns and comorbidity. J Stud Alcohol 2001;62(5):706–12.
20. Ellenbogen S, Gupta R, Derevensky JL. A cross-cultural study of gambling behavior among adolescents. J Gambl Stud 2007;23(1):25–39.
21. Stinchfield R, Winters KC. Gambling and problem gambling among youths. Ann Am Acad Pol Soc Sci 1998;556(1):172–85.
22. Wallisch L. Gambling in Texas: 1995 Texas survey of adolescent gambling behavior. Austin, TX: Texas Commission Alcohol Drug Abuse; 1996.
23. Breen RB, Zuckerman M. Chasing in gambling behavior: Personality and cognitive determinants. Pers Individ Dif 1999;27(6):1097–111.
24. Cyders MA, Smith GT. Clarifying the role of personality dispositions in risk for increased gambling behavior. Pers Individ Dif 2008;45(6):503–08.
25. Steel Z, Blaszczynski A. Impulsivity, personality disorders and pathological gambling severity. Addiction 1998;93(6):895–905.
26. Gupta R, Derevensky JL, Ellenbogen S. Personality characteristics and risk-taking tendencies among adolescent gamblers. Can J Behav Sci 2006;38(3):201–13.
27. Vitaro F, Arseneault L, Tremblay RE. Dispositional predictors of problem gambling in male adolescents. Am J Psychiatry 1997;154(12):1769–70.
28. Vitaro F, Arseneault L, Tremblay RE. Impulsivity predicts problem gambling in low SES adolescent males. Addiction 1999;94(4):565–75.
29. Vitaro F, Brendgen M, Ladouceur R, Tremblay RE. Gambling, delinquency, and drug use during adolescence: Mutual influences and common risk factors. J Gambl Stud 2001;17(3):171–90.
30. Vitaro F, Ferland F, Jacques C, Ladouceur R. Gambling, substance use, and impulsivity during adolescence. Psychol Addict Behav 1998;12(3):185–94.
31. American Psychiatric Association. Diagnostic and statistical manual of mental disorders. 4th ed, text rev. Washington, DC: Author; 2000.
32. Nower L, Derevensky J, Gupta R. The relationship of impulsivity, sensation seeking, coping and substance use in youth gamblers. Psychol Addict Behav 2004;18(1):49–55.
33. Breyer JL, Botzet, AM, Winters KC, Stinchfield RD, August G, Realmuto G. Young adult gambling behaviors and their relationship with the persistence of ADHD. J Gambl Stud. 2009;25(2):227–38.
34. Gillespie MA, Derevensky JL, Gupta R. The utility of outcome expectancies in the prediction of adolescent gambling behavior. J Gambl Issues 2007;19:69–85.
35. Wood RT, Griffiths MD. A qualitative investigation of problem gambling as an escape-based coping strategy. Psychol Psychother 2007;80(1):107–25.
36. Felsher JR, Derevensky JL, Gupta R. Young adults with gambling problems: The impact of childhood maltreatment. Int J Ment Health Addiction, in press.
37. Bergevin T, Gupta R, Derevensky J, Kaufman F. Adolescent gambling: Understanding the role of stress and coping. J Gambl Stud 2006;22(2):195–208.
38. Blaszczynski A, Nower L. A pathways model of problem and pathological gambling. Addiction 2002;97(5):487–99.
39. Ste-Marie C, Gupta R, Derevensky J. Anxiety and social stress related to adolescent gambling behavior and substance use. J Child Adolesc Subst Abuse 2006;15(4):55–74.
40. Delfabbro P, Lahn J, Grabosky P. Psychosocial correlates of problem gambling in Australian students. Aust NZ J Psychiatry 2006;40(6–7):587–95.

41. Carlton PL, Manowitz P. Behavioral restraint and symptoms of attention deficit disorder in alcoholics and pathological gamblers. Neuropsychology 1992;25(1):44–48.
42. Carlton PL, Manowitz P, McBride H, Nora R, Swartzburg M, Goldstein L. Attention deficit disorder and pathological disorder. J Clin Psychiatry 1987;48(12):487–88.
43. Hardoon K, Gupta R, Derevensky JL. Psychosocial variables associated with adolescent gambling. Psychol Addict Behav 2004;18(2):170–9.
44. Stewart SH, Kushner, MG. Recent research on the comorbidity of alcoholism and pathological gambling. Alcohol Clin Exp Res 2003;27(2):285–91.
45. Stinchfield R. A comparison of Gambling among Minnesota Public School Students in 1992, 1995 and 1998. J Gambl Stud 2001;17(4):273–96.
46. Volberg RA. Gambling and problem gambling among adolescents in Washington State. Olympia, WA: Washington State Lottery; 1993.
47. Welte JW, Barnes GM, Tidwell MC, Hoffman JH. Association between problem gambling and conduct disorder in a national survey of adolescents and young adults in the United States. J Adolesc Health 2009;45(4):396–401.
48. Gupta R, Derevensky JL. Adolescents with gambling problems: From research to treatment. J Gambl Stud 2000;16(2/3):315–42.
49. LaPlante DA, Shaffer HJ. Understanding the influence of gambling opportunities: Expanding exposure models to include adaptation. Am J Orthopsychiatry 2007;77(4):616–23.
50. Welte J, Barnes GM, Tidwell M, Hoffman J. The association of form of gambling with problem gambling among American youth. Psychol Addict Behav 2009;23(1):105–12.
51. Monaghan S, Derevensky J, Sklar A. Impact of gambling advertisements and marketing on children and adolescents: Policy recommendations to minimize harm. J Gambl Issues 2008;22:252–74.
52. Derevensky J, Sklar A, Gupta R, Messerlian C. An empirical study examining the impact of gambling advertisements on adolescent gambling attitudes and behaviors. Int J Ment Health Addiction [published online]. Available from doi:10.1007/ s11469–009–9211–7.
53. Raylu N, Oei TP. Role of culture in gambling and problem gambling. Clin Psychol Rev 2004;23(8):1087–1114.
54. Zitzow D. Comparative study of problematic gambling behaviors between American Indian and non-Indian adolescents within and near a northern plains reservation. Am Indian Alsk Native Ment Health Res 1996;7(2):14–26.
55. Derevensky JL, Gupta R. Internet gambling amongst adolescents: A growing concern. Int J Ment Health Addiction 2007;5(2):93–101.
56. Byrne A. An exploratory study of Internet gambling among youth. Dissertation. Montreal, QC: McGill University; 2004.
57. McBride J, Derevensky J. Internet gambling behavior in a sample of online gamblers. Int J Ment Health Addiction 2009;7(1):149–67.
58. Brounstein PJ, Zweig JM, Gardner SE. Understanding substance abuse prevention: Toward the 21st century – A primer on effective programs. Substance Abuse and Mental Health Services Administration, Center for Substance Abuse Prevention, Division of Knowledge Development and Evaluation; 1999.
59. Lussier I, Derevensky JL, Gupta R, Bergevin T, Ellenbogen S. Youth gambling behaviors: An examination of the role of resilience. Psychol Addict Behav 2007;21(2):165–73.
60. Parker JD, Taylor RN, Eastabrook JM, Schell SL, Wood LM. Problem gambling in adolescence: Relationships with Internet misuse, gaming abuse and emotional intelligence. Pers Individ Dif 2008;45(2):174–80.
61. Turner NE, Macdonald J, Somerset M. Life skills, mathematical reasoning and critical thinking: A curriculum for the prevention of problem gambling. J Gambl Stud 2008;24(3):367–80.
62. Delfabbro P, Lahn J, Grabosky P. It's not what you know, but how you use it: Statistical knowledge and adolescent problem gambling. J Gambl Stud 2006;22(2):179–93.

63. Moore SM, Ohtsuka K. Beliefs about control over gambling among young people, and their relation to problem gambling. Psychol Addict Behav 1999;13(4):339–47.
64. Brown SJ. The surge in online gambling on college campuses. New Directions for Student Services 2006;113:53–61.
65. Wood RT, Gupta R, Derevensky JL, Griffiths M. Video game playing and gambling in adolescents: common risk factors. J Child Adolesc Subst Abuse 2004;14(1):77–100.
66. Jessor R, ed. New perspectives on adolescent risk behavior. New York: Cambridge Univ Press; 1998
67. Ladouceur R, Vitaro F, Côté M. Parents' attitudes, knowledge, and behavior toward youth gambling: a five-year follow-up. J Gambl Stud 2001;17(2):101–16.
68. Campbell CA, Derevensky J, Meerkamper, E, Cutajar, J. Parents' perceptions of adolescent gambling behavior: a Canadian national study. J Gambl Iss 2011;25:36–53.

5 Defining and assessing binge gambling

Rina Gupta and Jeffrey L. Derevensky

Prevalence studies have shown that a significant proportion of adolescents and young adults engage in gambling activities, highlighting the need to identify risk factors that influence and impact the development of problem gambling. Recent research has also pointed to the need to help differentiate among a diversity of problem gamblers. As a result, subtypes of gamblers must be studied to help inform our prevention and treatment efforts. Research examining a particular subtype of problem drinking – binge drinking – has yielded important insights into its prevalence, causes, and associated problems. These findings have not only helped raise awareness about binge drinking as a serious, hazardous behavior; they have also contributed to the development of prevention and treatment approaches aimed at addressing this growing concern. Following the growing body of research focused on binge drinking, the current study explored the concept of binge gambling and its relationship to traditional conceptualizations of gambling severity as well as binge and problem drinking.

5.1 Introduction

Despite legal sanctions prohibiting youth gambling on regulated activities, prevalence studies have indicated that significant proportions of adolescents engage in gambling activities (1–6). Recently, results from two national surveys of gambling and alcohol use were combined to identify patterns of U.S. gambling and alcohol use across the lifespan. Results indicate that gambling, frequent gambling and problem gambling rates increase in frequency during adolescence, reaching their peak in an individual's 20s and 30s and then dropping off among those over 70 years (7).

High rates of gambling and problem gambling among youth and young adults highlight the necessity of identifying the factors that influence the development and/or maintenance of gambling. Of parallel importance, understanding differences in patterns of play allows for a deeper understanding of varying degrees of gambling participation and can inform the measurement of gambling behaviors and gambling severity. Though past studies have examined the prevalence of continuous or pathological gambling and its associated risk factors, virtually no studies have investigated the prevalence of episodic or "binge" gambling. This chapter is devoted to better understanding of the concept of binge behavior as it applies to gambling by presenting data collected on college students in Quebec, Canada, and by drawing parallels with the alcohol literature. Questions currently being asked in the field of gambling research are: Do young adolescents/young adults engage in binge gambling? What defines a binge episode? Does the presence of binge gambling affect prevalence rates of pathological gambling?

There is a growing need to examine and respond to the presence of risk and multiple risk behaviors in adolescents from prevention and public health perspectives.

Understanding the concept and experience of binge gambling and its relationship to other addictive behaviors will help inform policy and prevention initiatives by assisting in the design and implementation of targeted screening and interventions. Moreover, elucidation of the binge concept will further clarify potential disparities among subgroups of gamblers, namely those who binge with and without meeting traditional diagnostic criteria for gambling pathology. Differences among subgroups have clear implications for the content and marketing of prevention materials and the refinement of treatment strategies. Specifically, the co-occurrence of risk behaviors highlights the multidimensional nature of youth risk taking, thereby increasing the need for treatment strategies that account for the variability in at-risk groups. Overall, delineating the characteristics and prevalence of subpopulations of gamblers will better equip front-line workers and mental health professionals to identify youth who may be at risk for developing gambling problems and/or who may engage in binge behaviors.

The current chapter addresses the issues of screening and understanding binge gambling behavior among older adolescents and young adults and further explores the relationship of binge gambling to binge drinking and alcohol abuse disorders. A subgoal of the present study was to closely examine gender similarities and differences in regard to binge behavior.

5.2 Background

Though there is still controversy around the issue of problem/pathological gambling being an addictive behavior, a problem of cognitive distortion, or an impulse control disorder, an increasing number of researchers categorize pathological gambling as an addictive behavior comparable to chemical addictions and other behavioral addictions such as binge eating and sex addiction (8). Along the same lines of thought, because binge patterns are evident among other addictive behaviors, it likely occurs among those who gamble. There is currently sufficient reason to believe that gambling shares a relationship with binge patterns of involvement. For example, problem gambling has been associated with binge eating in a university sample (9).

According to our current conceptualization, the DSM-IV identifies pathological gambling as a disorder of impulse control that is generally characterized by a loss of control over gambling activities and a preoccupation with gambling that typically results in multiple harmful negative consequences for the individual (10). Although gambling urges may vary by intensity and duration, they are nevertheless assumed to be continuous. Conceptually, clinical and empirical research suggests that the development of pathological gambling is unremitting in nature and progressive in course, following a sequential path from early wins to devastating losses (11–13). In other words, it is assumed that problem gamblers are constantly moving along a continuum of behavioral severity.

This focus on progressive continuity has, in turn, shaped measurement of the disorder. The gambling assessment tools currently utilized screen for symptoms of impaired control and adverse behavioral consequences over a specific time frame – lifetime, past year, or past month prior to assessment. Consequently, these instruments focus on the presence of specific symptoms over time without identifying the specific duration, frequency, or intensity of those symptoms (13, 14). The omission of criteria to pinpoint the timeframe within which loss of control over gambling occurs is suspected of diminishing the ability of clinicians and researchers to determine the exact nature and progression of particular gambling behaviors. Moreover, the absence of specific items to assess the temporal features of gambling episodes within conventional screening instruments may increase the degree of overestimation for the prevalence of particular risk-taking behavior problems, which is typical of many self-report psychometric tools (15).

In contrast to traditional conceptualizations, Nower and Blaszczynski (13) have hypothesized the existence of a unique typology of gambler who clearly differs from others in the problem or pathological categories. They hypothesized this subpopulation of "binge gamblers" to participate in intermittent bouts of severe dyscontrol and excessive gambling coupled with intervening periods of abstinence characterized by an absence of persistent preoccupations and urges. Furthermore, these gamblers are presumed to experience rapid escalations of intense uncontrolled gambling binges that may result in important psychosocial consequences.

Several researchers support this notion of an alternative pattern for the emergence and progression of problem gambling. For instance, Rosenthal (16) and Shaffer and Hall (4) suggest that in selected cases, problem gambling may manifest itself as acute and transitory rather than chronic and enduring. Related to the idea of problem gambling as a transitory behavior, there has been speculation concerning screening outcomes. Though binge gamblers may meet diagnostic criteria if screened during a binge episode, they are likely to elude classification by traditional measures at other occasions because of the absence of significant symptoms during intervening periods of abstinence (13). Similarly, it may be the case that people having experienced a small number of binge episodes may meet diagnostic criteria during play periods when they should not, due to an ability to control their gambling behaviors between episodes. Both of the above outcomes highlight the importance of distinguishing patterns of gambling behavior, as it is unclear when binge gambling should be considered as undoubtedly distinct from pathological gambling, and when it should be considered a pattern of gambling play among pathological gamblers. Therefore, correct classification of these individuals will require evaluation of symptoms with respect to frequency, severity, and duration of occurrence in order to differentiate acute gambling episodes from chronic, progressive patterns of play.

Problem gambling, binge eating, and problem drinking have been previously linked to an underlying impulsivity trait (17, 18) although not always (19). Inconsistency in the link is probably due to different definitions and measurements of impulsivity (20, 21), but may also be due to how problem gambling is measured as well. Binge gambling may share a different relationship with impulsivity than does pathological gambling. When one measures problem gambling, it is possible that binge gamblers are being included, thus possibly dissolving the relationship between pathological gambling and impulsivity. Furthermore, broad impulsivity measures can lead to inaccurate results, with different impulsivity-related constructs surfacing as significant factors in different addictive behaviors (21).

Another factor that may link behaviors that are prone to addiction or binging patterns is one's coping style. Problem drinking, binge eating, and problem gambling have all been linked to attempts to alleviate stress and negative affect (22–24), linking back to Bandura's early work in social learning theory (25).

Binge gambling may be conceptualized in light of other binge behaviors such as substance abuse (26) and eating disorders (27, 28). Like gambling, periods of excessive abuse of alcohol and food involves a loss of control, preoccupation, escape, denial, secrecy, and persistence despite adverse consequences. There are, however, noticeable differences between these binge behaviors such that gambling can continue indefinitely without physical limitation, whereas it is not the case for eating and drinking alcohol (13). Specifically, food and alcohol are readily quantifiable, measured in terms of physical factors such as organ capacity, weight, and metabolic rate, and are therefore subject to physical limitation. In contrast, money spent gambling is highly individual, related to the gambler's income and access to money, and is limited by few external controls aside from time, fatigue, and lack of funds (13). As such, correctly identifying binge behavior will need to take into account numerous factors that diverge from those utilized in substance abuse and eating disorders.

At present, there are no known studies of binge gambling among adolescents or adults. Nower and Blaszczynski (13) were the first to explore the concept in a theoretical examination of the issue with two case histories. They hypothesized that gambling binges are characterized by six factors including: (a) the sudden onset of irregular or intermittent periods of sustained gambling; (b) involvement of excessive expenditures relative to income; (c) rapid spending over a discrete interval of time; (d) an accompanying a sense of urgency and impaired control; (e) result of marked intra- and interpersonal distress; and (f) the absence between bouts of any rumination, preoccupation, or cravings to resume participation in gambling. Although these defining characteristics make intuitive logical sense, they remain to be examined and established empirically.

Some of the characteristics proposed by Nower and Blaszczynski (13) as pertaining to binge gambling are not completely consistent with the literature on binge drinking. They perceive gambling binge episodes to be triggered by urges to gamble whereas binge drinking is more often engaged in as a result of planned activity (29). The issues of intensity, urgency, and impaired control are also not completely consistent with binge drinking literature, such that binge drinking, by definition only relates to the number of drinks consumed in one sitting; this amount being easily reached without the implication of intensity, urgency, or impaired control. Rather, binge drinking appears to present itself as planned behavior, with a clear beginning and end, that is engaged in for both social and environmental reasons (30–32). The issue of impaired control is more one that is reserved for alcohol dependency. In challenging propositions set by Nower and Blaszczynski (13), it is possible that a similar distinction applies to binge gambling and pathological gambling, such that impaired control and urgencies are not part of the defining criteria.

Regardless, one cannot argue that binge behaviors are necessarily harmless. Research into other binge behaviors suggests that binging is associated with increased pathology and adverse outcomes. For instance, binge drinking and substance abuse have been found to correlate with risky sexual behavior (33, 34) and to predict later substance use and dependence (35, 36). This has particularly significant implications for adolescents and young adults given that much mental health research has established that adolescent behavioral patterns often set the stage for adult maladaptive behaviors (37).

Therefore, the study of binge episodes is timely, important, and central to the goal of reducing harm associated with gambling involvement.

5.3 Context

A pilot project was conducted in 2009, whereby focus groups were conducted and six-item binge screen, developed by Nower and Blaszczynski (13), was administered to students at the high school level. Based on the findings of the 2009 project, a modified binge gambling screen was proposed. We recommended that the proposed six questions be reduced to four (Part A). In addition, questions 2–4 are only to be analyzed among those who endorsed question 1, because they are by their very nature conditional to answering yes to that question. We also recommended that a secondary set of questions (Part B) aimed at better understanding and defining the construct of binge gambling. Thus, the new questionnaire is composed of Part A and Part B (see Appendix A).

Because the first question pertains to experiencing a gambling episode with a clear beginning and end, endorsement of this question is an endorsement of having experienced at least one defined sustained period of time where gambling behavior was present. For simplicity, we are referring to these people who endorsed this question as our *potential binge gamblers*, as it represents the minimum necessary criteria from which we can build a definition of binge.

5.4 Our pilot study

The total sample includes 1,254 participants (507 males; 747 females), ranging in age from 17 to 23 (mean age 18.69). Respondents were asked to indicate their primary language spoken at home, with approximately 20% indicating French, 18% indicating English, 20% indicating Italian, and the remaining 40% indicating a blend of the three listed above or another language such as Portuguese, Russian, Chinese, or Tamil. With respect to household income levels, 27% reported income levels below $50,000 annually, with 73% indicating household income at $50,000 or more.

5.4.1 Instruments

Gambling Activities Questionnaire-Adapted (GAQ) (38). The GAQ is divided into four general domains related to gambling behavior. For this study, an adapted version of the GAQ was employed that focused on descriptive information of preferred types of gambling. Respondents were asked about their frequency of participation ("daily," "at least once a week," "at least once a month," "less than once a month," and "not at all") among different gambling activities.

DSM-IV-MR-J (14). This revised version of the DSM-IV-J provides an assessment of problem gambling among adolescents. It contains twelve questions, forming nine categories, and is designed specifically for use with individuals under the age of 18 years. Endorsement of ≥ 4 out of the 9 categories on the scale indicates a Probable Pathological Gambler (PPG), a score of 2 or 3 indicates an At-Risk Gambler, and a score of 0 or 1 indicates a Social Gambler.

DSM-IV-TR Pathological Gambling Criteria (10). This instrument has ten questions that query the presence of various symptoms of pathological gambling, including preoccupation with gambling, need to increase bet to achieve the same level of excitement (tolerance), loss of control, withdrawal symptoms, escape, chasing of losses, lying to family, illegal activities to pay for gambling, disruptions to family or job, and borrowing money to pay for gambling debts. Standard cut-off scores for problem gambling categorization were used to form three DSM categories of problem gambling that correspond to those of DSM-IV-MR-J. Participants who report five symptoms or more are categorized as PPGs, those who endorse three or four symptoms are categorized as At-Risk Gamblers, and those who report two symptoms or fewer are categorized as Social Gamblers.

Modified binge gambling screen. This screen consists of seven questions, four in Part A (yes/no format) and three in Part B (multiple choices). This screen is a modification of the original binge gambling screen (13) developed by Nower and Blaszczynski and is found in Appendix A.

Binge drinking screen: This consists of two questions, tapping into the occurrence of having consumed at least four or five alcoholic drinks in one sitting over the previous two week period of time. Females who indicated consuming four or more drinks in one sitting met the criteria for binge drinking, whereas males had to indicate five or more drinks to meet binge drinking criteria (32).

AUDIT: Alcohol Use Disorders Identification Test (AUDIT) (39). The AUDIT is a ten-item self-administered screening instrument designed to detect hazardous (score greater than or equal to 8) and harmful (score greater than or equal to 10) alcohol consumption over the previous year. Responses for each item are scored 0–4, with a maximum score of 40. The AUDIT is widely accepted and has been used in numerous alcohol use prevalence studies as it demonstrates sensitivities and specificities comparable, and typically superior, to those of other self-report screening measures. Test-retest reliability and internal consistency are good (40).

5.4.2 Data collection procedure

McGill University Ethics approval was obtained, and parental consent was obtained for all students under the age of 18. All participants were required to give personal consent as well, and were informed that they could withdraw from participating at any time. All participants were students attending one of six CEGEPs (equivalent to grades 12 and 13) in the greater Montreal area, and completed the questionnaire in their classrooms during class time. A research assistant was present at all times to respond to any questions.

5.5 Our findings

5.5.1 Gambling participation and classification

A large majority of the sample (98%) reported gambling within the previous 12 months; 734 females (59.7%) and 495 males (40.3%). Twelve types of gambling activities were listed in the questionnaire, along with an "other" category, and respondents indicated their frequency of participation (within the previous 12 months) by indicating *never, less than once a month, 1–3 times a month, 1–6 times a week,* or *daily* for each. Respondents who indicated *never* to all of the gambling activities were considered nongamblers. Anyone who indicated anything other than *never* to any of the activities was considered to have gambled in the previous 12 months and they were referred to as gamblers.

With respect to gambling severity, the rates of problem gambling among this sample are very low. Ninety-six percent of the total sample are considered to be social gamblers. This means that they endorse zero or one item on the DSM gambling screen. At-risk gamblers, defined as endorsing two or three items on the DSM, represent 3.3% of the total sample. Probable pathological gamblers, endorsing four or more items on the DSM gambling screen, are represented by less than 1% of the sample (.7%).

Problem gamblers are mostly represented by males, with 29 out of the 41 at-risk gamblers being male, and 7 out of the 9 PPGs being males.

The total sample from which we can run data on the question of binge gambling is 1162, as 92 people did not complete the binge questions on the questionnaire. In this sample, 191 (16.4%) endorsed question 1, while 971 (83.6%) did not.

5.5.2 Part A: Analysis of usefulness of questions

Part A, Question 1: I have episodes of gambling, over a sustained period of time, that seem to have a clear beginning and end

Among the sample of gamblers 16.4% (191/1162) responded positively to this question. In examining rates of endorsement of question 1 by classification of gambler, the distribution is reflective of the sample, such that 82% are social gamblers, 14% are at-risk gamblers, and 3.7% are PPGs. Therefore, all classifications of gamblers are represented among those who endorsed this question whereby they have some period of time where gambling is present, with a clear beginning and end.

However, to better understand how the notion of binge gambling applies to problem gambling, an examination of those who endorsed question 1 within each gambler subtype indicates that 22.4% of social gamblers, 69.2% of at-risk gamblers, and 77.8% of PPG's did so. The results suggest gambling severity is positively correlated with the occurrence of experiencing gambling episodes that have a clear beginning and end.

The following three questions in Part A are analyzed out of a total sample of 191 participants, as they were only relevant to individuals who endorsed question 1. This subgroup will be referred to as potential binge gamblers (see ▶Tab. 5.1).

Part A, Question 2: These gambling episodes begin with a sudden uncontrollable urge to gamble

With regard to question 2, the majority of potential binge gamblers (83%) did *not* report that their episodes begin with a sudden uncontrollable urge, suggesting that the criteria of binge gambling needing to begin with sudden urges is not a necessary prerequisite. It is highly plausible that gambling binges start with simple planned gambling opportunities such as a poker tournament, sports betting, or an occasional end-of-week trip to a casino among friends.

The issue of uncontrollable urges, or loss of control, is one that likely pertains to individuals experiencing gambling-related problems. In fact, only 10.3% of social gamblers endorsed this question, whereas 44.4% of at-risk, and 57% of PPGs indicated that their gambling episodes were launched by an uncontrollable urge. As such, it appears

Tab. 5.1: Endorsement of questions 2–4 by gambler subtype.

Part A	Social gambler (n = 155)	At-risk gambler (n = 27)	PPG Gambler (n = 7)	Total (n = 189)
Question 2	10.3% (16)	44.4% (12)	57.1% (4)	16.9% (32)
Question 3	28.6% (44)	66.7% (18)	71.4% (5)	35.6% (67)
Question 4	57.2% (87)	57.7% (15)	57.1% (4)	57.3% (106)

as though the issue of uncontrollable urges triggering gambling episodes can serve as a factor that distinguishes between binge gambling and problem gambling.

Part A, Question 3: These gambling episodes are best described by an increase in frequency and intensity of play

Approximately a third of the sample of potential bingers (35.6%) report that their gambling episodes are best described by an increase in frequency and intensity of play. It is possible that this subset represent the *true* binge gamblers, as the notion of binge usually implies an increase in frequency and/or intensity of an activity.

If we examine this issue of increased frequency and intensity as it relates to gambling severity, 29% of social gamblers, 67% of at-risk gamblers, and 71% of PPG gamblers endorse this construct. Though the overall sample size of problem gamblers is small, they do suggest that this notion of increased intensity and frequency applies to all potential bingers, and increases in a linear fashion as problem gambling severity increases.

Part A, Question 4: Between episodes, I do NOT have a persistent urge to resume gambling

The issue of not experiencing gambling urges between episodes is divided among the sample of potential binge gamblers. Slightly more than half (106/189) endorse this as being an adequate descriptor, whereas 43% do not.

An examination of this construct among gamblers with varying degrees of gambling severity does not reveal any meaningful relationship with gambling severity. Overall, 57% of social gamblers, 57% of at-risk gamblers, and 57% of PPG gamblers endorse this question. Therefore, it is difficult to determine whether this question was properly understood by respondents, as it may be confusing due to its focus on the lack of symptoms (I do NOT have a persistent urge).

5.5.3 Part A: Scale reliability

A Cronbach's Alpha of .547 (see ▶Tab. 5.2) suggests the scale is not very reliable. An examination of the inter-item correlation matrix reveals overall poor correlations with question 4 (coefficients ranging from .10 to .18), further supporting the idea that question 4 was not properly understood by respondents.

Factor analysis confirms the overall lack of cohesiveness of the scale. It is interesting to note that question 1 accounts for almost half the variance (see ▶Tab. 5.3).

The scale reliability of Part A is improved by removing question 4, the Cronbach's alpha increasing to .634 (▶Tab. 5.4.). Below are the results of the factor analysis run

Tab. 5.2: Reliability statistics for Part A, 4 question scale.

Reliability Statistics		
Cronbach's Alpha	Cronbach's Alpha Based on Standardized Items	N of Items
.547	.616	4

Tab. 5.3: Factor analysis results for Part A, 4 questions.

Factor Analysis			
Question #	Communalities	Eigenvalues	% of variance
1	.487	1.9	47.7
2	.547	.94	23.4
3	.696	.72	17.9
4	.180	.44	10.9

Tab. 5.4: Factor analysis results for Part A, question 4 removed.

Question #	Communalities	Eigenvalues	% of variance
1	.479	1.8	60.8
2	.608	.74	24.8
3	.737	.43	14.4

with the first three questions only. Question 1 accounts for approximately 61% of the variance, suggesting its usefulness. It should be noted that because question 2 was only endorsed by a small percentage of potential binge gamblers, a non-endorsement of the construct is most informative to the definition of binge gambling.

To summarize, the three remaining questions in Part A can serve as a quick binge gambling screen, thereby assessing three defining characteristics: (a) a clear gambling episode, (b) which begins with a planned activity, and (c) is characterized by an increase in frequency and intensity (see Appendix B).

5.5.4 Part B: Qualitative descriptors of binge gambling

Part B was developed in order to assist in the conceptualization and definition of binge gambling behavior. The three questions were designed to provide more detailed qualitative information on the nature of the episode(s) endorsed in part A; In particular, the reasons underlying why binges end, the length of each episode, and the period of time between episodes. Depending on the question, 10 or 11 respondents did not respond, resulting in a reduced sample of 180 participants for questions 1 and 2, and 179 for question 3.

5.5.5 Reasons why binges end

The two most endorsed reasons for why episodes come to an end were due to decreased urges, or a recognition that the gambling was becoming too risky (34.4% and 35.9% respectively). Other reasons included the ending of the gambling opportunity (18.2%) and the depletion of funds (11.6%). Given that they were not highly endorsed, they might not serve as adequate defining qualities (▶Tab. 5.5).

Keeping in mind that binge behavior might present differently for males and females, these questions were also examined for each gender. Gender distinctions were found such that females are more likely to stop gambling due to a reduction of urges (46% females, 28% males), whereas males were more likely to stop as a result of feeling the risks they were incurring were getting too high (40% males, 28% females).

An examination of why binges come to an end for individuals falling into the different gambling categories highlights meaningful differences between the three gambling groups. While social gamblers end their gambling episodes primarily due to decreased urges, at-risk gamblers are less likely to endorse decreasing urges as a reason, and PPGs do not endorse that reason at all. Furthermore, as gambling problem severity increases, so does the percentage of individuals endorsing either ending their gambling episode as a result of a lack of funds or as a result of the high level of risk they are incurring.

5.5.6 Episode duration

Overall, the majority of respondents indicated that their episodes lasted for a period of 3 days or less (79%), with an additional 14.4% endorsing a period of time lasting between 3 days and 2 weeks. Negligible amounts of respondents indicated lengths of time longer than 2 weeks (6.7%). Had we included a window of time slightly larger than 3 days (i.e, 5 days or a week) we may have captured up to 85% of responses. An examination of response patterns among males and females suggests that females are slightly more likely to end their episodes within the 3-day window (87% females, 75% males).

An examination of this construct among social gamblers, at-risk gamblers, and PPGs reveals an important distinction. The vast majority of social gamblers, 81%, indicate

Tab. 5.5: Reasons why binges end.

	Reasons Binges End			
	Social gamblers (n = 148)	At-Risk (n = 26)	PPG (n = 7)	Total (n = 181)
Decreased urge	38.5% (57)	19.2% (5)	0	34.3% (62)
Opportunity ends	18.2% (27)	23.1% (6)	0	18.2% (40)
Depleted funds	9.5% (14)	15.4% (4)	42.9% (3)	11.6% (24)
Too risky	33.8% (50)	42.3% (11)	57.1% (4)	35.9% (81)

their gambling episodes last less than 3 days. Though still a highly endorsed period of time among at-risk and PPGs, the percentages of those endorsing this small time frame decreases as the severity of gambling increases. Furthermore, they are more likely than social gamblers to indicate a larger time frame of gambling episode duration, with up to 14% of PPGs indicating times frames greater than a month (see ▶Tab. 5.6).

5.5.7 Length of time between episodes

Slightly more than half of the sample indicated at least one month between gambling episodes (56.4%), with another 22% endorsing a period of time lasting from a week to a month. Together, these categories capture over 75% of the responses. It should be noted that very few participants endorsed the option "a few days to a week," likely due to the fact that "a few days" is not concretely defined, thus making it difficult to differentiate a few days from a week. In hindsight and with respect to endorsement rates, it appears the wording was difficult for respondents to relate to (see ▶Tab. 5.7).

With respect to gender differences, females were more likely to endorse a period of time greater than a month than males (70.5% females, 49% males), whereas males were more inclined to indicate slightly shorter amounts of time between episodes (26% of males vs. 13 % of females indicating a week to a month).

The length of time between episodes is longer among those not experiencing gambling-related problems, with 62% of social gamblers indicating time frames greater than a month. At-risk gamblers were more likely to indicate a window of time varying from

Tab. 5.6: Duration of gambling episodes.

	Episode Duration			
	Social gamblers (n = 148)	At-Risk (n = 26)	PPG (n = 7)	Total (n = 181)
< 3 days	85.1% (126)	53.8% (14)	42.9% (3)	79% (143)
3 days–2 weeks	10.8% (16)	26.9% (7)	42.9% (3)	14.4% (26)
2 weeks–1 month	.7% (1)	7.7% (2)	0	1.7% (3)
> 1 month	3.4% (5)	11.5% (3)	14.3% (1)	5% (9)

Tab. 5.7: Length of time between episodes.

	Time Frame between Episodes			
	Social gamblers (n = 146)	At-Risk (n = 26)	PPG (n = 7)	Total (n = 179)
Few days	17.1% (25)	7.7% (2)	42.9% (3)	16.8% (30)
Few days–1 week	3.4% (5)	15.4% (4)	0	5% (9)
1 week–1 month	17.1% (25)	46.2% (12)	26.8% (2)	21.8% (39)
> month	62.3% (91)	30.8% (8)	26.8% (2)	56.4% (101)

one week to one month (46%), whereas PPGs were more inclined to indicate a shorter period of time of "a few days."

5.6 Prevalence of binge gambling

The preliminary study conducted in 2009 and the current results suggest that there are varying degrees of binge gambling. In the current sample, 191 individuals endorsed the first question on the binge screen, thus reporting gambling in episodes that have a clear beginning and end. This represents 15% of the total sample, and encompasses both light and heavy binge gamblers. One hundred of those bingers only endorsed the first question and not the other two (we are not taking into consideration that 4th question that was deemed problematic), so it can be argued that 8% of the total sample are light binge gamblers. If we apply stricter criteria whereby all three questions from Part A of the gambling screen are endorsed, 91 individuals, or 7% of the total sample, met the criteria for heavy binge gambling.

5.7 Relationship of binge gambling to binge drinking and heavy alcohol use

Binge drinking is defined in this sample as having consumed five or more drinks in one sitting in the previous two weeks for males, and four or more drinks in one sitting in the previous two weeks for females. In total, 40.8% of the sample reported at least one binge drinking episode in the previous two-week time frame. Binge drinking was slightly more prevalent among males, with 47.3% of males and 36.5% of females reporting the behavior among this college-age sample.

The relationship between binge gambling and binge drinking is evident, with 55% of binge gamblers also being identified as binge drinkers. This trend is more pronounced among males, with 67% of binge gamblers also reporting binge drinking. For females, 35% of those who report binge gambling also report binge drinking.

Among binge drinkers, 26% also report binge gambling. Therefore, from both perspectives, the occurrence of one form of binge behavior increases the likelihood of the other by approximately 10%.

Problem drinking, as assessed with the AUDIT (a score of 10 or more), yielded a similar pattern of results. Of the total sample, 27% met the criteria for problem drinking, with males slightly more represented than females (31% vs. 24%). Not surprisingly, problem drinking shares a stronger relationship with heavy binge gambling than with light binge gambling. Of those who endorse all three binge questions, 47.3% meet the criteria for problem drinking, compared to 28% of those who endorsed the first binge question but not all three.

Interesting gender differences surfaced, such that females who were heavy binge gamblers were more likely to experience problems with alcohol use as compared to males. Specifically, female heavy bingers were 1.93 times more likely to be heavy drinkers, whereas male heavy bingers were .65 times more likely to be heavy drinkers. It therefore appears that heavy binge gambling might represent a risk factors for females more than for males.

5.8 Toward building a construct of binge gambling

The results of the 2009 study and the current study support the idea that a meaningful percentage of the young adult population gamble in a defined period of time that has a clear beginning and end (16%). The idea put forth in the previous research, that binge gambling itself falls on a continuum, seems to be supported with the current data, such that a meaningful subset also report increased frequency and intensity of play during these episodes. Consistent with previous findings, these binge gambling episodes occur among social gamblers, or those who do not report significant gambling-related issues. Though binge patterns of gambling are also present among at-risk and PPG gamblers, they tend to take on a more intense quality, happen more frequently, and last longer.

Binge gambling, unlike binge drinking, is very difficult to define concretely. Binge drinking is defined as consuming five or more alcoholic drinks within one sitting. However, gambling behavior is not as quantifiable as to be able to define it as a number of hands played (primarily due to the fact that there are so many types of gambling activities with such varying lengths of time that "one game" can occur within) or amount wagered. A such, it is necessary to attempt a definition leaning more toward the occurrence of gambling episodes, the quality of the play within those episodes, approximate length of episodes, and reasons for engaging in these episodes.

Among social gamblers, it could be stated that gambling episodes are defined as being periods of time where gambling behavior started out as a planned activity and is sustained for a few days. These episodes typically end as a result of reduced urges or reduced desire to play, or because risks are too high. Periods of times between episodes are usually longer than a month. Males are more likely to end binges due to their perceptions that the risks of continuing are too high.

Arguably, gambling episodes among most of the PPGs in the current sample are better described as being part of the addiction cycle as opposed to binge gambling, given that they are more likely to start gambling as a result of uncontrollable urges, less likely to stop as a result of decreased urges, more likely to gamble until their funds are depleted, and more likely to endorse very short intervals of time between gambling episodes. Following this line of logic, only two or three individuals categorized as PPGs might have been falsely identified, and would better fit the criteria of binge gamblers due to the fact that their patterns of play and qualitative descriptors of their gambling episodes more resemble those of binge gamblers (i.e., not triggered by uncontrollable urges, short duration of episode, longer periods of time between episodes). The implication is that traditional screening instruments might be inaccurately (falsely) classifying people as being pathological gamblers when in fact they may be binge gamblers who have also experienced negative consequences as a result of their binge style of play. The difference between the two categorizations is one of impaired control, a construct not present in the current diagnostic criteria of pathological gambling.

5.9 Discussion

Although most individuals gamble without meeting the DSM-IV criteria for pathological gambling, many will experience significant problems related to binge gambling that remain unidentified. As such, the integration of a binge gambling screen within a diagnostic screen might prove to be clinically useful. The need for a different set of guidelines to identify binge gamblers and differentiate them from chronic pathological gamblers is becoming apparent. Such a process would allow for the development of appropriate strategies addressing binge gambling. In a similar way, many binge drinkers would never be categorized as having an alcohol use disorder according to DSM criteria and, at the very least, identifying binge drinking as a problem at a societal level has led to the development of several useful strategies for preventing and remediating binge drinking in particular (26).

Binge gambling remains of concern as this behavior also has the potential to result in severe psychosocial difficulties but likely remains undetected in individuals who do not fit the traditional criteria of a problem or pathological gambler. Future research examining the relationship between binge gambling and other psychosocial problems would be very informative. Reasons why individuals engage in binge gambling (i.e., to escape boredom, to relieve stress, as a social facilitator), and the risk factors that would result in binge gamblers progressing to pathological gamblers (i.e., impulsivity, poor coping skills, poor social skills) remain to be explored and better understood.

Urgency and lack of planning are also variables associated with behavioral addictions (41–43) but may not be applicable to binge gambling, with current results suggesting that binge gambling occurs as a result of planned behavior, or at minimum, not engaged in as a result of strong urges to gamble. This issue of why gambling is engaged in might be a major factor that differentiates pathological gamblers from binge gamblers.

An interesting finding, in line with research on binge drinking, was that gambling episodes did not appear to be triggered by uncontrollable urges, as was previously hypothesized by Nower and Blaszczynski (13). Instead, it appears that such activities are social in nature and planned ahead of time, but this assumption needs to be examined in future research on binge gambling. The Theory of Planned Behavior (TPB) was developed to explain the motivational determinants of behavior (44) and has been found useful in explaining binge drinking (29). This model postulates that the primary determinants of future behavior are one's intention to perform the behavior. A person's intentions are a function of three variables: attitudes, subjective norms, and perceived behavioral control (i.e., I want to gamble, it's a very enjoyable thing for me to do, and I have a plan on how I will do it). Johnston and White (45) found that intention actually explained 51% of the variance in binge drinking behavior. Furthermore, the perception of the drinking behaviors of one's peers appears to have a significant influence on drinking and binge drinking behavior (30, 31).

Anticipated regret is a variable that has also surfaced as a significant predictor of binge-drinking behavior (46). Cook et al. proposed an extension to the Theory of Planned Behavior, such that anticipation of negative consequences of binge drinking would influence the decision to perform the behavior. They reported that anticipated regret mediated the relationship between past binge-drinking behavior and intentions to binge drink in the future, and suggest that although past involvement in binge drinking and intentions predicts behavior, regret is a more important variable for binge-drinking intentions. If applicable to binge gambling, programs designed to foster anticipated regret could be beneficial to the gambling prevention arena and research is warranted to explore this possibility.

Binge drinking has been positively associated with easy access and opportunity. Students exposed to "wet" environments (drinking is prevalent, alcohol is cheap and easily accessible) were more likely to engage in binge drinking than those not exposed to such environments (32). One can extrapolate that with the proliferation and high accessibility of gambling (i.e., Internet gambling, sports pools, poker tournaments) and the ability to play at small stakes, the occurrence of binge gambling is to be expected as well. From a perspective of prevention, curtailing access to gambling, especially low stakes gambling, could prove beneficial. Though logical, such an approach is quite challenging to execute due to online access of gambling venues. Nonetheless, colleges and universities can and should adopt policies that limit gambling activities on their campuses. Furthermore, because binge gambling and binge/problem drinking share a relationship with one another, limiting access to one might in turn benefit a reduction in the other.

The current results identify gender trends, with males more likely to engage in binge gambling. Nonetheless, a significant percentage of females report engaging in binge patterns of play as well, and it is not known at this time if this set of females represents a group that is at heightened risk for other high-risk behaviors or behavioral addictions, although preliminary indications point to increased probability of being a problem drinker. Within the alcohol research, at-risk profiles differed for males and females in a university-based study, whereby binge drinking and other psychosocial correlates surfaced as risk factors for females only, arguing for gender-based prevention interventions (47).

Clearly, some individuals report engaging in binge-like gambling behavior but future research needs to clarify whether this behavior should necessarily be considered problematic. Binge behaviors were endorsed by both social and problem gamblers; thus a key first step in future research would be to determine if there are any particular qualities or characteristics inherent to binge behavior that are unique to gamblers falling within different categories of gambling severity. It may simply be that a higher number of endorsed binge behaviors differentiate pathological gamblers. Based upon the planned nature of the gambling episodes, the current data also suggest that positive expectancies may be key in determining the risk of binge gambling.

As shown in the current research, some criteria of binge gambling are regularly endorsed by pathological gamblers. This convergence inevitably makes it more difficult to generate a measure for reliably distinguishing binge gamblers from pathological gamblers. Gambling may be viewed as falling on two dimensions: "non-problem – problem" and "non-binging – binging." The problem dimension addresses persistent and recurrent maladaptive gambling behavior whereas the binging dimension addresses brief episodes of gambling. Future studies on binge gambling will benefit from examining individuals who are low on the problem dimension (i.e., nonproblem gamblers) but high on the binging dimension. Once a sufficiently large sample of these "pure" binge gamblers is identified and studied, a more complete profile of a typical binge gambler may be generated. This information would, in turn, aid in the development of assessment and preventive approaches.

Binge gambling has become a topic of concern because this behavior has the potential to result in severe psychosocial difficulties but likely remains undetected in individuals who do not fit the traditional criteria of a problem or pathological gambler. Thus, it will also be important to examine whether more symptoms of binge gambling coincide with other psychosocial problems such as relationship difficulties or missing work. Given that interpersonal, educational, and occupational problems are inherent in the definition of pathological gambling, it would be informative to treatment providers and public policymakers to show that these types of problems can also occur as a result of binge gambling, particularly in a sample of non-pathological gamblers. In order to make this connection, further research needs to establish an association between "pure" binge gambling and secondary problems. Subsequently, longitudinal data may clarify a causal link in which these problems follow the onset of binge gambling.

The current research is intended as a starting point for future research on a relatively new and unexplored topic. As an overarching goal, future research needs to address binge gambling as a unique construct and its associated problems on individual, interpersonal, and societal levels. The inroads achieved through these lines of inquiry will lead to practical treatment and prevention strategies aimed at benefiting individuals who remain misunderstood by current gambling researchers. Furthermore, focusing on binge gambling among adolescents and young adults may ultimately allow for a fuller understanding of the multiple pathways by which pathological gambling develops.

References

1. Adlaf EM, Ialomiteanu A. Prevalence of problem gambling in adolescents: Findings from the 1999 Ontario student drug use survey. Can J Psychiatry 2000;45:752–5.
2. National Research Council. Pathological Gambling: A Critical Review. Washington, DC: National Academy Press; 1999.
3. Jacobs DF, editor. Youth gambling in North America: Long-term trends and future prospects. New York: Kluwer Academic/Plemun; 2004.
4. Shaffer HJ, Hall MN. Estimating the prevalence of adolescent gambling disorders: A quantitative synthesis and guide toward standard gambling nomenclature. J Gambl Stud 1996;12:193–214.
5. Volberg R, Gupta R, Griffiths MD, Olason D, Delfabbro PH. An international perspective on youth gambling prevalence studies. Int J Adolesc Med Health 2010;22:3–38.
6. Gupta R, Derevensky J. Adolescent gambling behavior: A prevalence study and examination of the correlates associated with problem gambling. J Gambl Stu. 1998;14:319–45.
7. Welte JW, Barnes GM, Tidwell M-CO, Hoffman JH. Gambling and problem gambling across the lifespan. J Gambl Stud 2011;27:49–61.
8. Procopio M. Comment/Reply. Can J Psychiatry 2005;50(5):302–3.
9. Engwall D, Hunter R, Steinberg M. Gambling and other risk behaviors on university campuses. J Am Coll Health 2002;52(6).
10. American Psychiatric Association. Diagnostic and statistical manual of mental disorders: DSM-1V-TR (4th Edition). Washington, DC: APA; 2000.
11. Custer RL, Milt H. When lady luck runs out: Help for compulsive gamblers and their families. New York, NY: Warner; 1985.
12. Lesieur HR, Custer RL. Pathological gambling: Roots, phases, and treatments. Ann Am Acad Polit Soc Sci 1984;474:146–56.
13. Nower L, Blaszczynski A. Binge gambling: A neglected concept. Int Gambl Stud 2003;3(1):23–35.
14. Fisher S. Developing the DSM-IV-MR-J criteria to identify adolescent problem gambling in non-clinical populations. J Gambl Stud 2000;16:253–73.
15. Shakeshaft AP, Bowman JA, Sanson-Fisher RW. Comparison of three methods to assess binge consumption; One-week retrospective diary, AUDIT, and quantity/frequency. Subst Abuse 1998;19(4):191–203.

16. Rosenthal R, Lorenz V. The pathological gambler as criminal offender: Comments on evaluation and treatment. Psychiatr Clin North Am 1992;15(3):647–60.
17. Petry N. Substance abuse, pathological gambling, and impulsiveness. Drug Alcohol Depend 2001;63(1):29–38.
18. Grant JE, Kushner MG, Kim S. Pathological gambling and alcohol use disorder. Alcohol Res Health 2002;26:143–50.
19. McDaniel S, Zuckerman M. The relationship of impulsive sensation seeking and gender to interest and participation in gambling activities. Pers Individ Differ 2003;35(6):1385–400.
20. Evenden J. Impulsivity: A discussion of clinical and experimental findings. J Psychopharmacol 1999;13:180–92.
21. Fischer S, Smith G. Binge eating, problem drinking, and pathological gambling: Linking behaviour to shared traits and Social Learning. Pers Individ Differ 2008;44:789–800.
22. Gupta R, Derevensky J. Adolescent gambling behaviour: A prevalence study and examination of the correlates associated with problem gambling. J Gambl Stud 1998;14:319–45.
23. Nower L, Gupta R, Blaszczynski A, Derevensky J. Suicidality and depression among youth gamblers: A preliminary examination of three studies. Int Gambl Stud 2004;4(1):70–80.
24. Stice E. Risk and maintenance factors for eating pathology: A meta-analytic review. Psychol Bull 2002;128:825–48.
25. Bandura A. Principles of behavior modification. New York: Holt Rinehart Winston; 1969.
26. Wechsler H, Wuethrich B. Dying to drink: Confronting binge drinking on college campuses. New York, NY: Rodale; 2002.
27. Fairburn CG, Cooper Z, Doll HA, Norman P, O'Connor ME. The natural course of bulimia nervosa and binge eating disorder in young women. Arch Gen Psychiatry 2000;57:659–65.
28. Castonguay LG, Eldridge KL, Agras WS. Binge eating disorder: Current state and future directions. Clin Psychol Rev 1995;15:865–90.
29. Norman P, Conner M. The theory of planned behavior and binge drinking: Assessing the moderating role of past behaviour within the theory of planned behaviour. Br J Health Psychol 2006;11:55–70.
30. Campo S, Brossard D, Frazer MS, et al. Are social norms campaigns really magic bullets? Assessing the effects of students' misperceptions on drinking behavior. Health Commun 2003;15:481–97.
31. Kuntsche E, Rehm J, Gmel G. Characteristics of binge drinkers in Europe. Soc Sci Med 2004;59:113–27.
32. Weitzman ER, Nelson TF, Wechsler H. Taking up binge drinking in college: The influences of person, social group, and environment. J Adolesc Health 2003;32:26–35.
33. Langer LM, Tubman JG. Risky sexual behavior among sunstance-abusing adolescents: psychosocial and contextual factors. Am J Orthopsychiatr 1997;67:315–22.
34. Martin CS, Kaczynski NA, Maisto SA, Bukstein OM, Moss HB. Patterns of DSM-IV alcohol abuse and dependence symptoms in adolescent drinkers. J Stud Alcohol 1995;56:672–80.
35. Jennison KM. The short-term effects and unintended long-term consequences of binge drinking in college: A 10-year follow-up study. Am J Drug Alcohol Abuse 2004;30:659–84.
36. Yu J, Shacket RW. Alcohol use in high school: Predicting students' alcohol use and alcohol problems in four-year colleges. Am J Drug Alcohol Abuse 2001;27(4):775–93.
37. Resnick MD, Bearman PS, Blum RW, Bauman KE, Harris KM, Jones J, et al. Protecting adolescents from harm. Findings from the National Longitudinal Study on Adolescent Health. JAMA 1997;278(10):823–32.
38. Gupta R, Derevensky J. The relationship between gambling and video-game playing behavior in children and adolescents. J Gambl Stud 1996;12:375–94.
39. Saunders JB, Aasland OG, Babor TF, de la Fuente JR, Grant M. Development of the Alcohol Use Disorders Identification Test (AUDIT): WHO collaborative project on early detection of persons with harmful alcohol consumption-II. Addiction 1993;88:791–804.

40. Reinert DF, Allen JP. The Alcohol Use Disorders Identification Test (AUDIT): A Review of Recent Research. Alcohol Clin Exp Res 2002;26(2):272–9.
41. Fischer S, Smith GT, Anderson KG, Flory K. Expectancies influence the operation of personality and behavior. Psychol Addict Behav 2003;17:108–14.
42. Vitaro F, Brendgen M, Ladouceur R, Tremblay RE. Gambling, delinquency, and drug use during adolescence: Mutual influences and common risk factors. J Gambl Stud 2001;17:171–90.
43. Miller J, Flory K, Lynam D, Leukefeld C. A test of the four-factor model of impulsivity-related traits. Pers Individ Differ 2003;34(8).
44. Ajzen I. The theory of planned behavior. Org Behav Hum Decis Process 1991;50:179–211.
45. Johnston KL, White KM. Binge-drinking: A test of the role of group norms in the theory of planned behaviour. Psychol Health 2003;18(1):63–77.
46. Cooke R, Sniehotta F, Schüz B. Predicting binge-drinking behaviour using and extended TPB: Examining the impact of anticipated regret and descriptive norms. Alcohol Alcohol 2006;42(2):84–91.
47. DeMartini KS, Carey KB. Correlates of AUDIT risk status for male and female college students. J Am Coll Health 2009;58:233–9.

Appendix A Modified binge gambling screen for adolescents and young adults

Section A-Scored items (yes/no format)

*I have episodes of gambling, over a sustained period of time, that seem to have a clear beginning and end

These gambling episodes begin with a sudden uncontrollable urge to gamble

These gambling episodes are best described by an increase in frequency and intensity of play

Between episodes, I do not have a persistent urge to resume gambling.

* *only those indicating "yes" to the first item should be scored on the 3 proceeding items*

Section B-Qualitative information

These gambling episodes usually come to an end because
    There is a decrease in the urge to gamble
    The gambling opportunity came to an end
    I ran out of funds
    I realized it was too risky to continue in that fashion

These gambling episodes last for:
    Less than 3 days
    3 days to 2 weeks
    2 weeks to 1 month
    More than a month

The period of time *in between* these gambling episodes usually lasts:
    A few days
    A few days to a week
    A week to a month
    More than a month

Appendix B Quick binge gambling screen (Gupta & Derevensky)

1 I have episodes of gambling that seem to have a clear beginning and end, and last less than 2 weeks
2 These gambling episodes usually start as a result of planned activity
3 These gambling episodes are best described by an increase in frequency and / or intensity of play

   Note: Items 2–3 scored only if question 1 is endorsed

Scoring

Endorsement of question 1 only – mild binge gambling

Endorsement of 1, 2, and 3 – heavy binge gambler

Endorsement of 1 and 3 only (not 2) – should screen for problem / pathological gambling as gambling likely the result of a persistent gambling problem as opposed to binge behavior.

6 Positive youth development and intention to gamble

Daniel T. L. Shek and Cecilia M. S. Ma

This chapter explores the relationships between different aspects of positive youth development and intention to gamble among Chinese adolescents in Hong Kong based on six waves of longitudinal data over three years. Correlation analyses showed that a higher level of positive youth development was concurrently and longitudinally related to a lower level of behavioral intention to engage in gambling. Regarding predictors of adolescent intention to gamble, resilience, recognition for positive behavior, emotional competence, moral competence, prosocial attributes, and general positive youth development qualities negatively predicted intention to gamble, whereas social competence, self-determination, and positive identity positively predicted behavioral intention to gamble over time. The theoretical and practical implications of the findings are discussed.

6.1 Introduction

Gambling refers to "an activity that implies an element of risk, and that money, or something of sentimental or monetary value, could be won or lost by the participants" (p. 57, 1). Compared to other forms of adolescent risk behavior such as substance abuse, youth gambling is a relatively new research topic. Based on an extensive literature review, no articles in relation to adolescent gambling were found before 1985 (2). The paucity of this research area might be the result of invisible signs of addiction that makes it difficult to measure (3) and also the misconceptions as portrayed by the mass media (4, 5). Against this background, Derevensky, Shek, and Merrick (6) argued that there is a strong need to conduct more studies on adolescent gambling in different places throughout the world.

In Hong Kong, gambling venues and activities are restricted to adults aged 18 years or older. Recent surveys reveal that the most popular gambling activities in Hong Kong were Mark Six lottery, social gambling, horse racing, and football betting (7, 8). Although these activities were slightly different from those found in Western countries (9–11), researchers noted that the findings in this area might vary across cultural contexts (12, 13). In Chinese society, gambling activities are generally considered as a form of recreation and perceived as social gathering, such as dice games or playing mahjong and card games with friends or family members (8). Furthermore, people perceive problem gambling as prevalent only in adults, and pathological gambling is not normally considered as a psychiatric illness in Chinese society (14).

Based on the data from a sample of 2,088 Hong Kong people aged at 15 years or above, about 71% engaged in gambling in the past year, and over 30% took part in social gambling (8). About 34% of them reported that their onset age of gambling participation was before 18 years old (8), and often the first time they engaged in gambling activities was at the age of 10 (7). Although the prevalence of gambling is lower than those reported in Western countries (15, 16), these estimates are likely to increase with the continued growth in the accessibility and availability of different forms of gambling activities, such as online gambling and casinos in Macau.

In a recent study conducted among a sample of 4,734 students, about 30% of the students reported that they had engaged in gambling activities at least once in the past months, though only 1% were regarded as "pathological gamblers" based on the DSM-IV-J diagnostic criteria (17). Trends between 2001 and 2005 revealed an increase in the proportion of youth gambling from 78% to 81%. In particular, a sharp rise was found in football betting, from 5% in 2001 to 13% in 2005 (7). Although the proportion of youth gambling is low compared with the findings in Western countries (11,18), this phenomenon deserves our attention as problem gambling has been linked with adverse outcomes such as delinquency, poor academic performance, and high risk for depression and suicide ideation and attempts (3, 9, 19).

More importantly, adult problem gamblers were likely to report their gambling-related problems developed during their adolescence and early adulthood (20). Results showed that early onset of gambling was associated with an increased likelihood of problematic behaviors later in life (21–23). Given the age of onset is a significant risk factor associated with pathological gambling (9), early detection of the signs of problematic gambling and exploration of the determinants of this behavior are necessary.

Though most of the studies have examined the relationships between adolescent pathologies (e.g., mental health problems and delinquency) and problem gambling, there are few studies investigating the relationship between positive youth development and adolescent gambling. Scholars and practitioners advocated the adoption of a "positive youth development" approach to buffer against mental health and the risk of addictive behavior (24–28). In light of the paucity of empirical youth gambling research, more effort in examining possible factors that work against youth problem gambling is warranted (29).

Positive youth development can be defined as the growth, cultivation, and nurturance of developmental assets, abilities, and potentials in adolescents. It attempts to understand adolescents in terms of strengths, instead of problems or risky behaviors (30). There are views arguing that individuals' psychological well-being is likely to be improved by facilitating positive youth development in adolescents because the related qualities can serve as potent protective factors of risky behaviors (31, 32). Catalano and colleagues (33) reviewed 77 programs on positive youth development. The review showed that 25 programs were successful and the following 15 positive youth development constructs were identified in the successful programs. These constructs include promotion of bonding, cultivation of resilience, promotion of social competence, promotion of emotional competence, promotion of cognitive competence, promotion of behavioral competence, promotion of moral competence, cultivation of self-determination, promotion of spirituality, development of self-efficacy, development of a clear and positive identity, promotion of beliefs in the future, provision of recognition for positive behavior, provision of opportunities for prosocial involvement, and fostering prosocial norms. Obviously, it is interesting to ask whether these positive youth developmental qualities are related to adolescent gambling. The general hypothesis derived from the empirical literature is that positive youth development is expected to be negatively related to pathological gambling.

With reference to the Chinese culture, Shek (34) reported findings on the relationship between Chinese positive youth development and adolescent behavioral intention to gamble. Consistent with the general prediction and with the exception of social competence and positive and clear identity, results showed that positive youth development indexed by different indicators was negatively related to adolescent behavioral intention to gamble. As there are mixed findings and the study was based on the four waves of data collected over a period of 2 years (34), it would be helpful if more time points could be included in the analyses. Against this background, the primary goals of the study were a) to examine the relationship between positive youth development constructs and intention to gamble and b) to explore the predictive effect of these positive youth development constructs on behavioral intention to gamble across time.

6.2 Our experience

Our data for this chapter was part of a multi-year positive youth development program. Data were collected at September 2006 (Wave 1), May 2007 (Wave 2), September 2007 (Wave 3), May 2008 (Wave 4), September 2008 (Wave 5), and May 2009 (Wave 6). The majority of missing data were the result of participant absence at the day of data collection rather than attrition from the study. The numbers of collected questionnaires were 7,846 in Wave 1, 7,388 in Wave 2, 6,939 in Wave 3, 6,697 in Wave 4, 6,876 in Wave 5, and 6,733 in Wave 6. The numbers of successfully matched responses of the overall sample was 96% in Wave 2, 97% in Wave 3, 98% in Wave 4, 99% in Wave 5, and 97% in Wave 6. Participants completing all six waves were 4,712 (i.e., 60% of the sample). Details were shown in ▶Tab. 6.1.

The purpose of our study was mentioned, and confidentiality of the collected data was repeatedly emphasized to all students in attendance on the day of testing. Parental and student consent had been obtained prior to data collection. All participants responded to all scales in the questionnaire in a self-administration format. Adequate time was provided for the participants to complete the questionnaire. A trained research assistant was present throughout the administration process.

At different measurement points, participants were required to respond to different measures of positive youth development, including an objective outcome questionnaire which included the Chinese Positive Youth Development Scale (CPYDS, 35). The CPYDS is an 80-item self-report instrument developed to assess positive youth development. The CPYDS has 15 subscales, including bonding (6 items), resilience (6 items), social competence (7 items), recognition for positive behavior (4 items), emotional competence (6 items), cognitive competence (6 items), behavioral competence (5 items), moral competence (6 items), self-determination (5 items), self-efficacy (2 items), clear and positive identity (7 items), beliefs in the future (3 items), prosocial involvement (5 items), prosocial norms (5 items), and spirituality (7 items). The details of the items can be seen in Shek et al. (35). Using multigroup confirmatory factor analyses (MCFA), Shek and Ma (36) showed that 15 basic dimensions of the CPYDS could be subsumed under four higher-order factors (i.e., cognitive-behavioral competencies, prosocial attributes, positive identity, and general positive youth development qualities). Evidence of factorial invariance in terms of configuration, first-order factor loadings, second-order factor loadings, intercepts of measured variable, and intercepts of first-order latent factor, was found.

Tab. 6.1: Number of collected questionnaires across waves

	Wave 1	Wave 2	Wave 3	Wave 4	Wave 5	Wave 6
N (Schools)	48	47[a]	44[b]	44[c]	43	43
N (Participants)	7,846	7,388	6,939	6,697	6,876	6,733
Control Group	3,797	3,654	3,765	3,698	3,757	3,727
Male	1,936	1,876	1,896	1,888	1,874	1,894
Female	1,613	1,619	1,666	1,599	1,682	1,679
Experimental Group	4,049	3,734	3,174	2,999	3,119	3,006
Male	2,154	1,998	1,691	1,548	1,632	1,591
Female	1,745	1,571	1,283	1,259	1,312	1,278
% of successfully matched	98%	96%	97%	98%	99%	97%

[a]1 Experimental school (n = 207) had withdrawn after Wave 1.
[b]3 Experimental schools (n = 629) had withdrawn after Wave 2.
[c]1 Experimental school (n = 71) had withdrawn after Wave 4.

For behavioral intention to gamble, the respondents were asked to assess their intention to gamble in the next two years with reference to a question (*"From now on, will you engage in gambling activities in the next two years?"*). There are four response options (*"absolutely will not," "probably will not," "probably will,"* and *"absolutely will"*).

6.3 Our findings

Reliability analyses showed that all subscales, except the self-efficacy (SE) subscale, were highly reliable (i.e., alpha coefficients above .70, ▶Tab. 6.2). Generally speaking, the measures based on the primary- and second-order factors of the CPYDS were also found to be internally consistent.

As shown in ▶Tab. 6.3, analyses based on Pearson correlation showed that all variables were correlated in the expected directions. In general, a higher level of positive youth development was related to a lower level of behavioral intention to engage in gambling in the same year and at the end of the third year.

To examine the relative contribution of different aspects of positive youth development to behavioral intention to gamble, multiple regression analyses were performed with positive youth development measures at Time 1 as the predictors and intention to gamble at Wave 6 as the criterion variable. The findings based on multiple regression analyses can be seen in ▶Tab. 6.4. Results showed that bonding (BO), resilience (RE), recognition for positive behavior (PB), emotional competence (EC), moral competence (MC), prosocial norms (PN), spirituality (SP), prosocial attributes second-order factor (PA), and general positive youth development qualities second-order factor (GPYDQ)

Tab. 6.2: Internal consistency and mean inter-item correlations for all variables

	Wave 1		Wave 2		Wave 3		Wave 4		Wave 5		Wave 6	
	α	mean[a]	α	mean[a]	α	mean[a]	α	mean[a]	α	mean[a]	α	mean[a]
Subscales based on primary-order factors												
BO	.83	.45	.85	.49	.86	.51	.88	.54	.88	.55	.88	.55
RE	.82	.44	.86	.50	.88	.54	.88	.55	.89	.56	.88	.55
SC	.83	.42	.86	.47	.87	.51	.87	.50	.89	.53	.88	.52
PB	.76	.44	.80	.51	.83	.55	.83	.56	.85	.58	.84	.58
EC	.83	.44	.85	.48	.86	.51	.86	.51	.87	.52	.86	.51
CC	.84	.47	.86	.52	.87	.54	.88	.54	.88	.56	.88	.55
BC	.76	.38	.80	.44	.82	.47	.82	.48	.83	.49	.83	.50
MC	.78	.37	.79	.39	.81	.42	.80	.41	.82	.44	.82	.43
SD	.76	.40	.80	.44	.82	.48	.81	.47	.82	.47	.82	.48
SE	.50	.34	.56	.39	.58	.41	.59	.42	.61	.43	.61	.44
CPI	.84	.43	.85	.45	.87	.48	.86	.47	.87	.48	.87	.49
BF	.82	.61	.83	.62	.84	.64	.84	.65	.85	.66	.84	.65
PI	.83	.49	.83	.50	.86	.55	.85	.52	.86	.55	.86	.54
PN	.77	.40	.80	.45	.81	.46	.81	.46	.81	.46	.81	.47
SP	.88	.51	.89	.56	.91	.60	.91	.60	.92	.62	.91	.62
Subscales based on second-order factors												
CBC	.85	.66	.87	.69	.88	.71	.88	.71	.88	.72	.89	.72
PA	.79	.65	.77	.62	.79	.66	.78	.64	.79	.66	.77	.63
GPYDQ	.89	.52	.89	.53	.90	.55	.90	.54	.90	.57	.90	.55
PID	.83	.72	.84	.73	.85	.75	.85	.74	.86	.76	.86	.76

[a]Mean inter-item correlation.

BO: bonding; RE: resilience; SC: social competence; PB: recognition for positive behavior; EC: emotional competence; CC: cognitive competence; BC: behavioral competence; MC: moral competence; SD: self-determination; SE: self-efficacy; CPI: clear and positive identity; BF: beliefs in the future; PI: prosocial involvement; PN: prosocial norms; SP: spirituality; CBC: cognitive-behavioral competencies second-order factor; PA: prosocial attributes second-order factor; GPYDQ: general positive youth development qualities second-order factor; PID: positive identity second-order factor.

Tab. 6.3: Correlation coefficients on the relationships between positive youth development measures and behavioral intention to gamble

	Wave 1	Wave 2	Wave 3	Wave 4	Wave 5	Wave 6	Wave 1 and Wave 6
Subscales based on primary-order factors							
BO	−.19	−.16	−.17	−.17	−.19	−.16	−.13
RE	−.17	−.15	−.16	−.17	−.17	−.16	−.13
SC	−.12	−.09	−.09	−.11	−.12	−.09	−.07
PB	−.17	−.15	−.16	−.17	−.18	−.16	−.13
EC	−.15	−.13	−.14	−.16	−.15	−.15	−.13
CC	−.16	−.12	−.13	−.15	−.15	−.14	−.12
BC	−.16	−.12	−.14	−.16	−.15	−.13	−.11
MC	−.20	−.16	−.17	−.19	−.19	−.19	−.15
SD	−.13	−.10	−.11	−.13	−.14	−.12	−.07
SE	−.07	−.06	−.07	−.07	−.09	−.09	−.05
CPI	−.12	−.10	−.11	−.12	−.11	−.11	−.08
BF	−.14	−.13	−.13	−.15	−.13	−.12	−.08
PI	−.16	−.13	−.15	−.15	−.17	−.15	−.09
PN	−.21	−.20	−.19	−.22	−.22	−.20	−.12
SP	−.20	−.16	−.18	−.16	−.17	−.18	−.13
Subscales based on second-order factors							
CBC	−.17	−.13	−.14	−.16	−.16	−.14	−.12
PA	−.20	−.18	−.19	−.20	−.21	−.19	−.12
GPYDQ	−.21	−.18	−.19	−.20	−.20	−.19	−.15
PID	−.14	−.13	−.13	−.14	−.13	−.12	−.08

All correlation coefficients were significant ($p < .01$).
Wave 1, Wave 2, Wave 3, Wave 4, Wave 5, Wave 6 = cross-sectional correlation coefficients at each wave. Wave 1 and Wave 6 = longitudinal correlation coefficients on the relationship between positive youth development measures at Time 1 and behavioral intention to gamble at Wave 6. BO: bonding; RE: resilience; SC: social competence; PB: recognition for positive behavior; EC: emotional competence; CC: cognitive competence; BC: behavioral competence; MC: moral competence; SD: self-determination; SE: self-efficacy; CPI: clear and positive identity; BF: beliefs in the future; PI: prosocial involvement; PN: prosocial norms; SP: spirituality; CBC: cognitive-behavioral competencies second-order factor; PA: prosocial attributes second-order factor; GPYDQ: general positive youth development qualities second-order factor; PID: positive identity second-order factor.

negatively predicted intention to engage in gambling activities. However, it is noteworthy that social competence (SC), self-determination (SD), clear and positive identity (CPI), prosocial involvement (PI), cognitive-behavioral competencies second-order factor (CBC), and positive identity second-order factor (PID) positively predicted behavioral intention to gamble over time.

Tab. 6.4: Multiple regression analyses predicting behavioral intention to gamble

Predictor	Without Controlling BIG			Controlling Initial BIG		
	R	R^2	β^a	R	R^2	β^a
Subscales based on primary-order factors						
BO			−.04*			−.03
RE			−.05**			−.05*
SC			.11**			.10**
PB			−.06**			−.04*
EC			−.06**			−.06**
CC			−.04			−.04
BC			.00			−.01
MC			−.11**			−.08**
SD			.05*			.05*
SE			.02			.01
CPI			.06*			.04
BF			−.01			−.01
PI			.05*			.04
PN			−.05**			−.03
SP			−.06**			−.03
BIG at Wave 1						.24**
Model	.21	.04		.31	.10	
Subscales based on second-order factors						
CBC			.06*			.03
PA			−.12**			−.11**
GPYDQ			−.19**			−.14*
PID			.05**			.04*
BIG at Wave 1						.25*
Model	.21	.05		.32	.11	

*$p < .05$. **$p < .01$.
aStandardized coefficients.
BIG: behavioral intention to gamble; BO: bonding; RE: resilience; SC: social competence; PB: recognition for positive behavior; EC: emotional competence; CC: cognitive competence; BC: behavioral competence; MC: moral competence; SD: self-determination; SE: self-efficacy; CPI: clear and positive identity; BF: beliefs in the future; PI: prosocial involvement; PN: prosocial norms; SP: spirituality; CBC: cognitive-behavioral competencies second-order factor; PA: prosocial attributes second-order factor; GPYDQ: general positive youth development qualities second-order factor; PID: positive identity second-order factor.

Additional analyses were carried out to examine the relative influence of different positive youth development constructs on the changes in behavioral intention to gamble over time. For each equation, intention to gamble at Wave 6 was treated as the dependent variable and the corresponding Time 1 scores were entered in Step 1. In Step 2, different positive youth development measures were entered. Results showed that higher levels of resilience (RE), recognition for positive behavior (PB), emotional competence (EC), moral competence (MC), prosocial attributes second-order factor (PA), and general positive youth development qualities second-order factor (GPYDQ) at Wave 1 were associated with a drop in behavioral intention to gamble at Wave 6. However, the findings also showed that higher levels of social competence (SC), self-determination (SD), and positive identity second-order factor (PID) at Wave 1 were associated with a rise in behavioral intention to gamble at Wave 6.

6.4 Discussion

In this study, we examined the relationship between positive youth development and intention to gamble among Chinese adolescents in Hong Kong. There are several unique characteristics of our study. First, in view of the paucity of research in different Chinese contexts, Chinese adolescents were recruited. Second, a large sample size was employed. Third, with reference to the limitations of cross-sectional research design, longitudinal data based on six waves of data were collected, a feature unique in the field. Finally, a validated measure of positive youth development in Chinese adolescents was used. This study is a positive response to the scarcity of gambling research in the Chinese context. It provides insights into the adolescents' intentions to gamble and design of appropriate prevention strategies for Chinese young people.

The findings are generally consistent with a growing body of literature suggesting that the association of positive youth development qualities in reducing the youth risk behaviors (37–40). The associations between three positive youth development subscales (i.e., resilience, moral competence, and prosocial attributes second-order factor) and intention to gamble support the notion that negative attitude toward deviance would be a protective factor toward risky behaviors (41). The result of this socially unacceptable attitude toward gambling may be related to the recent adoption of "restricted gambling" policy and a massive government advertising campaign that emphasized the negative impacts brought by gambling not only on the gamblers themselves, but also their families. In a city-wide survey of 2,093 Hong Kong people aged from 15 to 64 about their awareness of problem gambling, about 88% of them reported that TV commercials and docu-drama are their major sources for receiving the relevant information (7). The impact of this media-based campaign might have led to a decrease in the prevalence of gambling behavior from 78% in 2001 to 71% in 2008 (8, 42). Dickson et al. (29) developed a framework that integrated risk and protective factors across multiple levels (e.g., individual, peer, family, school, community, society). They suggested public education and social policy were effective ways for changing public attitude and raising awareness toward problem and pathological gambling. Messerlian and Derevensky (43) advocated the use of social marketing techniques in portraying the negative consequences of problem gambling to the public. The influence of social norms and policies is particularly salient when it incorporates prevention services and programs among students, as shown in empirical prevention research (44, 45). The findings of the study highlight the importance of building a protective social environment in minimizing youth gambling problems.

Consistent with both current gambling literature conducted in Chinese (34) and Western samples (46, 47), scores on the bonding subscale were positively related to the decrease of intention to gamble. Connectedness (i.e., bonding) exerts a protective function for multiple problem behaviors (48–50). Feelings of bonding with one's family and school have been shown to reduce the strength of the relation between individual vulnerabilities and a number of risk behaviors, such as youth gambling, delinquency, alcohol and substance abuse (41, 51, 52).

Also, the negative relationship between emotional competence and intention to gamble is in line with prior work that demonstrated high emotional competence (i.e., affect regulation abilities) was likely to reduce the risk of problem gambling (53–55), smoking and alcohol use (56), and deviant school behavior (57). The findings of the present study note the importance of promoting emotional competence in prevention of adolescent gambling.

Interestingly, although correlation analyses showed negative relationships among social competencies, self-determination, positive identity second-order factor, and intention to gamble, multiple regression analyses indicated that these positive youth development subscales were associated with an increased likelihood to gamble in the future. There are several explanations for this unexpected finding, which appears to be at odds with the general hypothesis.

First, it is important to note that higher scores in these constructs might only reflect their psychosocial maturity and intention to gamble, but not a direct link to problem gambling. In fact, researchers argue that gambling might be a healthy part of adolescent development as it provides pleasure and arousal of playing when they gamble in a safe-level or low-risk manner (58–63). "The lure of excitement, entertainment and financial freedom accompanying gambling is particularly attractive to youth" (p. 70, 4). One of the common reasons for adolescents engaging in addictive behaviors is to escape from stressful realities (64). Very often, adolescents view gambling as a form of coping strategy for reducing tension. They might perceive it as a way to reduce boredom and loneliness. As shown in a recent study (7), Chinese adolescents perceived gambling as a way to "kill time" and "escape from boredom."

Second, adolescent gambling may serve an instrumental function to enhance their identification with adult life. They are likely to perceive gambling as a symbol of adulthood and also to gain social support from their peers (62, 65). Youth gambling is influenced by socialization (13). Gambling is perceived as a form of entertainment or leisure activities during family gathering events (8) and considered as a quick-fix approach to have money (7). Under this atmosphere, Hong Kong adolescents might overestimate their ability to win. This is supported by a survey of 2,019 Hong Kong people (aged 15–64 years old), in which about 12% reported that their family members reacted calmly and provided advice when they knew they gambled (7). In the same study involving 2,095 secondary school students, nearly 40% of the sample reported that their first gambling experience was invited by their friends/schoolmates and family members. "Hoping to win money" was one of the most common reasons for them to engage in gambling activities. Clearly, more research in this area is needed in the future to understand the relationships of these factors with youth gambling.

Finally, it is possible that the present "odd" findings are due to methodological limitation of the measurement of intention to gamble. In the current study, behavioral intention to gamble instead of actual gambling behavior was measured. It is noteworthy that the intention to gamble may not have high correlation with actual gambling behavior. In addition, as only one item was used to assess intention to gamble, it is not possible to assess the reliability of the measure. It is suggested that more items should be used to examine this behavioral outcome in the future. Nevertheless, in view of such odd findings, it is suggested that more studies should be carried out to clarify this issue.

"Treatment is not just fixing what is broken; it is nurturing what is best" (28, p. 7). More empirical support for the positive youth development approach is needed for helping youths to stretch their full potential when they enter into adult society (66, 67). Previous prevention study demonstrated the importance of using school as a basis for promoting social and personal competence to minimize adolescent problem behavior via the school setting. Given the severe negative consequences of gambling on youth, their families, and communities, more research in this area for increasing knowledge of youth gambling is warranted.

There are several limitations to our study. First, it did not distinguish between gambling forms, types, or activities (e.g., Mark Six lottery, card games, horse racing, dice games, football betting). It is noteworthy that various forms of gambling activities exist, ranging from asking friends to place bets on Mark Six lottery to more formal types found in mahjong houses or casinos, and illegal gambling activities. As noted by Raylu and Oei (13), "very little research exists that explores why different groups of individuals choose different forms of gambling and the processes that are involved in determining which forms of gambling are chosen" (p. 1015). More information would be obtained by distinguishing different types of gambling in future research.

Future studies might examine the longitudinal effects of positive youth development subscales on a specific behavioral outcome. As little empirical work has addressed the systematic changes of correlates and consequences of youth gambling across time, especially in the Chinese context, it would be desirable to examine the generalizability of the study across multiple ethnic groups.

The current study might provide useful insights when designing gambling prevention programs among youths. In particular, researchers noted the importance of understanding the underlying psychological, familial, social, and cultural factors causing, or preventing, youth problem gambling (13). Future studies are needed to examine the effects of positive youth development constructs on other addiction-related behaviors.

Acknowledgements

Preparation of this chapter and the project P.A.T.H.S. were financially supported by The Hong Kong Jockey Club Charities Trust.

References

1. Ladouceur R, Boudreault N, Jacques C. Pathological gambling and related problems among adolescents. J Child Adolesc Subst Abuse 1999;84:55–68.
2. Blinn-Pike L, Worthy SL, Jonkman JN. Adolescent gambling: A review of an emerging field of research. J Adolesc Health 2010;47:223–36.

3. Gupta R, Derevensky JL. Adolescent gambling behavior: A prevalence study and examination of the correlates associated with excessive gambling. J Gambl Stud 1998;14:319–45.

4. Messerlian C, Derevensky J, Gupta R. Youth gambling problems: A public health perspective. Health Promot Int 2005;20(1):69–79.

5. Zangeneh M, Griffiths M, Parke J. The marketing of gambling. In: Zangeneh M, Blaszczynski A, Turner NE, eds. In the pursuit of winning: Problem gambling theory, research and treatment. New York: Springer; 2008: 135–53.

6. Derevensky J, Shek DTL, Merrick J. Adolescent gambling. Int J Adolesc Med Health 2010; 22(1):1–2.

7. Home Affairs Bureau. Study on Hong Kong peoples' participation in gambling activities. The Hong Kong Special Administration Region, P.R.C.: Author; 2005.

8. Home Affairs Bureau. Final report: Evaluation study on the impacts of gambling liberalization in nearby cities on Hong Kong peoples' participation in gambling activities and development of counseling and treatment services for problem gamblers. The Hong Kong Special Administration Region, P.R.C.: Author; 2008.

9. Derevensky J, Gupta R. Adolescents with gambling problems: A synopsis of our current knowledge. e-Gambling: The Electronic Journal of Gambling Issues 2004;10:119–40.www.camh.net/egambling/issue10/ejgi_10_derevensky_gupta.html. Accessed November 2010.

10. Derevensky J, Gupta R, Messerlian C, Gillespie M. Youth gambling problems: A need for responsible social policy. In: Derevensky J, Gupta R, eds. Gambling problems in youth: Theoretical and applied perspectives. New York: Kluwer Academic/Plenum Publishers; 2004: 231–52.

11. Jacobs DF. Youth gambling in North America: Long term trends and future prospects. In: Derevensky J, Gupta R, eds. Gambling problems in youth: Theoretical and applied perspectives. New York: Kluwer Academic/Plenum Publishers; 2004: 1–24.

12. Gupta R, Derevensky JL. A treatment approach for adolescents with gambling problems. In: Derevensky J, Gupta R, eds. Gambling problems in youth: Theoretical and applied perspectives. New York: Kluwer Academic/Plenum Publishers; 2004: 165–88.

13. Raylu N, Oei TPS. Pathological gambling: A comprehensive review. Clin Psychol Rev 2002;22(7):1009–61.

14. Chinese Medical Associations & Nanjing Medical University. Chinese classification of mental disorders. 2nd ed. China: Dong Nan University Press; 1995.

15. Ladouceur R. Prevalence estimates of pathological gamblers in Quebec, Canada. Can J Psychiatry 1991;36:732–34.

16. Shaffer HJ, Hall MN, Vanderbilt MN. Estimating the prevalence of disordered gambling behavior in the United States and Canada: A meta-analysis. Boston: Harvard University; 1997.

17. Cheung NWT, Cheung YW. Pathological gambling of marginal youths and students in Hong Kong. http://www.cuhk.edu.hk/cpr/pressrelease/100628e.htm. Accessed November 2010.

18. Jacobs DF. Juvenile gambling in North America: An analysis of long term trends and future prospects. J Gambl Stud 2000;16:119–52.

19. Marget N, Gupta R, Derevensky J. The psychosocial factors underlying adolescent problem gambling. Poster presented at the annual meeting of the American Psychological Association, Boston; 1999.

20. Custer RL. An overview of compulsive gambling. In: Carone PA, Yoles SF, Kieffer SN, Krinsky L, eds. Addictive disorders update: Alcoholism, drug abuse, gambling. New York: Human Services Press; 1982: 107–24.

21. Lynch WJ, Maciejewski PK, Potenza MN. Psychiatric correlates of gambling in adolescents and young adults group by age at gambling onset. Arch Gen Psychiatry 2004;61(11):1116–22.

22. Welte JW, Barnes GM, Tidwell MCO, Hoffman, JH. Association between problem gambling and conduct disorder in a national survey of adolescents and young adults in the United States. J Adolesc Health 2009;45(4):396–401.

23. Winters KC, Stinchfield RD, Botzet A, Anderson N. A prospective study of youth gambling behaviors. Psychol Addict Behav 2002;16(1):3–9.
24. Catalano RF, Berglund ML, Ryan JAM, Lonczak HS, Hawkins JD. Positive youth development in the United States: Research findings on evaluations of positive youth development programs. Prev Treatment 2002;5:article 15.
25. Benson P, Mannes M, Pittman K, Ferber T. Youth development, developmental assets and public policy. In: Lerner RM, Steinberg L, eds. Handbook of adolescent psychology. New York: Wiley; 2004: 781–814.
26. Lerner RM, Benson PL, eds. Developmental assets and asset-building communities: Implications for research, policy, and practice. New York: Kluwer Academic/Plenum Publishers; 2003.
27. Rich GJ. The positive psychology of youth and adolescence. J Youth Adolesc 2003;32(1):1–3.
28. Seligman MEP, Csikszentmihalyi M. Positive Psychology. Am Psychol 2000;55(1):5–14.
29. Dickson LM, Derevensky JL, Gupta R. The prevention of gambling problems in youth: A conceptual framework. J Gambl Stud 2002;18(2):97–159.
30. Amodeo M, Collin ME. Using a positive youth development approach in addressing problem-oriented youth behavior. Fam Soc 2007;88(1):75–85.
31. Klein JD, Sabaratnam P, Auerbach MM, Smith SM, Kodjo C, Lewis K, Ryan S, Dandino C. Development and factor structure of a brief instrument to assess the impact of community programs on positive youth development: The Rochester Evaluation of Asset Development for Youth (READY) Tool. J Adolesc Health 2006;39:252–60.
32. Seligman MEP. Comment on "priorities for prevention research at NIMH". Prev Treatment 2001;4:article 21.
33. Catalano RF, Berglund ML, Ryan JAM, Lonczak HS, Hawkins JD. Positive youth development in the United States: Research findings on evaluations of positive youth development programs. Ann Am Acad Pol Soc Sci 2004;591(1):98–124.
34. Shek DTL. Positive youth development and behavioral intention to gamble among Chinese adolescents in Hong Kong. Int J Adolesc Med Health 2010;22(1):163–72.
35. Shek DTL, Siu AMH, Lee TY. The Chinese Positive Youth Development Scale: A validation study. Res Soc Work Pract 2007;17:380–91.
36. Shek DTL, Ma CMS. Dimensionality of the Chinese Positive Youth Development Scale: Confirmatory factor analyses. Soc Indic Res 2010;98:41–59.
37. Catalano RF, Berglund ML, Ryan JAM, Lonczak HS, Hawkins JD. Positive youth development in the United States: Research findings on evaluations of youth development programs. Washington, DC: U.S. Department of Health and Human Services; 1999.
38. Drug Strategies. Making the grade: A guide to school drug prevention programs. Washington, DC: Author; 1996.
39. Drug Strategies. Safe schools, safe students: A guide to violence prevention strategies. Washington, DC: Author; 1998.
40. Durlak JA, Wells AM. Evaluation of indicated preventive intervention (secondary prevention) mental health programs for children and adolescents. Am J Community Psychol 1998;26:775–802.
41. Jessor R, Van Den Bos J, Vanderryn J, Costan FM, Turbin MS. Protective factors in adolescent problem behavior: Moderator effects and developmental change. Dev Psychol 1995;31:923–33.
42. Home Affairs Bureau. Study on Hong Kong peoples' participation in gambling activities. The Hong Kong Special Administration Region, P.R.C.: Author; 2001.
43. Messerlian C, Derevensky JL. Social marketing campaigns for youth gambling prevention: lessons learned from youth. Int J Ment Health Addict 2006;4:294–306.
44. Brown JH, D'Emidio-Caston M. On becoming 'at-risk' through drug education: How symbolic policies and their practices affect students. Eval Rev 1995;19(4):451–92.

45. Gorman DM. The irrelevance of evidence in the development of school-based drug prevention policy, 1986–1996. Eval Rev 1998;22(1):118–46.
46. Barber BK, Buehler C. Family cohesion and enmeshment: Different constructs, different effects. J Marriage Fam 1996;58:433–43.
47. Barrera M, JR, Li SA. The relation of family support to adolescents' psychological distress and behavior problems. In: Pierce GR, Sarason BR, Sarason IG, eds. Handbook of social support and the family. New York: Plenum; 1996: 313–43.
48. McNeely CA, Nonnemaker JM, Blum RW. Promoting school connectedness: Evidence from the national longitudinal study of adolescent health. J Sch Health 2002;72(4):138–46.
49. Dornbusch SM, Erickson KG, Laird J, Wong CA. The relation of family school attachment to adolescent deviance in diverse groups and communities. J Adolesc Res 2001;16(4):396–422.
50. Springer JF, Wright LS, McCall GJ. Family interventions and adolescent resiliency: The southwest Texas state high-risk youth program. J Community Psychol 1997;25(5):435–52.
51. Dickson L, Derevensky JL, Gupta R. Youth gambling problems: Examining risk and protective factors. International Gambl Studies 2008;8(1):25–47.
52. Kaufman ED. The relationship between gambling activity, the occurrence of life stress, and differential coping styles in an adolescent sample. Unpublished doctoral dissertation, McGill University, Montreal, Quebec, Canada; 2002.
53. Coman GJ, Burrows GD, Evans BJ. Stress and anxiety as factors in the onset of problem gambling: Implications for treatment. Stress Med 1997;13:235–44.
54. Lumley MA, Roby KJ. Alexithymia and pathological gambling. Psychother Psychosom 1995;63:201–6.
55. Taylor GJ, Bagby RM, Parker JDA. Disorders of affect regulation: Alexithymia in medical and psychiatric illness. Cambridge: Cambridge University Press; 1997.
56. Trinidad DR, Johnson CA. The association between emotional intelligence and early adolescent tobacco and alcohol use. Pers Individ Dif 2002;32:95–105.
57. Petrides KV, Fredrickson N, Furnham A. The role of trait emotional intelligence in academic performance and deviant behavior at school. Pers Individ Dif 2004;36:277–93.
58. Ackerman D. Deep play. New York: Random House; 1999.
59. Anderson G, Brown RIF. Real and laboratory gambling, sensation seeking and arousal. Br J Clin Psychol 1984;75(3):401–10.
60. Driver B, Brown P, Peterson G. Benefits of Leisure. Pennsylvania: Venture Publishing Inc.; 1991.
61. Korn DA, Shaffer HJ. Gambling and the health of the public: Adopting a public health perspective. J Gambl Stud 1999;15:289–358.
62. Moore SM, Ohtsuka K. Gambling activities of young Australians: Developing a model of behavior. J Gambl Stud 1997;13(3):207–36.
63. Weiss MR. Children in sport: An educational model. In: Murphy SM, ed. Sport psychology interventions. Champaign, IL: Human Kinetics; 1995: 39–70.
64. Jacobs DF. A general theory of addictions: A new theoretical model. J Gambl Behavior 1986;2(1):15–31.
65. Delfabbro P, Thrupp L. The social determinants of youth gambling in South Australian adolescents. J Adolesc 2003;26:313–30.
66. Rich GJ. Positive psychology: An introduction. J Hum Psych 2001;41(1):8–12.
67. Roth J, Brooks-Gunn J, Murray L, Foster W. Promoting healthy adolescents: Synthesis of youth development program evaluations. J Res Adolesc 1998;8:423–59.

7 Relationship between positive youth development and intention to gamble among Chinese adolescents in Hong Kong

Daniel T. L. Shek and Rachel C. F. Sun

This chapter examines the relationship between positive youth development and behavioral intention to gamble among Chinese adolescents in Hong Kong. Over a period of two years, four waves of data were collected from Chinese secondary school students, who responded to validated measures of Chinese positive youth development and adolescent behavioral intention to gamble. Consistent with the general prediction, results showed that positive youth development indexed by different indicators was negatively related to adolescent behavioral intention to gamble, except for social competence and positive and clear identity. Multiple regression analyses showed that positive youth development measures predicted adolescent intention to gamble and their changes over time. The present findings suggest that promoting positive youth development is a possible strategy that can help to prevent adolescent problem gambling.

7.1 Introduction

There are studies in the literature proposing that there are risk factors associated with adolescent problem gambling. For example, Gupta and Derevensky (1) identified several risk factors for youth with serious gambling problems and highlighted several observations: (a) gambling is more popular among males; (b) gambling is greater in risk takers; (c) youth problem gamblers have relatively lower self-esteem but higher rates of depression, suicidal ideation, and suicidal attempts; (d) loss of quality friendships and relationships and a higher number of gambling associates are common in youth problem gamblers; and (e) youth problem gamblers have poorer general coping skills. In a detailed review of risk and protective factors of youth problem gambling using an ecological model, Shead, Derevensky, and Gupta (see this book) concluded that different individual, relationship, community, and societal factors were associated with adolescent gambling problems.

Nevertheless, there are three limitations intrinsic to the existing studies on risk factors and adolescent problem gambling behavior. First, most of the studies have examined the relationships between adolescent pathologies (such as mental health problems and delinquency) and adolescent problem gambling, and there are few studies investigating the relationship between positive youth development and adolescent problem gambling. According to Damon (2), in contrast to the "traditional" approach, which focuses on youth developmental problems such as substance abuse and mental health problems, the field of positive youth development emphasizes talents, strengths, interests, and future potentials of each child. Pittman, Irby, Tolman, Yohalem, and Ferber (3) argued that "prevention alone is not enough" and "problem free is not fully prepared" (p. 6). In other words, problem-free youth (via reduction of school drop out, poor work habits, problem health behavior, social/emotional problems, and civic apathy) is not enough and fully prepared youth (having assets such as high academic motivation and aspirations, positive attitudes toward work, healthy life style, supportive relationships, and civic awareness) as well as fully engaged youth are important. Lerner and Dowling (4) similarly suggested that the thriving process involves the growth of functionally valued behaviors across development (including competence, character, connection, confidence, and caring and compassion) and their impacts on the attainment of structurally valued behaviors (including contribution to self, family, community, and civil society).

Catalano, Berglund, Ryan, Lonczak, and Hawkins (5) reviewed 77 programs on positive youth development. The review showed that 25 programs were successful, and the following 15 positive youth development constructs were identified in the successful programs: promotion of bonding, cultivation of resilience, promotion of social competence, promotion of emotional competence, promotion of cognitive competence, promotion of behavioral competence, promotion of moral competence, cultivation of self-determination, promotion of spirituality, development of self-efficacy, development of a clear and positive identity, promotion of beliefs in the future, provision of recognition for positive behavior, provision of opportunities for prosocial involvement, and fostering prosocial norms. Obviously, it is interesting to ask whether these positive youth development constructs are related to adolescent gambling.

There are theoretical propositions maintaining that positive youth development influences the well-being and health outcomes of an individual, and lack of that positive development would eventually contribute to problem behavior such as problem gambling in adolescents. According to Lent (6), positive development attributes such as self-efficacy affect life satisfaction. For existential theorists such as Victor Frankl, meaning in life fills "existential vacuum" thus leaving no space for the development of psychopathology. Empirically, there are research findings showing that positive youth development attributes, such as owning bonding and social roles, were closely related to adolescent life satisfaction. Several positive youth development constructs, including social and emotional competencies, academic and social self-efficacy, prosocial motivation and behavior, spirituality and religiosity, and mastery and ethnic identity, were found to act as significant predictors of life satisfaction (7).

As an adolescent, having weak resilience, poor psychosocial competencies, blurred self-identity, and low self-efficacy is likely to have poor developmental outcomes, and there are theoretical accounts regarding the influence of positive youth development on mitigating adolescent problem behavior. Based on the concepts of protective factors in resilience literature, it can be conjectured that internal resources such as psychosocial competencies and external resources such as bonding (8) would protect individuals from life stresses, thus minimizing the occurrence of problem behavior. There is research showing that positive youth development is negatively related to problem behavior, such as substance abuse and delinquency (7).

The second limitation is that most of the existing studies have been conducted in Western societies, and published scientific studies in this area are almost nonexistent in non-Western contexts, including the Chinese context. From a cross-cultural perspective, the lack of related research data in the Chinese context would motivate one to ask whether risk and protective factors related to Chinese adolescent gambling differ from those phenomena observed in the Western culture. This question should be addressed, as Chinese people generally endorse gambling as a way to get rich and as a recreational activity across different Chinese societies. Against such a cultural background, it would be interesting to ask whether positive youth development characteristics are related to gambling in Chinese adolescents (9).

The third observation is that with a few exceptions, existing findings on the factors related to adolescent gambling are mainly based on cross-sectional data. To understand the causal effect of positive youth development on adolescent gambling, longitudinal study is indispensable. In particular, longitudinal design can enable researchers to examine how positive youth development contributes to change in adolescent gambling over time.

To overcome the limitations of the literature, this chapter reports longitudinal findings to clarify the relationship between positive youth development and adolescent gambling in a large sample of Chinese adolescents over time. The general expectation is that positive youth development is negatively related to adolescent gambling behavior and intention. The findings reported in this chapter are based on an evaluation study of the Project P.A.T.H.S., which is a multi-year universal positive youth development program in Hong Kong (10–11). As the primary focus of the present chapter is on the relationship between positive youth development and adolescent gambling intention, the evaluation findings are not presented and discussed.

7.2 Our research design

The data for this chapter were derived from the first four waves of data of the P.A.T.H.S. Project. At Wave 1, a total of 48 schools (24 experimental groups, 24 control groups) from different parts of Hong Kong participated in the study. The participants could be considered heterogeneous, as they came from different areas and socioeconomic classes in Hong Kong. The number of participants generating data at different waves for the present analyses can be seen in ▶Tab. 7.1.

During the data collection process, the purpose of the study was mentioned and confidentiality of the data collected was repeatedly emphasized to all students in attendance on the day of testing. Parental and student consent had been obtained prior to data collection. All participants responded to all scales in the questionnaire in a self-administration format. Adequate time was provided for the subjects to complete the questionnaire. A trained research assistant was present throughout the administration process.

In the context of evaluation, participants responded to the measures of positive youth development and adolescent developmental problems, including behavioral intention to gamble. Positive youth development was measured by the Chinese Positive Youth Development Scale (CPYDS). The CPYDS is an 80-item self-report instrument developed to assess positive youth development. The CPYDS has 15 subscales, including bonding (6 items), resilience (6 items), social competence (7 items), recognition for positive behavior (4 items), emotional competence (6 items), cognitive competence (6 items), behavioral competence (5 items), moral competence (6 items), self-determination (5 items), self-efficacy (2 items), clear and positive identity (7 items), beliefs in the future (3 items), prosocial involvement (5 items), prosocial norms (5 items), and spirituality

Tab. 7.1: Number of participants and completed questionnaires collected at Year 1 (Wave 1 and Wave 2) and Year 2 (Wave 3 and Wave 4)

Cases	Year 1 (Waves 1 and 2)			Year 2 (Waves 3 and 4)		
	Experimental	Control	Total	Experimental	Control	Total
Pretest questionnaire collected	4,121	3,854	7,975	3,290	3,861	7,151
Pretest questionnaire available for matching	4,050	3,795	7,845	3,276	3,845	7,121
Posttest questionnaire collected	3,914	3,770	7,684	3,047	3,764	6,811
Posttest questionnaire available for matching	3,880	3,728	7,608	3,047	3,763	6,810
Successfully matched	3,312	3,363	6,675	2,784	3,401	6,185

Note. The number (percentage) of the successfully matched cases across Waves 1–4 is 5,054: experimental group, 2,236; control group, 2,818.

(7 items). The details of the items can be seen in Shek, Siu, and Lee (12). Using multigroup confirmatory factor analyses (MCFA), Shek and Ma (13) showed that the 15 basic dimensions of the CPYDS could be subsumed under 4 higher-order factors (i.e., cognitive-behavioral competencies, prosocial attributes, positive identity, and general positive youth development qualities). Evidence of factorial invariance in terms of configuration, first-order factor loadings, second-order factor loadings, intercepts of measured variable, and intercepts of first-order latent factor, was found.

For behavioral intention to gamble, the respondents were asked to assess their intention to gamble in the next two years with reference to a question ("from now on, will you engage in gambling activities in the next two years?"). There are four response options ("absolutely will not," "probably will not," "probably will," and "absolutely will").

7.3 Our findings

The number of participants whose data were included in the analyses can be seen in ▶Tab. 7.1. Reliability analyses showed that all the scales and subscales except the self-efficacy subscale were highly reliable, i.e., they had alpha coefficients of .75 or above (▶Tab. 7.2). Generally speaking, the measures based on the primary and second-order factors (13) were found to be internally consistent.

Tab. 7.2: Cronbach's alphas and mean inter-item correlations for positive youth development measures across waves

	Wave 1		Wave 2		Wave 3		Wave 4	
	α	mean[a]	α	mean[a]	α	mean[a]	α	mean[a]
Subscales based on primary factors								
BO	.83	.45	.85	.48	.86	.51	.88	.54
RE	.82	.44	.86	.50	.88	.54	.88	.55
SC	.83	.42	.86	.47	.87	.51	.87	.50
PB	.76	.44	.80	.51	.83	.55	.83	.56
EC	.83	.44	.85	.48	.86	.51	.86	.51
CC	.84	.47	.86	.52	.87	.54	.88	.54
BC	.76	.38	.80	.44	.82	.47	.82	.48
MC	.78	.37	.79	.39	.81	.42	.80	.41
SD	.76	.40	.80	.44	.82	.48	.81	.47
SE	.50	.34	.56	.39	.58	.41	.59	.42
CPI	.84	.43	.85	.45	.87	.48	.86	.47
BF	.82	.61	.83	.62	.84	.64	.84	.65
PI	.83	.49	.83	.50	.86	.55	.85	.52
PN	.77	.40	.80	.45	.81	.46	.81	.46
SP	.88	.51	.89	.56	.91	.60	.91	.60
Subscales based on second-order factors								
CBC	.85	.66	.87	.69	.88	.71	.88	.71
PA	.79	.65	.77	.62	.79	.66	.78	.64
PID	.83	.72	.84	.73	.85	.75	.85	.74
GPYDQ	.89	.52	.89	.53	.90	.55	.90	.54
TOTAL	.97	.32	.98	.34	.98	.37	.98	.36

[a]Inter-item correlations

BO: bonding; RE: resilience; SC: social competence; PB: recognition for positive behavior; EC: emotional competence; CC: cognitive competence; BC: behavioral competence; MC: moral competence; SD: self-determination; SE: self-efficacy; CPI: clear and positive identity; BF: beliefs in the future; PI: prosocial involvement; PN: prosocial norms; SP: spirituality; CBC: cognitive-behavioral competencies second-order factor; PA: prosocial attributes second-order factor; PID: positive identity second-order factor; GPYDQ: general positive youth development qualities second-order factor.

As shown in ▶Tab. 7.3, analyses based on Pearson correlation showed that all variables were correlated in the expected directions. Generally speaking, a higher level of positive youth development was related to a lower level of behavioral intention to engage in gambling in the next two years. Both cross-sectional and longitudinal correlation coefficients showed this pattern.

Tab. 7.3: Correlation coefficients on the relationship between positive youth development measures and behavioral intention to gamble

	Wave 1	Wave 2	Wave 3	Wave 4	Wave 1 and Wave 4
Subscales based on primary factors					
BO	−.19	−.16	−.17	−.17	−.14
RE	−.17	−.15	−.16	−.17	−.14
SC	−.12	−.09	−.09	−.11	−.07
PB	−.17	−.15	−.16	−.17	−.12
EC	−.15	−.13	−.14	−.16	−.14
CC	−.16	−.12	−.13	−.15	−.13
BC	−.16	−.12	−.14	−.16	−.11
MC	−.20	−.16	−.17	−.19	−.16
SD	−.13	−.10	−.11	−.13	−.09
SE	−.07	−.06	−.07	−.07	−.06
CPI	−.12	−.10	−.11	−.12	−.09
BF	−.14	−.13	−.13	−.15	−.12
PI	−.16	−.16	−.15	−.15	−.12
PN	−.21	−.20	−.19	−.22	−.14
SP	−.20	−.16	−.18	−.16	−.13
Subscales based on second-order factors					
CBC	−.17	−.13	−.14	−.16	−.13
PA	−.20	−.18	−.19	−.20	−.15
GPYDQ	−.21	−.18	−.19	−.20	−.16
PID	−.14	−.13	−.13	−.14	−.11

All correlation coefficients were significant ($p < .01$).

Wave 1, Wave 2, Wave 3, and Wave 4 = cross-sectional correlation coefficients at each wave. Wave 1 and Wave 4 = longitudinal correlation coefficients on the relationship between positive youth development measures at Time 1 and behavioral intention to gamble at Wave 4. BO: bonding; RE: resilience; SC: social competence; PB: recognition for positive behavior; EC: emotional competence; CC: cognitive competence; BC: behavioral competence; MC: moral competence; SD: self-determination; SE: self-efficacy; CPI: clear and positive identity; BF: beliefs in the future; PI: prosocial involvement; PN: prosocial norms; SP: spirituality; CBC: cognitive-behavioral competencies second-order factor; PA: prosocial attributes second-order factor; GPYDQ: general positive youth development qualities second-order factor; PID: positive identity second-order factor.

In order to examine the relative contribution of different aspects of positive youth development to intention to gamble, multiple regression analyses were performed with positive youth development measured at Time 1 as the predictors and intention to gamble at Time 4 as the criterion variable. The findings based on multiple regression analyses can be seen in ▶Tab. 7.4. Analyses showed that bonding (BO),

Tab. 7.4: Multiple regression analyses predicting behavioral intention to gamble (using Enter method)

Predictor	Without Controlling BIG			Controlling Initial BIG		
	R	R^2	β[a]	R	R^2	β[a]
Subscales based on primary factors						
BO			−.05*			−.03
RE			−.06**			−.06**
SC			.12**			.10**
PB			−.02			.00
EC			−.07**			−.07**
CC			−.01			−.01
BC			.02			−.01
MC			−.11**			−.09**
SD			.03			−.03
SE			.02			−.00
CPI			.07**			.06*
BF			−.05*			−.04
PI			.00			−.01
PN			−.05**			−.02
SP			−.04*			−.01
BIG at Wave 1						.26**
Model	.21	.05		.33	.11	
Subscales based on second-order factors						
CBC			.04			.02
PA			−.07**			−.04*
GPYDQ			−.16**			−.11**
PID			.02			.01
BIG at Wave 1						.27**
Model	.17	.03		.32	.10	

*$p < .05$. **$p < .01$.

[a]Standardized coefficients.

BIG: Behavioral intention to gamble; BO: bonding; RE: resilience; SC: social competence; PB: recognition for positive behavior; EC: emotional competence; CC: cognitive competence; BC: behavioral competence; MC: moral competence; SD: self-determination; SE: self-efficacy; CPI: clear and positive identity; BF: beliefs in the future; PI: prosocial involvement; PN: prosocial norms; SP: spirituality; CBC: cognitive-behavioral competencies second-order factor; PA: prosocial attributes second-order factor; GPYDQ: general positive youth development qualities second-order factor; PID: positive identity second-order factor.

resilience (RE), emotional competence (EC), moral competence (MC), prosocial norms (PN), and spirituality (SP) at Wave 1 were negatively related to intention to gamble at Wave 4. However, it is noteworthy that social competence (SC) and clear and positive identity (CPI) predicted intention to gamble in a *positive* manner.

Additional analyses were carried out to examine the relative influence of different positive youth development constructs on the changes in behavioral intention to gamble over time. For each equation, intention to gamble at Wave 4 was treated as the dependent variable and the corresponding Time 1 scores were entered in Step 1. In Step 2, different positive youth development measures were entered. Results showed that higher levels of resilience, emotional competence (EC), and moral competence (MC) at Wave 1 were associated with a drop in behavioral intention to gamble at Wave 4. However, the findings also showed that higher levels of social competence (SC) and clear and positive identity (CPI) at Wave 1 were associated with a rise in behavioral intention to gamble at Wave 4.

7.4 Discussion

The main goal of the present study was to examine the relationship between positive youth development and gambling in Chinese early adolescents. There were several unique features of this study. First, the present study is a positive response to the observation that there are few related studies in this area, particularly in the Chinese context (14). Second, because of the paucity of studies on Chinese gambling behavior, Chinese adolescents were recruited in the present study. Third, a large sample was employed in this study. Fourth, a validated assessment tool of positive youth development was employed. Finally, longitudinal data with four waves were collected. This is the first published scientific study on positive youth development and adolescent gambling in the Chinese culture.

Consistent with our expectation, the findings showed that positive youth development predicted adolescent intention to gamble and its change over time. Theoretically speaking, there are models proposing that a higher level of positive youth development should be related to a lower level of problem gambling. For example, Victor Frankl's logotherapy would predict that a higher level of life meaning would be related to a lower level of adolescent problem behavior. In the self theories (e.g., theory proposed by Carl Rogers), it is also commonly hypothesized that higher self-concept is related to fewer adolescent developmental problems. Finally, positive youth development constructs can be regarded as protective factors inhibiting the development of problem behavior, as proposed in the resilience literature on risk and protective factors (8).

The present findings are also consistent with the observation that positive youth development was negatively associated with problem behavior, such as substance abuse and delinquency. For example, according to Catalano et al.'s review (5) on 25 well-evaluated positive youth development programs, about three-quarters of the programs increased adolescents' positive behavior and almost all programs reduced adolescent delinquency. Based on the present and previous findings, the possibility of launching positive youth development programs to tackle adolescent problem behavior should be considered. The basic argument is that by strengthening the competencies of adolescents, the development of adolescent problem behavior will be inhibited.

To our surprise, the present findings showed that both social competence (SC) and clear and positive identity (CPI) were *positively* related to intention to gamble over time. There are several explanations for this observation. First, higher social competence does not necessarily mean that young people understand the problems of gambling. In fact, with good social competence, they may get support from their friends to gamble. Second, better self-concept may mean more self-confidence, which will motivate young people to gamble. Finally, higher scores in these two constructs may simply mean psychosocial maturity, which may motivate young people to try what adults are doing (i.e. intention to gamble is not problem gambling). Nevertheless, as the effect size of the beta values of these two constructs is not high, further studies should be conducted to replicate the findings.

A survey of the literature shows that there are many intervention programs that have utilized positive youth development constructs. For example, Guerra and Williams (15) described a multi-year project in which an integrated health promotion and prevention program was developed, implemented, and evaluated. In the project, five core competencies for healthy youth development were emphasized, including positive identity (positive self-concept, hopefulness, future goals), personal agency (self-efficacy, effective coping, locus of control, attributional style), self-regulation (affective, behavioral, and cognitive self-regulation, impulse control), social relationship skills (social problem-solving skills, empathy, conflict resolution, capacity for intimacy), and prosocial system of beliefs (attitudes, norms, values, moral engagement). As pointed out by Dickson, Derevensky and Gupta (16), "despite increased awareness of the need to begin educating young children about the potential dangers of gambling, empirical knowledge of the prevention of adolescent gambling and its translation into science-based prevention initiatives is scarce" (p. 97). Therefore, it is worthwhile to examine how positive youth development constructs can help to prevent gambling problem in adolescents.

There are several limitations of the present study. First, although the present study was based on a large sample collected in the Hong Kong Chinese context, the generalizability and replicability of the findings should be further examined. Second, it is noteworthy that as the amount of variance explained in the various models was not high, there is a need to take into account the influence of other factors as well. Third, as the data were collected by students' self-reporting, the possibility that the statistically significant findings were due to social desirability and self-serving biases exists. Despite these limitations, the present study demonstrates that positive youth development plays a role in intention to gamble in Chinese adolescents. The present findings represent an important advance in the literature on positive youth development, particularly in the Chinese context. In particular, the findings related to social competence and clear and positive identity demand replication and further exploration.

Acknowledgements

Preparation of this chapter and the Project P.A.T.H.S. were financially supported by The Hong Kong Jockey Club Charities Trust.

References

1. Gupta R, Derevensky JL. Adolescents with gambling problems: From research to treatment. J Gambl Stud 2000;16:315–42.
2. Damon W. What is positive youth development? Ann Am Acad Pol Soc Sci 2004;591:13–24.
3. Pittman KJ, Irby M, Tolman J, Yohalem N, Ferber T. Preventing problems, promoting development, encouraging engagement: Competing priorities or inseparable goals? The Forum for Youth Investment. 2003 Mar 1; [about 38 screens]. http://www.forumforyouthinvestment.org/preventproblems.pdf
4. Lerner RM, Dowling EM. Positive youth development: Thriving as the basis of personhood and civil society. In: Taylor CS, von Eye A, eds. Pathways to positive development among diverse youth. San Francisco: Jossey-Bass; 2002:11–34.
5. Catalano RF, Berglund ML, Ryan JAM, Lonczak HS, Hawkins JD. Positive youth development in the United States: Research findings on evaluations of positive youth development programs. Ann Am Acad Pol Soc Sci 2004;591:98–124.
6. Lent RW. Toward a unifying theoretical and practical perspective on well-being and psychosocial adjustment. J Consult Psychol 2004;51:482–509.
7. Sun RCF, Shek DTL. Life satisfaction, positive youth development, and problem behaviour among Chinese adolescents in Hong Kong. Soc Indic Res 2010;95:455–74.
8. Jessor R, Turbin MS, Costa FM, Dong Q, Zhang H, Wang C. Adolescent problem behavior in China and the United States: A cross-national study of psychosocial protective factors. J Res Adolesc 2003;13:329–60.
9. Shek DTL, Yiu ITL, Chan EML, eds. Inaugural Asian Pacific Problem Gambling Conference 2005: Conference Proceedings. Hong Kong: Tung Wah Group Hospitals, Soc Welfare Pract Res Centre, Chinese Univ Hong Kong; 2005.
10. Shek DTL. Effectiveness of the Tier 1 Program of Project P.A.T.H.S.: Findings based on the first 2 years of program implementation. ScientificWorldJournal 2009;9:539–47.
11. Shek DTL, Sun RCF. Development, implementation and evaluation of a holistic positive youth development program: Project P.A.T.H.S. in Hong Kong. Int J Disabil Hum Dev 2009;8:107–17.
12. Shek DTL, Siu AMH, Lee TY. The Chinese Positive Youth Development Scale: A validation study. Res Soc Work Pract 2007;17:380–91.
13. Shek DTL, Ma CMS. Dimensionality of the Chinese Positive Youth Development Scale: Confirmatory factor analyses. Soc Indic Res 2010;98:41–59.
14. Shek DTL, Chan YK, Lee PSN. Quality of life in the global context: A Chinese response. Soc Indic Res 2005;71:1–10.
15. Guerra NG, Williams KR. Implementation of school-based wellness centres. Psychol Sch 2003;40:473–87.
16. Dickson LM, Derevensky JL, Gupta R. The prevention of gambling problems in youth: A conceptual framework. J Gambl Stud 2002;18:97–159.

Technological changes in youth gambling

8 Remote gambling in adolescence

Mark D. Griffiths, Jonathan Parke, and Jeffrey L. Derevensky

Remote gambling, particularly via the Internet, continues to grow at an unprecedented rate. Though economic uncertainly and legal impediments still remain in some jurisdictions, the number of countries regulating and/or operating sites continues to rapidly increase. The widespread social acceptance of gambling in general, and the adoption of technological advances associated with the Internet and mobile phones are likely to have been important contributing factors in gambling's growth and popularity. Yet, remote gambling in general, and in particular how it impacts young people, remains a relatively under-researched area. Our current knowledge remains in its infancy and the prevalence rates remain relatively low (1), but policy experts, researchers, and clinicians are predicting greater involvement among youth as more countries legalize, license, or operate this form of gambling and alternative methods of payment are developed.

8.1 Introduction

This chapter provides a review of the relevant literature relating to remote gambling, with a particular emphasis on Internet gambling among youth. The chapter comprises five sections: (a) the empirical studies on adolescent Internet gambling, (b) online gambling-like experiences during adolescence, (c) adolescent gambling via social networking sites, (d) adolescent gambling via online penny auction sites, and (e) adolescent gambling via the use of mobile phones. Age verification in relation to prevention and regulation are also briefly examined. A cautionary note is important when examining the research in this chapter. The studies presented vary in terms of the methodological procedures used to collect data, cultural and geographical differences, and the year the data was collected, all of which likely influences their results.

8.2 Background

There is little doubt that youth gambling prevalence rates in most jurisdictions have increased as availability, accessibility, and social acceptance have risen (2). On an international level, gambling has become normalized and widely accepted. As such, it should come as no great surprise that it is viewed as a popular form of entertainment for adolescents and adults alike. The proliferation of both land-based and Internet gambling continues at an unprecedented rate. Studies on youth gambling in more traditional, non-online, settings generally reveal that the predominant reasons for engaging in this behavior are for entertainment and enjoyment, excitement and to make money (3). Though questions as to the effectiveness of legal statutes prohibiting underage gamblers from accessing government-regulated forms of gambling (e.g., lottery playing, casinos, electronic gambling machines) have been raised, procedures are in fact in place to limit accessibility. Nevertheless, there is ample evidence that youth are engaged in both regulated and nonregulated forms of gambling.

Gambling via online gambling sites takes many different forms, whether wagering on more traditional types of gambling (e.g., sports events, casino-style games, poker, bingo, lotteries, skill-based activities, betting exchanges, etc.) or nontraditional activities (e.g., the outcome of a political race, spelling bee contest, hot dog eating contest, nomination of Supreme Court judges, winners of reality shows, personal academic performance, celebrity marriages, whether celebrities will become incarcerated and locations of where they will adopt a child, etc.). An examination of the activities found on Internet gambling sites reveals significant diversity, to appeal to any age group, gender, and cultural group.

Internet gambling, though similar in many ways to land-based forms of gambling, has notable features that make it highly appealing. Motivations for engaging in online gambling include convenience, availability, ease of access, multiple games, entertainment, enjoyment, excitement, anonymity, and privacy (4–8). Other less frequently reported reasons include an aversion to the clientele and atmosphere of land-based venues and the ability to assume opposite sex roles (8, 9). A disturbing trend among youth seems to suggest that Internet gambling is now perceived to be a functional way to relieve boredom (7, 10).

Given online gambling's popularity, are youth particularly vulnerable to Internet gambling? An early national Internet gambling prevalence survey of 2,098 people in the United Kingdom (119 adolescents; aged 15 to 19 years) by Griffiths (11) suggested that at that time no teenagers reported gambling on the Internet, but 4% of teenagers indicated they would like to try online gambling. There is little doubt that this generation of youth have spent most of their lives embracing the Internet for multiple reasons (e.g., education, purchasing items, acquiring information, playing games, etc.). Gambling can best be viewed as just one extension of its use.

There is a growing body of adult research suggesting that Internet gambling may be problematic. Such findings have been made in nationally representative adult surveys (12, 13) and those of young adults (7), with children and adolescents commonly thought to be more susceptible and vulnerable in terms of developing a gambling problem (3, 14). The question remains, will Internet gambling result in increased problem gambling prevalence rates? This is a serious concern among policymakers, legislators, regulators, public health officials, and treatment providers.

8.3 Empirical studies on adolescent Internet gambling

Though virtually all Internet gambling sites have some age restrictions, the enforcement of these restrictions is highly variable. An early study in the United Kingdom found that a 16-year-old was able to place bets online on 81% (30 out of 37) sites tested and a European survey reported that 17% of visitors to online gambling sites were under the age of 18 (15, 16). Among a sample of online gamblers, there was widespread belief that underage players are gambling online and several participants in their focus groups reported noticing fellow gamblers soliciting help for their homework via chat boxes (17). Early studies of online gambling have suggested that in spite of legal or social responsibility prohibitions, many online gambling sites fail to provide stringent age checks, age verification procedures, and the enforcement of age restrictions (18). There are further suggestions that though the current situation has improved considerably as a result of regulatory provisions of Internet gambling sites in some jurisdictions, age verification procedures are often limited at best, with many sites not having any verification procedures in place. Online gambling by underage minors remains of significant concern. Furthermore, it has been noted that the distinction between gambling and video gaming is becoming ever more blurred and that gaming convergence is widespread (19–22). For example, many gaming sites incorporate technology similar to video games, have similar graphic features, and offer rewards in the form of "tokens" or "credits," which gamblers can exchange for a monetary prize.

Given the concern among policymakers and clinicians it is surprising that there have only been a limited number of studies examining youth Internet gambling. The following review focuses on studies examining the impact of Internet gambling on adolescents and young adults. Brunelle and her colleagues (23, 24) carried out a study comparing the profiles of young nongamblers, gamblers, and Internet gamblers in relation to severity of substances use (25), impulsivity, and risk taking among Quebec adolescents. They surveyed 1,876 high school students (46% male; 54% female), aged 14 to 18 years (mean = 15.4 years), and reported that 93.5% of adolescents (95% male; 92% female) reported having gambled in the previous 12 months, with 8% (13% males; 3% females) having gambled on the Internet during the same time period. They also reported that 35% of youth (49% males; 21% females) had played the "free play"/"demo" mode on Internet gambling sites. Males were significantly more likely than females to gamble in general, gamble on the Internet, and play the 'free play' modes on Internet gambling sites. Using the DSM-IV-J, 3% of their participants were found to be problem gamblers. They also found significantly more problem gamblers among those individuals reporting gambling on the Internet (11%) compared to those who did not gamble on the Internet (1.5%), with no gender differences found for any type of problem gambling. Further findings revealed that nearly 7% of the participants had a substance use problem and that those with problematic substance use were also more likely to be Internet gamblers (4% nongamblers, 8% gamblers, 18% Internet gamblers) (see ▶Tab. 8.1). In relation to impulsivity, Internet gamblers and non-Internet gamblers had significantly higher scores on measures of impulsivity and risk-taking than nongamblers. As expected, problem gamblers also had significantly higher scores on impulsivity and risk taking than nonproblem gamblers.

Using the same data set, Brunelle and her colleagues (23, 24) examined some of the contextual elements surrounding Internet gambling among adolescents. They explored the types of Internet games, Internet gambling initiation contexts, and Internet gambling contexts in general (e.g., when, where, with whom, how long, etc.). Of the 137 Internet gamblers, only 0.8% had regularly played for money at an online casino, whereas 1.9% had regularly played for money on online poker sites (see ▶Tab. 8.2). However, the 'play for free' modes were played more regularly in both online casinos (8.9%) and online poker (13.8%; see ▶Tab. 8.2). The results revealed that 37% of online gambling was done primarily with friends, 34% with an immediate family member, 23% with other family members, 2% alone, and 4% with others.

Brunelle and her colleagues (23, 24) in a qualitative examination interviewed 37 adolescent online gamblers and reported that the primary types of online gambling carried out were poker, blackjack, electronic gambling (slot) machines, bingo, and

Tab. 8.1: Substance use by gamblers, Internet gamblers, and nongamblers (n = 1,876) (adapted from Brunelle, Gendron, et al., 2009)

Type of substance use	Nongambler (%)	Gambler (%)	Lifetime Internet gambler (%)
Alcohol**	76.9	91.3	96.3
Tobacco**	26.3	42.6	51.5
Cannabis**	26.8	40.6	55.1
Hallucinogens**	5.4	10.0	12.5
Speed	6.3	13.1	19.9
Cocaine**	1.0	3.8	5.9
Solvents	0.2	1.0	1.5
Heroin*	0.6	1.0	3.7

Comparison between gamblers and nongamblers: *p < 0.05. **p < 0.001.

Tab. 8.2: Types of Internet games played in the last 12 months (n = 137) (adapted from Brunelle, Cousineau, Dufour, et al., 2009)

	Never (%)	Once (%)	Occasionally (%)	Regularly (%)
Internet casino (for money)	95.4	2.3	1.5	0.8
Internet casino ("free play" mode)	75.2	8.5	7.4	8.9
Internet poker (for money)	94.7	1.7	1.7	1.9
Intenet poker ("free play" mode)	71.9	8.0	8.0	13.8

sports betting. Most of the gambling was done either at home or in school, but because the vast majority was played in the evening it is unlikely that playing at school was highly prevalent. Those who played for more than two hours at a time were most likely to engage in this behavior on their own, whereas playing socially with others was more likely to be done for much less time per session. Most online gamblers found the atmosphere exciting and pleasant (rather than stressful or serious). Brunelle and her colleagues concluded that (a) poker was the most popular form of online gambling, (b) adolescent online gamblers were more likely to be problem gamblers compared with those who did not gamble online, (c) most initiation of online gambling took place with family members, (d) most adolescent online gamblers began by playing in the "free play" mode, and (e) for many adolescents, online gambling was a way to make money, occupied them when they had nothing else to do, and allowed them to socialize. Two points are noteworthy: (a) Internet gambling was done on offshore sites and (b) all students were underage.

Olason and his colleagues (26, 27) reported two studies examining gambling behavior among Icelandic adolescents that included questions relating to Internet gambling. The first in-class study comprised 1,513 adolescents aged 16 to 18 years (730 males; 783 females). The second school-based study comprised 1,537 adolescents aged 13 to 18 years (768 males; 747 females). The surveys included questions relating to gambling on Icelandic Internet Web sites (lotto, sports pools, sports betting) and on foreign Web sites (poker, casino games, sports betting, and 'free play' modes). In addition to assessing their gambling behavior, students completed the DSM-IV-MR-J (28), a gambling screen assessing severity of gambling and gambling-related problems.

With respect to participation, Olason (26) reported that in the first study, 62% of the participants had gambled, 11% were regular gamblers, 20% had gambled on the Internet, and just under 4% were regular Internet gamblers. In the second study, 57% of the participants had gambled, 8% were regular gamblers, 24% had gambled on the Internet, and just over 4% were regular Internet gamblers. ▶Tab. 8.3 outlines in more detail the findings in relation to Internet gambling. In both studies, males were significantly more likely than females to gamble on the Internet (32% boys vs. 9% girls in study I; 37% boys vs. 11.5% girls in study II). The results in relation to problem gambling revealed a prevalence rate of 3% problem gambling in the first study and 2.2% in the second study. However, among those who had gambled on the Internet, the problem gambling prevalence rates were significantly higher, 10.1% and 7.5% respectively. The results also revealed that 11.5% of the adolescents had used their own personal credit card, 23.1% had used their personal debit card, 15.4% had used a parents' credit card, and 50% had used another method of payment (e.g., brother's credit card, loans from friends, electronic cash, PayPal, Neteller, bonus money, etc.).

In the United Kingdom, Griffiths and Wood (29) surveyed 8,017 young people between 12 and 15 years of age about their Internet gambling behavior. Like the studies

Tab. 8.3: Types of games played on the Internet by Icelandic adolescents (adapted from Olason, 2009)

	Study 1: Regular Gamblers (n = 1,513)	Study 1: Total Gamblers (n = 1,513)	Study 2: Regular Gamblers (n = 1,537)	Study 2: Total Gamblers (n = 1,537)
Icelandic Web sites				
Lotto	0.6	2.4	0.5	8.7
Sports pools	0.7	3.4	0.9	8.5
Sports betting	0.8	2.9	1.2	6.2
Foreign Web sites				
Online poker	0.6	1.9	1.8	6.5
Casino games	2.2	15.8	1.8	12.3
Sports betting	–	–	0.5	1.9
"Free play" modes	3.3	28	–	–

by Olason and his colleagues (27), their survey included the DSM-IV-MR-J screen to identify problematic gambling behavior. The study examined remote gambling in relation to use of the National Lottery products online. Adolescents were asked "Have you ever played any National Lottery game on the Internet?" Those who reported having gambled on the Internet were also asked "Which, if any, of the following games have you played in the past 7 days?" Students were presented with the following options: (a) instant win games for money, (b) free instant win games, (c) lotto, and (d) one of the other lottery draw games. Those who had experience of gambling online were also asked how they accessed and played the National Lottery games on the Internet (the minimum age for gambling was 16). The following options were presented: (a) the system let me register, (b) I played along with my parents, (c) another adult let me play, (d) I used my parent's/guardian's online National Lottery account with their permission, (e) I used my parent's/guardian's online National Lottery account without their permission, and (f) played free games.

The results revealed that approximately one in twelve young people (8%), age 12 to 15 years, reported having played a National Lottery game via the Internet. Boys were more likely than girls to endorse playing the National Lottery games via the Internet (10% vs. 6%), as were young people who were Asian and black. Not surprisingly, young people identified as "problem gamblers" on the DSM-IV-MR-J were more likely than "social gamblers" to have played a National Lottery game on the Internet (37% compared with 9%). Of those who had gambled on the Internet, a quarter of the adolescents revealed they had played free instant win games (24%), nearly one in five had played instant win games for money (19%) or the Lotto (18%), and 10% had played another draw. Problem gamblers were more likely to have played every game in the past week, compared with social gamblers, who were less likely to recall the games they played during the same time period. Young people with parents who approved of their gambling were more likely to have played online instant win games for money (35% vs. 19%), Lotto (40% vs. 15%), or other draw games (22% vs. 6%). Not surprisingly, the results clearly suggest that youth with parental consent were more likely to gamble online.

Griffiths and Wood (29) also noted that among youth who gambled online, 29% reported playing free games, 18% reported that the system let them register, 16% played along with their parents, 10% used their parent's online National Lottery account either with their permission (10%), or without (7%). However, it should be noted that one third of online players reported they "couldn't remember" (35%) the method used for payment. Overall, among all young people (not just players), 2% played National Lottery games online with their parents and 2% had played independently without their parents. Those who played independently are most likely to have played free games, with just 0.3% of young people having played National Lottery games on their own for money. More recently, Ipsos MORI (30) in a survey of 8,598 students, aged 11–15 years, from 201 schools reported that overall, 1% of youth had gambled on the Internet for money in the past week.

In the United States, Welte, Barnes, Tidwell, and Hoffman (31) assessed the relationship between specific types of gambling and the extent of problem gambling reported by American adolescents and young adults using data from the National Survey of Youth and Gambling, comprising 2,274 youth age 14–21 years. They reported that 2% of respondents (3% males; 0% females) reported gambling online in the past twelve months, with respondents having gambled online an average of 48 days per year. They also noted that 65% of respondents who gambled on the Internet reported having at least one symptom on the South Oaks Gambling Screen Revised for Adolescents (SOGS-RA) (32), which again was the highest of the 15 forms of gambling being considered. Statistical analyses revealed that when participating in other forms of gambling was controlled, the link between Internet gambling and problem gambling among youth was no longer significant. In other words, they concluded that young Internet gamblers were likely to experience more problem gambling symptoms by virtue of gambling on multiple gambling activities as opposed to the properties of Internet gambling itself.

A more recent report by the Annenberg Foundation suggests that despite efforts by the U.S. government to impose restrictions on Internet gambling, college age youth have little difficulty accessing online gambling sites. Based on the latest National Annenberg Survey of Youth, monthly use of Internet gambling sites dramatically increased from 4.4% to 16.0% between 2008 and 2010 (33). Projecting onto the national sample, the results suggest that more than 400,000 young adult males between age 18 and 22 gamble on Internet gaming sites at least weekly. Rates among adolescent males are considerably lower but they report a significant number accessing gambling sites monthly. Though card playing remains the predominant online gambling activity, it is suggested that youth are engaged in multiple forms of online gambling. Even though the overall rate of increase in Internet gambling was not as pronounced for females, the rates tripled for female adolescents (0.5% in 2008 to 1.5% in 2010) and increased fourfold for young female adults (0% in 2008 to 4.4% in 2010).

An early study in Canada by Byrne and Messerlian, Byrne, and Derevensky (34, 35) of 2,087 adolescents and young adults found that more adolescents (under the age of 18 years) than 18 to 24-year-olds played "free play" games on Internet gambling sites (43% vs. 33% for males; 42% vs. 29% for females). The most popular form of "free play" activity for both groups was card playing (poker and blackjack), with less frequent gamblers (i.e., those gambling less than once per month) playing slot machines or other forms of online gambling machines.

Over the past year, almost one in twenty (4.6%) of the participants (7.8% males; 2.3% females) had gambled online with their own money. When examined by age, those under 18 years were more likely to be male (8.6%; over 18 years 6.8%) than female (3.2%; over 18 years 1.3%). The two most popular forms of Internet gambling for youth were card playing (online poker) and sports betting, similar to the recent results reported by Romer (33). For those who gambled online for money, Byrne (34) reported that many did so with a family member (i.e., parent or older sibling). Among Internet gamblers, the prevalence rate of problem gambling was almost 19%. Although very high, similar rates of problem gambling prevalence among self-selected samples have been reported by other research studies on youth gambling (5, 8, 36, 37). Though Byrne reported no significant gender differences, she noted that the younger the person gambling online, the more likely they were to exhibit problem gambling.

Meerkemper (38), in a recent survey of 569 Canadian youth (age 15–18 years) reported 8% had gambled online with their own money, with most reporting using personal savings (63%), previous winnings (30%), PayPal account (16%), loans from friends or family members (16%), a personal credit card (7%), or parents' credit card (5%) to fund their playing behavior.

In addition to the studies of Byrne (34) and Meerkamper (38), there have also been some smaller more locally based studies conducted in Canada. For instance, Meerkamper (39) reported that more than one in twenty teenagers in Nova Scotia aged 15 to 17 years reported playing online poker for money. Poulin and Elliot (40) reported that in the past year, 4.2% of adolescents had gambled for money online in Atlantic Canada, and in Montreal, almost one in ten teenagers (9%) reported having gambled online for money (10). A summary of the main findings of multiple current surveys concerning online gambling can be found in ▶Tab. 8.4. As can be seen in the table, males are significantly more likely to gamble online when compared to females.

Tab. 8.4: Summary of main findings of studies investigating online gambling in youth

Researcher (Year)	Country	Age (Number)	Prevalence of Online Gambling; Gender Differences	Problem Gambling
Byrne (2004)	Canada	16–24 years (n = 2,087)	4.6% past year; 7.8% male/2.3% female	Prevalence rate of problem gambling in Internet gamblers was almost 19%.
Griffiths and Wood (2007)	UK	12–15 years (n = 8,017)	8% past year; 10% male/6% female	Problem gamblers more likely than social gamblers to gamble on the Internet (37% vs. 9%).
Welte et al. (2009)	USA	14–21 years (n = 2,274)	2% past year; 3% male/0% female	Internet gamblers were likely to experience more problem-gambling symptoms by virtue of gambling on more forms of gaming, as opposed to the properties of Internet gambling itself.
Olason (2009)	Iceland	16–18 years (n = 1,513)	20% ever; 4% regularly; 32% male/9% female	Problem gambling among gamblers was 3%. Among Internet gamblers it was significantly higher at 10.1%.
Olason et al. (2010)	Iceland	13–18 years (n = 1,537)	24% ever; 4% regularly; 37% male/11.5% female	Problem gambling among gamblers was 2.2%. Among Internet gamblers it was significantly higher at 7.5%.
Ipsos MORI (2009)	UK	11–15 years (n = 8,598)	1% past week	Not reported.
Brunelle et al. (2009)	Canada	14–18 years (n = 1,876)	8% past year; 13% male/3% female	Significantly more Internet gamblers (11%) were likely to be problem gamblers than those who did not gamble on the Internet (1.5%).
Meerkamper (2010)	Canada	15–21 years (n = 1,000)	8% past year	Not reported.

8.4 Online gambling-like experiences among adolescents

Over the last decade, there have been a number of published reports examining gambling-like experiences engaged in by adolescents, including instant win games in children's snacks such as crisps and chocolate (41), and money-free gambling that could include "free play," "practice," and "demo" games on Internet gambling sites (29). North American studies have reported that anywhere between 25% and 50% of teenagers have played "free play" games on Internet gambling sites (7, 10, 23, 34, 40). In the study by Griffiths and Wood (29) outlined earlier, of the 8% of youth who had gambled online, a quarter (24%) of respondents reported they had played free instant win games.

Ipsos MORI (30) reported that 28% of their sample of youth ($N = 8,598$) in the United Kingdom had participated in money-free gambling of some sort in the week preceding the survey. As depicted in ▶Fig. 8.1, just over a quarter of adolescents had played in "money-free mode" in the week preceding the survey, with opportunities on the social networking sites four or five times more popular than those presented on actual gambling sites. Using statistical modeling to further examine the same data, Forrest and colleagues (42) reported that gambling in money-free modes was the single most important predictor of whether the adolescent had gambled for money, and was one of the most important predictors of problem gambling. However, it should be noted that this relationship is correlational and not necessarily causal. The possibility and extent to which money-free gambling is responsible for actual gambling participation and gambling-related risk and harm needs to be confirmed through longitudinal research. Ipsos MORI (30) also found that those youth who reported being male, having a black or white ethnic background, earning or receiving £30 in the last week, and having parents who were gamblers were all significantly more likely to have gambled in money-free mode in the specified time period.

Meerkamper (38) reported that 33% of 388 underage minors (aged 15 to 18 years) had reported having gambled online using the "free play" modes and/or via online social networking sites. Reasons suggested for playing online free (gambling) games were to relieve boredom (59%), for fun (49%), for the excitement (thrill) (15%), because their friends play (14%), and because it was perceived to be a good way to improve their skills before they start to play with real money. A significant minority (22%) also reported they played because it was easily accessible on a social networking site (e.g., Facebook). The survey also asked what the adolescents had learned from playing online for free. The most popular responses were that they learned how to manage risk (24%), learned how to play better (18%), had increased confidence by playing (10%), and it had prepared them for playing online with money. It was also reported that 8% of these youth had been invited to gamble for real money while playing in the free play mode.

A number of clinical researchers have asserted that youth gambling in money-free mode may be a cause for significant concern (3, 9, 10, 29, 35, 43). It has been alleged that such opportunities encourage teenagers to practice before "graduating" to playing for money games at online casinos (44) and that a "precautionary principle" should be applied that prevents adolescents from being exposed to gambling-like experiences (45). However, the specific impact of money-free play remains unclear. Despite the strong correlation of money-free play with both gambling participation and problem gambling (42), there is currently no conclusive evidence to suggest that money-free play causes individuals to start gambling for actual money or to be more at risk of experiencing

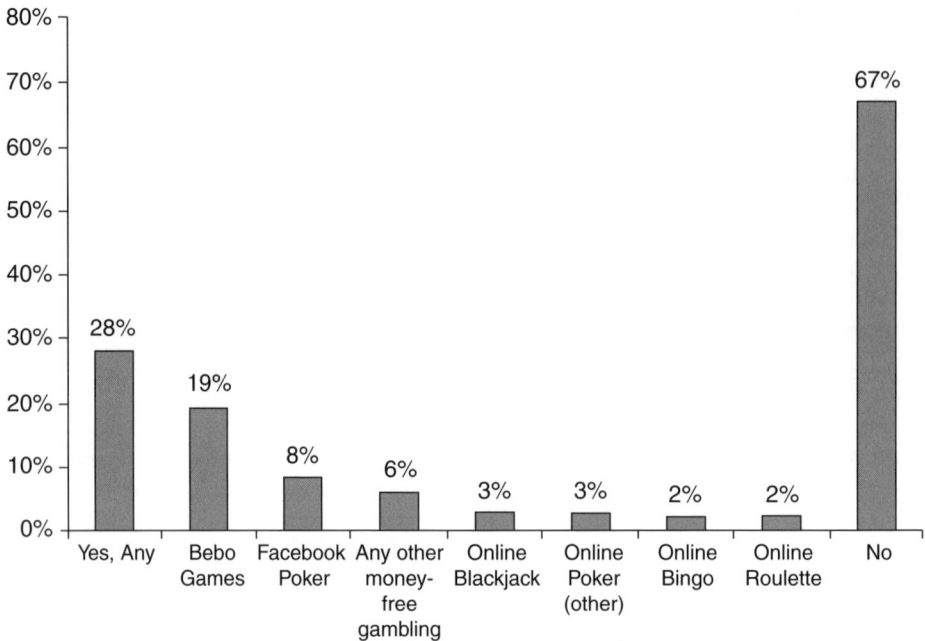

Fig. 8.1: Money-free gambling in the last 7 days (adapted from Ipsos MORI 2009)

gambling-related harm, although there is a growing body of correlational evidence. Clearly, with the growing popularity of such sites, further research is warranted.

The use of "free play" sites is not the only type of online gambling-like experience in which adolescents can now engage. Griffiths, King, and Delfabbro (46) identified other types of gambling-like experiences including gambling via social networking sites and gambling via online penny auction sites.

8.4.1 Adolescent gambling via social networking sites

Across the world, the social networking phenomenon has spread rapidly. Despite the fact that the minimum age for most major social networking sites is usually 13 years (and 14 years on MySpace), a study by the Office of Communications (47) in the United Kingdom reported that just over a quarter (27%) of 8- to 11-year-olds who are aware of social networking sites said that they had a profile on a social networking site. A recent report by Meerkamper (38) revealed that poker groups have grown exponentially since Facebook's inception and that they have become the number one favorite sites among Facebook users. The most popular social networking site used by children was Bebo (63%).

Recently, Downs (48) noted that content-generated risks from this new leisure activity have not been investigated in any detail, yet young people using these sites are able to easily gain access to gambling activities. Downs claimed that the potential of social networking sites to "normalize" gambling behaviors may change the social understandings and perceptions of the role of gambling among young people. For example, while socially responsible gambling emphasizes that money spent gambling may not offer a return other than the pleasure gained from the game, the social networking utilities can present gambling as a viable route for the acquisition of scarce virtual goods. According to Downs' pilot research, there were 25 poker applications on *Bebo* (and over 500 separate poker groups) and in excess of 100 poker applications on *Facebook* (and over 1,000 separate poker groups). These poker sites featured some with real prizes, others with cash-play options, and all easily downloadable by underage minors along with many free trial games. The largest of these poker groups had in excess of several thousand members and in one group surveyed, 15% of those in the group declared they were under the age of 18 years. Furthermore, gambling applications typically contain sidebar advertisements and hyperlinks to actual gambling sites.

Downs (48) also reported a type of pseudo-gambling among "Fluff Friends" that has over 100,000 active users monthly. In this social networking forum, users (typically young girls) create "Fluff Art." To do this they have to earn "munny"—a type of virtual money through pet racing. Pet racing costs 1 point per race and winnings can be up to 4,000 points. Though there is no actual money exchanged, it has been argued that young children are learning the mechanics of gambling, and Downs asserts there are serious questions about whether gambling with virtual money encourages enhanced positive attitudes toward gambling in young people. For instance, does gambling with virtual money lead to an increased prevalence of actual gambling? She also asks to what extent are gambling-related groups on social networking sites being used by underage minors (under 18 years) and whether membership within such groups facilitates access to commercial gambling sites. It also seems only natural for youth to question whether they should gamble on Internet sites if they were winning "play money" (49).

8.4.2 Adolescent gambling via online penny auction sites

Another gambling-like activity is participation in online penny auctions such as "Madbid," "Swoopo," "Bid Boogie," "Rapid Bargain," and "Budson" (50). In order to participate in online penny auctions, the individual needs to place a bid on an ongoing auction site. Bids can only be made in one penny (or one Euro cent) increments. This can be done by (a) placing a bid via a text message from a mobile phone (at £1.50 or €1.50 a bid plus operator's costs), or (b) placing a bid through the creation of an online account, where the person purchases a "bundle" of bids (at 75 pence/75 cents to £1.40/€1.40 a bid depending on how big a bundle they buy in advance). To bid by text message, a person sends a message with the code for the specific product that they want to bid on. There is no limit to how many bids can be submitted on the same auction product and no limit on how many different products can be bid on at any one time. For example, Griffiths (50) noted a PlayStation videogame console (retail price of £310) was recently won in a penny auction for £8.34. To the winner of the auction this was won at a hugely discounted price. However, what this really means is that there were 834 separate bids for this item, all costing up to £1.50 per bid (depending whether it was done online or via mobile phone). Looking at the "bid history," most of the final 50 bids were made by just two individuals, who at a minimum spent at least £30 in their final bids trying to secure the item. Although one person won the console, the other person spent a considerable amount of money and received nothing in return. Griffiths (50) has argued that this is a form of Internet gambling under another name. Anyone with a mobile phone (e.g., the vast majority of teenagers) can participate in such an activity, and it could be argued that many of the items in the auctions appeal particularly to teenage audiences (video game consoles, MP3 players, laptops, iPads, tablets, etc.). To what extent this new form of online activity with gambling-like experiences is impacting youth is as yet undetermined, but this is an area where further research is needed.

8.5 Adolescent gambling via mobile phone

The mobile phone industry has grown rapidly over the past decade. The number of international mobile phone users is already thought to have passed the two billion mark, with many people giving up their traditional land lines (51). At present, though Internet gambling lends itself most naturally to casino-style games such as slot machines, blackjack, roulette, poker, these games require more in the form of graphics, sounds, and interactivity. These types of gambling are not ideal for mobile devices but have now been introduced on some of the latest mobile phone applications (51). In various parts of Europe (the United Kingdom, Germany, Sweden, Austria, Holland) individuals can purchase national lottery tickets and wager on sports via their mobile phones (this has also recently been approved in Nevada). Market research suggests that Asia will become the largest market segment for mobile phone gambling, reaching $6.7 billion in 2011 (52). However, market research by Gartner (53) reported 2009 global mobile gambling revenues already to be $4.7 billion, and forecast $5.6 billion for 2010 and $11.4 billion by 2014.

At present, it is unlikely that mobile phone graphics and technology can compete with Internet web browsers (although the technology is improving all the time). Intuitively, Griffiths (51) argues that mobile phone gambling is best suited for sports and event betting. With mobile phone betting, all that is required is real-time access to data about the event (e.g., a horse race, a football match), and the ability to make a bet in a timely fashion. However, the limiting aspects of the technological and protocol demands of mobile gambling (graphics, sound, and visual displays) are largely being resolved through technological advances. Like Internet gambling, mobile phone gambling has completely changed the way some people think about betting. Mobile phones provide the convenience of making bets or gambling from wherever the person is located. This will be further increased by iPads, Playbooks, and so on, with enhanced graphics and cell phone and Internet capability.

There is a paucity of reliable data about mobile gambling, although the latest British Gambling Prevalence Survey reported that 4% of British adults (aged 16 years and over) had bet via phone in the previous week of the survey (54). Statistics collated by the British Gambling Commission (55) reported that 2.8% of British adults had gambled via their mobile phone. However, to date, no empirical research has been carried out into mobile phone gambling by adolescents, although anecdotal evidence suggests that this is not yet an activity that many youth engage in. Press reports have claimed older age adolescents are using their mobile phones to place bets on sporting events, but such speculation has not been substantiated empirically. As with all new forms of technological gambling, ease of use is paramount to success. In the early days of mobile phones, programming the phone to use various protocols was very difficult. However, mobile phones are becoming increasingly user-friendly, with many adolescents already downloading free and commercially available applications from service provider stores. More and more Internet gaming operators are creating "apps" for easy access.

Griffiths (51) claims that gambling companies think mobile gambling via smart phones is likely to attract a younger audience of gamblers. In fact, some companies are deliberately targeting the under-16 market with mobile phones specially designed for them, although they are not targeting gambling per se. This is certainly an area that needs to be monitored and empirically researched. Age restrictions will be difficult to monitor and enforce. However, the gaming industry claims one way to tackle underage use is through a pre-paid card system. Pre-pay systems are bound by the same security and accounting best practices currently employed within land-based casinos. This may potentially minimize problem gambling and prevent access to minors because its distribution is controlled by the operator.

8.6 Conclusions

Though there is some variation in participation rates reported in the studies considered in this review, the limited number of surveys reveal that a small but significant minority of adolescents can and do gamble via the Internet. Studies relating to mobile phone gambling have yet to be carried out. Several of the studies reported a past year Internet gambling prevalence rate of approximately 4% (34, 39, 40), though some reported a lower figure (2%) (31) and others report the rate as being considerably higher (e.g., 8%, [38, 56]; 9% [10]; and 20–24% [26, 27]). Interestingly, lower rates of participation were found in the United States (although the recent research by Romer [33] with a limited number of adolescents and young adults suggests significant increases) and English-speaking Canadian provinces, with higher rates being reported in Quebec and Europe.

Adolescent Internet gamblers were significantly more likely to be problem gamblers (7, 27, 56). It may be the case that problem gamblers are more susceptible and/or vulnerable to gambling online and the fact that it is easily accessible with few verification checks in place for underage gambling is a cause for concern. To make matters worse, there appears to be little concern among parents about youth gambling (57). However, it may also be that adolescent problem gamblers gravitate to the Internet, adding it as an additional mode of gambling to their general repertoire of gambling behaviors, as suggested by Wood and Williams (58). Consistent with findings reported in this review, Wood and Williams (58) reported a higher rate of problem gambling among Internet gamblers compared to non-Internet gamblers. Importantly, they noted that because other modes of gambling (other than Internet) were reported by participants as the main cause of their gambling problems, it was most likely that Internet gamblers were already heavy gamblers to begin with and that this was simply a new venue to play to complement their existing gambling activities. This is also consistent with initial conclusions by Welte and his colleagues (31) and McBride and Derevensky (7), who suggested the increased risk is the consequence of wide-ranging participation in gambling activities rather than being a direct causal link between Internet gambling and problem gambling.

Given the complexity of the available evidence, the role of remote gambling in creating adolescent problem gamblers should be treated with caution. However, it is clear that research that can help to identify the impact of remote gambling on either creating or facilitating gambling-related harm among adolescents should be made a research priority. The incidence of youth engaging in free play gambling sites is also a serious concern. As Derevensky (3) noted, this may be a training program for future gamblers. There is also clinical evidence that youth are prone to stealing their parents' credit cards to engage in this behavior. Such research should consider the potentially different roles that Internet gambling may play in creating new forms of harm and in exacerbating existing forms of harm.

Another interesting theme to emerge was that friends and family were reported to play an important role in the online gambling experience among adolescents. For example, Brunelle and colleagues (23, 24) reported that only 2% of Internet gambling was done with the adolescent playing alone. The fact that 57% of youth reported gambling with a family member and 37% with friends typifies the social acceptability and nature of Internet gambling among adolescents; an activity that has been traditionally noted as being an asocial activity. Similar findings were also reported by Griffiths and Wood (29) and Campbell et al. (57). These figures appear to be significantly different to trends among adults, with one study reporting that 59% of adult respondents indicated that they always gambled alone (59). There are two potential implications of these findings. Firstly, future research must explore the nature and the specific impact of the social processes in adolescent Internet gambling. The role of family may be particularly important in this regard. Secondly, parents clearly need to be educated about gambling (and its potential problems) in the same way as other potentially addictive behaviors (e.g., drinking, smoking, drug taking, etc.). Such findings are corroborated by both adolescent and parent studies.

With respect to regulation, there seem to be significant developments in trying to prevent underage individuals gambling online with clear licensing conditions and codes of practice being recommended, implemented, and regular compliance checks being performed for a number of sites (e.g., see guidelines by the Global Gambling Guidance Group [G4; http://www.gx4.com/], or e-Commerce Online Gaming Regulation and Assurance [e-COGRA; http://www.ecogra.org/]). However, with at least one in three regulated sites still permitting easy access to underage players, it is clear that there is still much work to be done. Some operations must tighten their age verification systems by using more sophisticated cross-referencing options and stricter criteria, even at the risk of losing customers. As well, even though there is some evidence, at least in the United Kingdom, that access to gambling online may prove more difficult relative to securing offline access, underage Internet gamblers may only need to get through the hurdles once. In other words, once an adolescent has managed to get through age verification systems and register, they can gamble again repeatedly. This differs from offline facilities, where adolescents would have to deceive the "gatekeepers" on each separate visit.

It should be emphasized that regulatory performance and compliance is only one aspect of preventing underage remote gambling. It seems that with only 23% of underage Internet gamblers using their own debit cards to register and pay for their gambling, most are being assisted in some way with their payment (i.e., using friends, family or sponsored credit cards, prepaid credit cards). In one survey, 17% of those that had played the lottery on the Internet had accessed their parents' accounts (either with or without their permission) (29). This places a significant level of responsibility with older friends and family members, either in terms of refusing assistance in accessing actual gambling opportunities or in closely monitoring the use of credit cards for which they have ultimate responsibility.

There appear to be two challenges in relation to parents preventing underage remote gambling. Firstly, parents must have the appropriate knowledge, attitudes, awareness, and intentions to prevent underage gambling. Parents may permit or assist their child as result of viewing such behavior as a harmless and/or fun activity. Secondly, even if parents are motivated to prevent underage remote gambling, they must be prepared to monitor their child's Internet and mobile phone usage, and where made available, spending on credit and debit cards and other types of accounts should be monitored. Educating parents should be one of the key components of any strategy aimed at preventing or minimizing underage remote gambling. Innovative anti-gambling software has been developed and in some jurisdictions has been offered without cost (e.g., the BetStopper program in Nova Scotia and British Columbia).

The issue of payment is perhaps one of the most important areas for further research. More work is needed to explore the relationship between underage payment mechanisms and the development of problem gambling. Derevensky (60), reporting results from a study of youth (aged 17 to 20 years), noted that 44% of youth used a personal credit card, 6% used a family member's credit card with permission, 4% used a family member's credit card without permission, 26% used a debit card, 6% used personal checks, and 27% used a wire or bank transfer to pay for their Internet wagering. What if an adolescent is gambling using someone else's credit or debit card and they are not winning or losing their own money? Will this have the same implications for developing or facilitating problem gambling? Factors that have been linked to the development and facilitation of problem gambling (e.g., the big win, chasing, arousal) could be argued to be dependent on the extent to which a gambler is winning or losing his or her own money.

Finally, there is evidence to suggest that "money-free" gambling plays a critically important role for adolescents in conceptualizing and experiencing remote gambling, particularly Internet gambling. Over one in three adolescents have been reported to gamble in a money-free mode (34, 56) with Ipsos MORI (30) reporting that 28% of 11- to 15-year-olds in a recent U.K. sample had done so within the last week. It is argued that it is through money-free gambling (using social networking sites or "demo" modes of real gambling sites) that children are being introduced to the principles and excitement of gambling without experiencing the consequences of losing actual money. Early research has shown it is significantly more commonplace to win while 'gambling' on the first few goes on a "demo" or "free play" game (49), although this is not the case for all games (e.g., U.K. National Lottery games). The same study also reported that it was commonplace for gamblers to have extended winning streaks during prolonged periods while playing in the "demo" modes. However, there have been significant regulatory developments in recent years with improved codes of practice requiring that age verification also applies to "demo modes" and that such modes should be an accurate representation of the actual playing experience including the probability of winning and the rate of return to the player (see U.K. Gambling Commission [61]).

Based on the available literature, it may be important to distinguish between the different types of money-free gambling being made available – namely social networking modes and "demo" or "free play" modes. Initial considerations suggest that these may be different both in nature and in impact. For example, as Downs (48) argues, players gambling in social networking modes may experience a different type and level of reinforcement than those gambling in "demo" mode. On some social networking sites the accumulation of "play money" or "points" may have implications for buying virtual goods or services or being eligible for certain privileges. This may increase the value and meaning of the gambling event to the individual. Second, when considering the "flow" and intention of individuals accessing such sites, it could be argued that individuals accessing money-free gambling through social networking sites may be more likely to be induced or persuaded to play given that these Web site visitors' primary intention may have been social interaction (i.e., the primary function of the Web site) in contrast to those playing in "demo" mode, where gambling is the primary function of the Web site. Interestingly, four or five times more children report playing money-free gambling on social networking sites compared to "demo" or "free play" modes on gambling Web sites. It is suggested that the nature and impact of various forms of money-free gambling should be the subject of further research and empirical investigation.

Some experts claim that "the exposure of children to gambling-like activities, games of chance with fake money, and play with materials of potential financial value should be seen as risks that need to be controlled" (45). However, to date, such individuals have failed to give an adequate explanation for the underlying reasons. No evidence or speculation are provided regarding the process by which gambling-like experiences may increase risk as opposed to moderating the risk or having no effect on potential risk.

There is ever-increasing social acceptance and multi-media integration between the Internet, mobile phones, and interactive television. Furthermore, young people are very proficient in using and accessing these media tools and are likely to be increasingly exposed to remote gambling opportunities. Of concern is the research suggesting that youth engage in many of these activities to relieve "boredom." These young people with expertise in this technology, perceived invulnerability, and belief that they are more intelligent than their adult counterparts will therefore require education and guidance to enable them to cope with the challenges of convenience gambling in all its guises. The same information also needs to be made available to parents, teachers, health professionals, and other practitioners.

References

1. Griffiths MD. Gambling addiction on the Internet. In: Young K, Nabuco de Abreu C, eds. Internet addiction: A handbook for evaluation and treatment. New York: Wiley; 2010.
2. Volberg R, Gupta R, Griffiths MD, Olason D, Delfabbro P. An international perspective on youth gambling studies. Int J Adolesc Med Health 2010;22:3–38.
3. Derevensky J. Gambling behaviors and adolescent substance use disorders. In: Kaminer Y, Buckstein OG, eds. Adolescent substance abuse: Psychiatric comorbidity and high risk behaviors. New York: Haworth Press; 2008:403–33.
4. American Gaming Association. State of the States 2006: The American Gaming Association survey of casino entertainment 2006. americangaming.org/surevy/2006/reference/ref.html.
5. Griffiths MD, Barnes A. Internet gambling: An online empirical study among student gamblers. Int J Ment Health Addict 2008;6:194–204.
6. Griffiths MD, Parke J. The social impact of Internet gambling. Soc Sci Comput Rev 2002;20:312–20.

7. McBride J, Derevensky J. Internet gambling behaviour in a sample of online gamblers. Int J Ment Health Addict 2009;7:149–67.

8. Wood R, Griffiths MD, Parke J. The acquisition, development, and maintenance of online poker playing in a student sample. Cyberpsychol Behav 2007;10:354–61.

9. Griffiths MD. Internet gambling: Issues, concerns, and recommendations. Cyberpsychol Behav 2003;6:557–68.

10. Derevensky J, Gupta R. Internet gambling amongst adolescents: A growing concern. Int J Ment Health Addict 2007;5:93–101.

11. Griffiths MD. Internet Gambling: Preliminary results of the first UK prevalence study. J Gambl Issues 2001;5.

12. Griffiths MD, Wardle J, Orford J, Sproston K, Erens B. Socio-demographic correlates of Internet gambling: Findings from the 2007 British Gambling Prevalence Survey. Cyberpsychol Behav 2009;12:199–202.

13. Griffiths MD, Wardle J, Orford J, Sproston K, Erens B. Internet gambling, health. Smoking and alcohol use: Findings from the 2007 British Gambling Prevalence Survey. Int J Ment Health Addict 2010;9:1–11.

14. Meyer G, Hayer T, Griffiths MD. Problem Gambling in Europe—Challenges, prevention and interventions. New York: Springer; 2009.

15. Net Value. Europeans take a Gamble Online. Net Value Survey. June 2002.

16. National Children's Home. Children as young as 11 can set up gambling accounts at the click of a button. July 27, 2004, press release by NCH, GamCare and CitizenCard. http://www.nch.org.uk/information/index.php?i=77&r=288.

17. Cotte J, Latour K. Blackjack in the kitchen: Understanding inline versus casino gambling. J Consum Res 2009;35:742–58.

18. Smeaton M, Griffiths MD. Internet gambling and social responsibility: An exploratory study. Cyberpsychol Behav 2004;7:49–57.

19. Griffiths MD. Digital impact, crossover technologies and gambling practices. Casino Gambl Int 2008;4(3):37–42.

20. Griffiths MD. Convergence of gambling and computer game playing: Implications. E-commer Law Policy 2008;10(2):12–3.

21. de Freitas S, Griffiths MD. The convergence of gaming practices with other media forms: What potential for learning? A review of the literature. Learning Media Technol 2008;33:11–20.

22. King DL, Delfabbro P, Griffiths MD. The convergence of gambling and digital media: Implications for gambling in young people. J Gambl Stud 2010;26:175–87.

23. Brunelle N, Cousineau M-M, Dufour M, Gendron A, Leclerc D. A look at the contextual elements surrounding Internet gambling among adolescents. Paper presented at the 8th Annual Conference of Alberta Gaming Research Institute, Banff Center, Alberta, Mar 2009.

24. Brunelle N, Gendron A, Dufour M, Leclerc D, Cousineau M-M. Gambling among youth in relation with alcohol and drug use, delinquency and psychological distress. Paper given at the International Centre for Youth Gambling Problems and High-Risk Behaviors, McGill University, Canada, Feb 2009.

25. Germain M, Guyon L, Landry M, Tremblay J, Brunelle N, Bergeron J. DEP-ADO. Detection of alcohol and drug prevention in adolescents (Version 3.2): Recherche et intervention sur les substances psychoactives-Quebec (RISQ); 2007.

26. Olason D. Internet gambling and problem gambling among 13–18 year adolescents in Iceland. Paper presented at the 7th SNSUS Conference (The Big Picture: Gambling in Perspective), Helsinki, Finland, Apr 2009.

27. Olason D, Kristjansdottir E, Einarsdottir H, Haraldsson H, Bjarnason G, Derevensky J. Internet gambling and problem gambling among 13–18 year old adolescents in Iceland. Int J Ment Health Addict 2011;9:257–63.

28. Fisher S. Developing the DSM-IV-MR-J criteria to identify adolescent problem gambling in non-clinical populations. J Gambl Stud 2000;16:253–73.
29. Griffiths MD, Wood R. Adoelscent Internet gambling: Preliminary results of a national survey. Educ Health 2007;25:23–7.
30. Ipsos MORI. British Survey of Children, the National Lottery and Gambling 2008–09: Report of a quantitative survey. London: National Lottery Commission, 2009.
31. Welte J, Barnes GM, Tidwell MO, Hoffman JH. The association of form of gambling with problem gambling among American youth. Psychol Addict Behav 2009;23:105–12.
32. Winters KC, Stinchfield RD, Fulkerson J. Toward the development of an adolescent gambling problem severity scale. J Gambl Stud 1993;9:63–84.
33. Romer D. Internet gambling grows among male youth ages 18 to 22 gambling also increases in high school age female youth.2010: http://www.annenbergpublicpolicycenter.org/Down loads/Releases/ACI/Card%20Playing%202010%20Release%20final.pdf.
34. Byrne A. An exploratory study of Internet gambling among youth. [Unpublished Master's thesis]. Montreal, Canada: McGill University, 2004.
35. Messerlian C, Byrne A, Derevensky J. Gambling, youth and the Internet: Should we be concerned? Can Child Adolesc Psychiatr Rev 2004;13(1):3–6.
36. Griffiths MD, Parke J, Wood R, Rigbye J. Online poker gambling in university students: Further findings from an online survey. Int J Ment Health Addict 2010;8:82–9.
37. Matthews N, Farnsworth WF, Griffiths MD. A pilot study of problem gambling among student online gamblers: Mood states as predictors of problematic behavior. Cyberpsychol Behav 2009:741–6.
38. Meerkamper E. Youth gambling 2.0: Understanding youth gambling, emerging technologies, and social platforms. Nova Scotia Gaming Corportaion 6th Annual Responsible Gambling Conference, Halifax, Nova Scotia, Oct 2010.
39. Meerkamper E. Decoding risk: Gambling attitudes and behvaiours amongst youth in Nova Scotia: Report prepared for Nova Scotia Gaming Commission, 2006.
40. Poulin C, Elliot D. Student drug use survey in the Atlantic Provinces: Atlantic Technical Report. Halifax: Dalhousie University, Community Health and Epidemiology, 2007.
41. Griffiths MD. Instant-win promotions: Part of the gambling environment? Educ Health 1997;15:62–3.
42. Forrest DK, McHale I, Parke J. Appendix 5: Full report of statistical regression analysis. In Ipsos MORI (2009) British Survey of Children, the National Lottery and Gambling 2008–09: Report of a quantitative survey. London: National Lottery Commission, 2009.
43. Mitka M. Win or lose, Internet gambling stakes are high. JAMA 2001;285(8):1005.
44. Kelley R, Todosichuk P, Azmier J. Gambling@home: Internet gambling in Canada. Gambling in Canada Research Report No. 15. Calgary, Alberta: Canada West Foundation, 2001.
45. Hyder A, Juul NH. Games, gambling and children: Applying the precautionary principle for child health. J Child Adolesc Psychiatr Nurs 2008;21:202–4.
46. Griffiths MD, King D, Delfabbro P. Adolescent gambling-like experiences: Are they a cause for concern? Educ Health 2009;27:27–30.
47. Office of Communications. Social Networking: A quantitative and qualitative research report into attitudes, behaviours and use. 2008: www.ofcom.org.uk.
48. Downs C. The Facebook phenomenon: Social networking and gambling. The Gambling and Social Responsibility Forum Conference, Manchester Metropolitan University, Manchester, Sep 2008.
49. Sevigny S, Cloutier M, Pelletier M, Ladouceur R. Internet gambling: Misleading payout rates during the "demo" period. Comput Hum Behav 2005;21:153–8.
50. Griffiths MD. Online "penny auction" sites: Regulation needed. E-Finance Payments Law Policy 2008;2(12):14–6.

51. Griffiths MD. Mobile phone gambling. In: Taniar D, ed. Encyclopedia of Mobile Computing and Commerce. Pennsylvania: Information Science Reference; 2007:553–6.

52. Online Casino Sniper. The Mobile Gambling Sector? What does the future hold for online gaming? 2011: http://onlinecasinosniper.net-genie.co.uk/casino-stocks/253999/the_mobile_gambling_sector.html.

53. Gartner. Gartner says worldwide mobile gaming revenues to grow 19% in 2010. Press release. 2010: http://www.gartner.com/it/page.jsp?id=1370213.

54. Wardle H, Moody A, Spence S, Orford J, Griffiths MD, Volberg R, et al. British Gambling Prevalence Survey 2010. London: The Stationery Office. 2011.

55. Gambling Commission. Industry statistics. 2010: http://www.gamblingcommission.gov.uk/pdf/Gambling%20Industry%20Statistics%202009%202010%20WEB%20-%20January%202011.pdf.

56. Gendron A, Brunelle N, Leclerc D, Dufour M, Cousineau M-M. Comparison of the profiles of young non-gamblers, gamblers and Internet gamblers relative to psychological distress, severity of substances use and impulsivesness/risk taking. Poster presented at The 8th Annual Conference of Alberta Gaming Research Institute, Banff Center, Alberta, Mar 2009.

57. Campbell C, Derevensky J, Meerkamper E, Cutajar J. Parents' perceptions of adolescent gambling: A Canadian national study. JGI, in Press.

58. Wood R, Williams R. Internet Gambling: Prevalence, Patterns, Problems, and Policy Options. Final Report prepared for the Ontario Problem Gambling Research Centre. 2009. http://hdl.handle.net/10133/693.

59. Valentine G, Hughes K. New forms of gambling participation: Problem Internet gambling and the role of the family: Report prepared for the Responsibility in Gambling Trust, 2008.

60. Derevensky J. Internet Gambling: The tip of the iceberg. The New York Council on Problem Gambling Annual Convention, Albany, Mar 2010.

61. Gambling Commission. Remote gambling and software technical standards. Technical Standards Paper. 2007. http://www.gamblingcommission.gov.uk/UploadDocs/publications/Document/Remote%20Gambling%20and%20Software%20Technical%20Standards.pdf.

Assessment Tools

9 A critical review of adolescent problem gambling assessment instruments

Randy Stinchfield

The field of youth gambling assessment is in its infancy. Currently, four youth problem gambling instruments have been used to identify adolescent problem gamblers: (a) South Oaks Gambling Screen-Revised for Adolescents (SOGS-RA), (b) DSM-IV-Juvenile (DSM-IV-J) and the related DSM-IV-Multiple Response-Juvenile (DSM-IV-MR-J), (c) Massachusetts Gambling Screen (MAGS), and (d) Canadian Adolescent Gambling Inventory (CAGI). Three of the four are adaptations of adult instruments, and none has undergone rigorous psychometric evaluation. Though these instruments are used with varying populations in divergent settings, the psychometric properties for their use in these populations and settings are unknown. This review provides information about the instruments and makes suggestions for further instrument development and refinement. Each instrument is described in terms of its development, content, intended purpose, psychometric properties, administration method, scoring instructions, and interpretation. Strengths and limitations of each instrument are compared for both research and clinical purposes. Existing instruments are used to make clinical, scientific, and public policy decisions, and therefore, it is critical that these instruments demonstrate evidence of reliability, validity, and accuracy. It is recommended that the field adopt testing standards for the development and use of adolescent problem gambling scales, and generate a body of rigorous psychometric research that demonstrates reliability, validity, and classification accuracy. Ultimately, the goal is to improve measurement precision in identifying youth problem gamblers.

9.1 Introduction

This chapter describes the instruments currently used to identify adolescent problem gamblers, compares the advantages and disadvantages of existing instruments, and makes recommendations for future instrument refinement and development. Three instruments are commonly used to measure adolescent problem gambling. All three are adaptations of adult instruments: (a) South Oaks Gambling Screen–Revised for Adolescents (SOGS-RA); (b) DSM-IV-Juvenile (DSM-IV-J) and its revision, DSM-IV-Multiple Response-Juvenile (DSM-IV-MR-J); and (c) Massachusetts Gambling Screen (MAGS). A fourth instrument currently under development is the Canadian Adolescent Gambling Inventory (CAGI).

The South Oaks Gambling Screen (SOGS) is the most commonly used adult problem gambling screening instrument. The SOGS is a 20-item instrument developed to screen for probable pathological gambling in adult clinical samples, which has demonstrated satisfactory reliability, validity, and classification accuracy (1–3). Winters, Stinchfield, and Fulkerson (4, 5) adapted the SOGS for an adolescent gambling survey in Minnesota in 1990. The DSM-IV (6) lists ten diagnostic criteria for pathological gambling (PG), with five or more of these criteria being present to diagnose PG. Fisher (7) adapted the DSM-IV diagnostic criteria for adolescent surveys in the U.K. and developed two forms, one with a yes/no response option, DSM-IV-J (7), and one with a multiple response option, DSM-IV-MR-J (8). Shaffer, LaBrie, Scanlon, and Cummings (9) attempted to improve on the existing instruments and developed the MAGS. Though not specifically an adolescent instrument, the MAGS was developed on an adolescent sample and adapted items from the Short Michigan Alcoholism Screening Test (SMAST), an adult alcoholism screen (10). A fourth instrument, currently under development, is the Canadian Adolescent Gambling Inventory (CAGI) (11, 12, 13).

This review serves as a resource for investigators and mental health professionals who are involved in the screening and assessing of adolescent problem gambling. Most adolescent problem gambling instruments have not undergone rigorous reliability, validity, and classification accuracy evaluation (14). The assessment of adolescent problem gambling has been conducted either by assuming that existing adult instruments are appropriate for adolescents (which is a questionable assumption) or by making revisions to adult instruments in order to make them developmentally appropriate. The literature on adolescent development would suggest that the phenomenology of problem gambling has a different appearance in youth than among adults, and therefore neither of these approaches seem ideal. Both investigators studying problem gambling and mental health professionals need to select from among existing instruments, which have little, if any, psychometric information for the adolescent population or the settings in which they are administered.

The primary aim of evaluating any instrument (see ▶Tab. 9.1 for the description of each instrument) is to determine whether it measures accurately the characteristics of interest (15). Therefore, the instrument is considered satisfactory if the scores are shown to reflect important features of gambling behavior. Instrument evaluations are dependent on the adequacy of their psychometric properties, including reliability, validity, and classification accuracy. Reliability is often defined as consistency, repeatability, and stability (16). Reliability can be influenced by factors such as the number of items in the scale, number of respondents used in the evaluation, and the types of respondents utilized in the development and evaluation of the instrument. There are two types of reliability – temporal stability and internal consistency. Temporal stability, measured by test-retest procedures and reported as correlation coefficients, involves administering the test to the same individual at two points in time, typically within a few days or a week. (It is assumed that the characteristics of interest have not changed over this brief time period.) This mathematical construct, usually shown as "r," expresses the extent of correspondence or magnitude of the relationship between two scores. It ranges from 0, indicating no relationship, to 1, indicating perfect correspondence between the two scores. In order to demonstrate satisfactory temporal stability, a test-retest correlation of $r = .70$ or higher typically needs to be obtained.

Reliability is also measured by looking at the internal consistency of the test items. Internal consistency is the concept that a set of items are all measuring the same construct. One way of measuring internal consistency is by comparing the score on half of the items to the score on the other half of the items. This split-half reliability is measured in terms of the correlation coefficient r. Another approach to measuring internal consistency is to utilize statistical techniques that measure the homogeneity of the scale,

Tab. 9.1: Descriptions of instruments

Name of Instrument (year)	Content Areas	Number of items; response options; time frame	Administration time and method	Scoring instructions, score range, cut-scores, interpretation of scores	Psychometrics		Classification Accuracy Indices
					Reliability	Validity	Sample characteristics, criterion, base rate, sensitivity, specificity, and hit rate
SOGS-RA (1990)	Signs and symptoms of problem gambling; negative consequences	12 items; yes/ no; past year	10 minute paper and pencil questionnaire	Each item is one point; score range 0-12; 0-1 = no problem; 2-3 = at risk gambling; 4+ = problem gambling;	alpha = .80; Two-week test-retest kappa = .57 and alpha of .81 and .76 for males and females respectively (Poulin, 2000); alpha of .74 (Welte et al., 2008)	Gambling activity ($r = .39$), gambling frequency ($r = .54$), and amount of money gambled in past year ($r = .42$)	Using a criterion of DSM-IV-J, 97% true positive; 0.5% false negative; and 2.4% false positives (Derevensky and Gupta, 2000); using two criteria of self-identified need for help and receipt of help, 96% were correctly classified, however, sensitivity was about 60% and specificity was 96% for both proxies (Boudreau and Poulin, 2007).

(Continued)

Tab. 9.1: Descriptions of instruments *(Continued)*

Name of Instrument (year)	Content Areas	Number of items; response options; time frame	Administration time and method	Scoring instructions, score range, cut-scores, interpretation of scores	Psychometrics Reliability	Validity	Classification Accuracy Indices
							Sample characteristics, criterion, base rate, sensitivity, specificity, and hit rate
DSM-IV-J and DSM-IV-MR-J (1992; 2000)	DSM-IV diagnostic criteria	9 criteria measured by 12 items; yes/no (DSM-IV-J) and multiple response options (DSM-IV-MR-J); past year	5–10 minute paper and pencil questionnaire	Each item is one point; score range is 0-9; score of 4 or more is classified as a problem gambler	alpha = .75	Significantly different mean scores between regular and nonregular gamblers and between problem and social gamblers. DSM-IV-MR-J problem gamblers also tended to play more games regularly, spend more money, borrow to fund their gambling, and sell their possessions to fund their gambling; DSM-IV-J related to the SOGS-RA (r = .67) and GA 20 (r = .68) (Derevensky and Gupta, 2000)	NA

| MAGS (1994) | Psychological and social problems associated with gambling | 14 items; 7 items are scored in a scale based on item weights from a discriminant function analysis; yes/no; past year time frame | 5–10 minute interview or paper and pencil questionnaire | Each item is scored 0 for no and 1 for yes. Each item score is multiplied by a weight and then summed along with a constant using a weighted scoring algorithm derived from a discriminant function analysis. The MAGS classifies respondents into nonpatho logical gambling, transitional gambling, or pathological gambling | alpha = .83 | MAGS score obtained a high correlation ($r = .76$) with DSM-IV score | Sample was 589 Boston, MA, high school students who reported gambling in the past year. Criterion was DSM-IV diagnostic criteria as measured by a 12-item instrument. See development article for classification accuracy indices. Note that these classification accuracy indices are based on a discriminant function analysis computed on the development sample and therefore other MAGS users are not likely to obtain as high an accuracy. |

(Continued)

Tab. 9.1: Descriptions of instruments *(Continued)*

Name of Instrument (year)	Content Areas	Number of items; response options; time frame	Administration time and method	Scoring instructions, score range, cut-scores, interpretation of scores	Psychometrics		Classification Accuracy Indices
					Reliability	Validity	Sample characteristics, criterion, base rate, sensitivity, specificity, and hit rate
CAGI (2007)	Gambling frequency; time spent gambling; money spent gambling; gambling problem severity (behaviors and consequences)	45 items measuring five domains: (a) gambling problem severity; (b) psychological consequences; (c) social consequences; (d) financial consequences; and (e) loss of control; four-point multiple response options; past three months time frame	20 minutes; paper and pencil questionnaire	9-item gambling problem severity subscale has a score range of 0 to 27	alphas range from .74 to .88; test-retest ranged from $r = .60$ to .91	Correlated with gambling frequency ($r = .32$ to $r = .55$) and money spent gambling ($r = .12$ to $r = .50$).	NA

commonly measured by Cronbach's alpha (17), a coefficient that ranges from 0 to 1. The higher the *alpha*, the greater the internal consistency of the scale. As a criterion, Nunnally (16) recommends that an *alpha* of .90 be used as the minimum standard and an alpha of .95 is desirable in applied settings where a test score is used to make important decisions.

Validity is defined as whether the instrument measures the construct it purports to measure (15). One type of validity is content validity, that is, do the scale items cover the various features of the construct being measured. A second type of validity is criterion-related validity. Criterion-related validity is commonly assessed by measuring correlations between the scale of interest and other scales that measure the same construct. In order to demonstrate validity, a new scale should be correlated with existing scales of the same construct that have already demonstrated satisfactory psychometric properties. For example, a new scale to measure problem gambling may be correlated with the SOGS, an instrument with demonstrated satisfactory psychometric properties.

Nunnally (16) and Cicchetti (18) suggested that validity correlations greater than $r = .30$ provide support for convergent validity. Finally, another validity indicator is how well the instrument is able to discriminate between two target samples. For example, a new measure of problem gambling should obtain high scores when administered to a sample of gambling treatment clients and low scores when administered to a sample from the general population.

Another measure of an instrument's utility and performance is referred to as classification accuracy (19, 20), that is, how well the instrument identifies those with and without the disorder. Classification accuracy is typically assessed with a number of coefficients, including *sensitivity, specificity, false positive rate, false negative rate, positive predictive power, and negative predictive power. Sensitivity* is the true positive rate, that is, the rate of positive test results among those with the disorder, and *specificity* is the true negative rate, that is, the rate of negative test results among those without the disorder. *False positive rate* represents the percent of positive test results among individuals without the disorder and *false negative rate* is the percent of negative test results among those with the disorder. *Positive predictive power* is the rate of true-positive results among all positive test results. *Negative predictive power* is the rate of true-negative results among all negative test results.

9.2 South Oaks Gambling Screen – Revised for Adolescents (SOGS-RA)

Given the widespread use of the SOGS, Winters, Stinchfield, and Fulkerson (4) revised the adult SOGS for an adolescent problem gambling survey in Minnesota. At the time (1989), there was no instrument to identify adolescent problem gamblers. Jacobs (21) had used the Gamblers Anonymous 20 questions in a youth study and Lesieur and Klein (22) had used DSM-III-based questions for their adolescent survey, but neither study reported detailed psychometric information on either instrument. As a result, Winters, Stinchfield, and Fulkerson (4) adapted the most commonly used adult instrument, the SOGS, for adolescents and referred to it as the SOGS-*Revised for Adolescents* (SOGS-RA). The investigators revised the original SOGS by changing the lifetime time frame to a "past 12 months" time frame, which seemed more developmentally appropriate for adolescents as they do not have as much life experience as adults and they tend to live more in the present than adults. Other revisions included changing the wording of items and response options to better reflect adolescent gambling behavior and youth reading levels, eliminating two items that were viewed as having poor content validity for adolescents, and retaining only one item for sources of borrowed money (rather than nine items as is done with the SOGS). The SOGS-RA consists of 12 items, and a copy of the SOGS-RA as well as a detailed description of the revisions can be found in Winters, Stinchfield, and Fulkerson (4). Reliability and validity coefficients were computed on 460 males aged 15–18 years, and the internal consistency reliability was alpha = .80. In terms of validity, the SOGS-RA was correlated with gambling activity ($r = .39$), gambling frequency ($r = .54$), and amount of money gambled in past year ($r = .42$) (4). The SOGS-RA was able to discriminate between youth who gambled regularly and those who did not. Since its development, the SOGS-RA has been used in a number of adolescent gambling surveys (14, 23).

Two scoring procedures have been used with the SOGS-RA, yet neither system has received extensive psychometric and classification accuracy analyses. These two scoring systems have come to be referred to as the SOGS-RA "broad" and "narrow" criteria (24). The broad criteria are based on a combination of gambling frequency and SOGS-RA score. To be classified as a problem gambler under the broad criteria, the respondent has to either gamble at least weekly and obtain a SOGS-RA score of two or more or gamble daily, regardless of SOGS-RA score (5). Under the SOGS-RA narrow criteria, a cut score of 4 or more indicates a problem gambler, a score of 2–3 indicates an at-risk gambler, and a score of 0–1 is a nonproblem gambler (24).

Because these two sets of SOGS-RA scoring criteria have caused some confusion, the problems associated with the broad criteria will be addressed. The SOGS-RA broad criteria are problematic for a number of reasons. First, Winters and Stinchfield (24) moved from the broad criteria in 1993 to the more narrow criteria in 1995 because of the low threshold for problem gambling of the broad criteria. Second, the broad criteria are not exhaustive of all patterns of gambling problem severity because not all patterns were present in the original data and the response options for gambling frequency items were limited to either daily, weekly, monthly, less than monthly, and not at all. Gambling more often than weekly and less often than daily is missing from the broad criteria (i.e., gambling between two and six days per week). Third, most recent studies that have used the SOGS-RA have used the narrow criteria and there appears to be a consensus among users of the SOGS-RA that the narrow criteria are preferred over the broad criteria.

Fourth, the broad criteria are probably "too broad." The SOGS-RA broad criteria define problem gambling as daily gambling and this is a questionable criterion for problem gambling – it is not found in either the SOGS or the DSM criteria. Does daily gambling indicate problem or pathological gambling? Not necessarily. The broad criteria considers a score of 2 as problem gambling and given that it is fairly easy to endorse two SOGS-RA items, particularly the subjective items, this also seems to be too low a threshold for problem gambling. The narrow criteria cut score of 4 is similar to the SOGS and DSM-IV cut scores of 5. Fifth, the SOGS was originally intended to correlate with diagnostic criteria for pathological gambling, and this is how most users interpret a SOGS cut score, whereas, the SOGS-RA broad criteria are not close to that level of problem severity. Sixth, although some convergent validity information was reported for the broad criteria in the original SOGS-RA study, it did not provide any classification accuracy information. Seventh, a minor additional point about the SOGS-RA broad criteria is that the category "no problem gambling" is misleading, as it suggests that all cases in this category are gamblers when in fact this category includes nongamblers. For these reasons, it is recommended that the SOGS-RA narrow criteria rather than the broad criteria be used for identifying adolescent problem gamblers, at least until further research on the classification accuracy of the SOGS-RA is conducted.

A few studies have examined the psychometric properties and cut score of the SOGS-RA. In terms of the cut score, some investigators have chosen to raise it above 4. Govoni, Rupcich, and Frisch (25) rejected the broad criteria as yielding "unreasonable estimates of problem and at risk gambling" and raised the cut score to 5 or more to reflect the same cut score that is used with the adult SOGS. However, they did not have a criterion to compare against and they gave no classification accuracy information for this new cut score.

Derevensky and Gupta (26) compared the SOGS-RA with the DSM-IV-J and GA 20. The authors noted some item content differences between these scales and found the DSM-IV-J to have obtained the more conservative estimate of problem gambling prevalence (3.4%) as compared to the SOGS-RA (5.3%). There was a fairly high degree of classification agreement between the SOGS-RA and DSM-IV-J. The SOGS-RA when compared to the DSM-IV-J as the criterion, yielded 97% true positive; 0.5% false negative; and 2.4% false positives.

Ladouceur et al. (27) raised the question as to whether adolescents understand SOGS-RA items. It should be noted that there are some errors in their description of the SOGS-RA. Ladouceur et al. describe the SOGS-RA as having 19 scored items when it actually only has 12, but the table provided indicated they only scored 12 items. The authors indicated that the cut score is 5 and this indicates probable pathological gambling, when the published cut score is 4 indicating problem gambling. They found that adolescents misunderstood SOGS-RA items and that after clarification their SOGS-RA score was lower on retest. The authors conclude that this misunderstanding of item content could cause inflated prevalence rates (see Derevensky, Gupta, and Winters [28] for a critical review of this study).

Wiebe, Cox, and Mehmel (29) examined the psychometric properties of the SOGS-RA in a community sample of adolescents. The authors found over- and under-endorsement of some items by problem gamblers versus at-risk gamblers, suggesting that item weighting, deleting items, or rewriting items may improve the classification accuracy of the SOGS-RA. They also found a two-factor solution that was interpretable as gambling consequences and lack of control over gambling.

Poulin (30) used the SOGS-RA in a survey of adolescents in the Atlantic provinces of Canada and found the broad criteria to be "complex and ambiguous" and not "exhaustive and mutually exclusive." She also found the narrow criteria to be problematic because of the lack of an adequate rationale for a cut score of 4 or more to define problem gambling. Poulin (31) also used this same survey data to conduct a psychometric study of the SOGS-RA and found three factors, which she labeled "self-awareness of one's problem gambling, insight into others' assessment of one's problem gambling, and expedient measures to address the negative financial consequences of problem gambling." Two-week test-retest stability showed fair to good agreement, with a kappa for the narrow criteria of .57. Internal consistency was satisfactory with a Cronbach's alpha of .81 and .76 for males and females respectively. She also notes that the cut point may be too high because it only classified 26% of male daily gamblers and 9%

of female daily gamblers as problem gamblers. However, I would contend that there is not a perfect relationship between gambling frequency and problem gambling and therefore, this failure to classify daily gamblers as problem gamblers should not be a concern.

Derevensky, Gupta, and Winters (28) addressed the issue of high prevalence rates, the arguments that they are inflated, and the role of the SOGS-RA in this debate. The authors concluded that most arguments against the high prevalence rates, some of which are measured with the SOGS-RA, do not hold up, but more psychometric research is needed.

Langhinrichsen-Rohling, Rohling, Rohde, and Seeley (32) examined the SOGS-RA cut score as it compares to the MAGS. The author found a lack of congruence between the SOGS-RA and the MAGS for classifying problem gamblers. The SOGS-RA classified 80 of 1,395 high school students who had gambled in the past year as problem gamblers using a cut score of 4 or more, and the MAGS classified only 26 as problem gamblers. The authors concluded that the prevalence estimates of adolescent problem gambling vary as a function of the instrument used. In response to this disparity, they suggested creating a fourth category for the SOGS-RA, using a cut score of 6 or more to indicate probable pathological gambling, which improved the agreement rate between the SOGS-RA and MAGS. This study exhibited some limitations, including the use of different time frames for SOGS-RA (past 12 months) versus the MAGS (lifetime), however, the MAGS development article used a past 12 months time frame (9). The authors report that the MAGS item "arrested for gambling" was the best item for discriminating the "probable pathological gamblers from all the other groups," but this raises a question as to the validity of this response. How many high school students get arrested for gambling?

Ladouceur et al. (33) compared the SOGS-RA to DSM-IV criteria in a sample of 631 adolescents. The SOGS-RA identified 93 adolescents as problem gamblers. Of those 93, only 7 were confirmed as pathological gamblers through clinical interviews conducted 1 or 2 weeks later. Though this study shows evidence of the likely discordant results obtained from the SOGS-RA versus DSM-IV diagnostic criteria, numerous weaknesses limit the validity of the results. One of the weaknesses is the 1- to 2-week time delay between the administration of the SOGS-RA and the clinical interview, which itself can lead to disagreement. Another weakness is that the two measures were administered by different methods (self-administered paper-and-pencil questionnaire in a classroom setting versus face-to-face interview), therefore the method of test administration becomes a confound and possible alternative explanation for the discordant results. Another weakness is the lack of details about the clinical interview content, reliability, validity, and classification accuracy. The clinical interview was deemed the criterion or gold standard for this study, however, no information about the reliability, validity, or classification accuracy of this "gold standard" was provided. Still further, the investigators failed to score the DSM-IV criteria, but rather used another party who listened to the recorded interviews and made a diagnosis. This diagnostician was not the interviewer and therefore could not probe or clarify any criteria that may have been vague or ambiguous. Though the authors' provide a Cohen's *kappa* of .74, it is not clear which two classifications are being compared nor how discrepancies between diagnosticians were resolved, because the classifications were not in perfect agreement. The authors call for a consensus on a definition of adolescent pathological gambling. This study raises questions about the classification accuracy of the SOGS-RA, but it is in no way a conclusive study. The SOGS-RA is not likely to match up perfectly with DSM-IV criteria, but this study does not rigorously demonstrate that likelihood.

Olason, Sigurdardottir, and Smari (34) compared the SOGS-RA with the DSM-IV-MR-J in a prevalence survey of 750 adolescents in Iceland. The authors computed a Principal Components Analysis and reported a one-factor solution accounting for 37% of the variance and a coefficient alpha of .81. The correlation between the SOGS-RA and DSM-IV-MR-J was $r = .79$. They reported that the SOGS-RA identified 2.7% with problem gambling, which was slightly more than the 2% identified by the DSM-IV-MR-J and a concordance rate of kappa = .62.

Boudreau and Poulin (35) compared the SOGS-RA cut score of 4 or more to indicate problem gambling to two gold standard proxies of self-identified need for help with gambling and receipt of help for gambling. This was a very creative study in its use of criteria other than DSM-IV, however, the criteria items are of unknown validity. The investigators found the SOGS-RA, using a cut score of 4, correctly classified 96% of these two proxies, however, the SOGS-RA demonstrated poor sensitivity at about 60% for both proxies. The SOGS-RA identified 59% of those 80 youth who self-identified as needing help (0.9%) and 62% of those 54 youth who received help (0.7%). In other words, the SOGS-RA did not identify 41% of those youth who self-identified as needing help and did not identify 38% of those youth who reported receiving help. Specificity was 96% for both proxies. To improve sensitivity, the authors suggest that the cut score should be lowered; however, this study was the only one that suggested lowering the SOGS-RA cut score to improve accuracy.

Welte et al. (36) used the SOGS-RA in a national survey of 2,274 U.S. respondents who were 14–21 years old and found the SOGS-RA had a Cronbach's *alpha* of .74, indicating satisfactory internal consistency. Using the SOGS-RA and a cut score of 4 or more they reported a 2.1% rate of problem gambling. The authors also measured DSM-IV diagnostic criteria by administering the Diagnostic Interview Schedule (DIS), and reported a 0.4% rate of pathological gambling. They did not directly compare the SOGS-RA to the DIS, but the SOGS-RA obtained a higher rate of problem gambling than the DSM-IV rate of pathological gambling.

9.3 DSM-IV-J and DSM-IV-MR-J

Fisher (7) developed a 12-item questionnaire to measure 9 of 10 DSM-IV diagnostic criteria of PG in juvenile fruit machine players in the United Kingdom. It was the first adaptation of DSM-IV criteria for youth. The DSM-IV-J (J = juvenile) response options are "yes" or "no." The DSM-IV-J has been used in a number of studies around the world to measure problem gambling among adolescents, including the United Kingdom (37–42). The DSM-IV-J has been revised by changing the phrase "playing fruit machines" to "gambling" and by using multiple response options in the DSM-IV-MR-J (8) (MR = multiple response).

The DSM-IV-MR-J also has 12 items to measure 9 of the 10 DSM-IV criteria, and the items are adapted from the DSM-IV criteria to reflect the developmental stage of youth. Fisher simplified the language and omitted details that were less relevant for youth. She excluded criterion 10, because "young problem gamblers tend to resolve desperate financial situations caused by gambling by illegal methods (incorporated in item 8)" (8). Eleven of the twelve items have four response options: never, once or twice, sometimes, and often. Fisher (8) has a scoring system for the set of response options for each item to match the nine DSM-IV criteria. The score range is from 0 to 9, and a score of 4 or more is classified as a problem gambler. A factor analysis indicated a unidimensional scale with satisfactory internal consistency reliability (alpha = .75). In terms of validity, the DSM-IV-MR-J had significantly different mean scores between regular and nonregular gamblers and between problem and social gamblers. Respondents classified as problem gamblers by the DSM-IV-MR-J also tended to play more games regularly, spend more money, borrow to fund their gambling, and sell their possessions to fund their gambling; no correlation coefficients were provided however. The readability of the DSM-IV-MR-J test questions was at grade level 4.8, using the Fleisch-Kincaid Grade Level Test.

The DSM-IV-J does not match up identically with the DSM-IV-MR-J in that the DSM-IV-J is missing an item to measure the DSM-IV criterion for loss of control, that is, making repeatedly unsuccessful efforts to control, to cut back, or to stop gambling. Furthermore, the DSM-IV-J measures the criterion for financial bailout whereas the DSM-IV-MR-J does not. So, the DSM-IV-J and DSM-IV-MR-J measure somewhat different DSM-IV criteria. As such, neither scale measures all ten DSM-IV criteria and the scales are not identical, which causes confusion by test users. Jacques and Ladouceur (43) report that this limitation may have occurred because Fisher was not working from the official DSM-IV criteria but rather a pre-DSM-IV version outlined by Lesieur and Rosenthal (44). Though this was true for the DSM-IV-J published in 1992, Fisher did have the official criteria when the DSM-IV-MR-J article was published in 2000.

There are four concerns about the DSM-IV-MR-J. First, item 3 does not appear to match or concur with the DSM-IV criterion it is intended to measure. The DSM-IV criterion is "Made repeated unsuccessful efforts to control, cut back, or stop gambling"; and the item to measure this criterion is "In the past year have you ever spent much more than you planned to on gambling?" This item appears to be more closely aligned to the earlier DSM-III-R criterion 2, "frequent gambling with larger amounts of money or over a longer period of time than intended." Second, the exclusion of criterion 10 seems premature, given that clinicians and the media have reported that parents have paid the gambling debts of their children. Criterion 10 seems relevant for youth and until proven otherwise, it should not be excluded from an instrument intended to measure DSM-IV diagnostic criteria. Therefore, the DSM-IV-MR-J appears to measure eight of the ten DSM-IV criteria and lacks items to measure criteria 3 and 10. Third, multiple response options were included in the DSM-IV-MR-J, but these multiple response options appear to be ignored when it comes to scoring. The scoring instructions collapse the multiple response options into a dichotomous scoring of 0 or 1 for each item and therefore do not use the multiple response options in the scoring system (8). Why provide multiple response options if they will not be used to score the scale? Fourth, there is a lack of evidence of validity and no estimates of classification accuracy are provided by Fisher. The developer states that there is evidence of validity (significant differences between groups), however, insufficient detail is provided to judge the value of this evidence. For example, we do not know how the groups (problem gamblers versus social gamblers) were selected or identified or what criteria were used to classify them as problem gamblers versus social gamblers.

Derevensky and Gupta (26) compared the DSM-IV-J with the SOGS-RA and GA 20. The authors found the DSM-IV-J to yield the lowest estimate of problem gambling of the three measures. In terms of convergent validity, they found the DSM-IV-J to be related to the SOGS-RA ($r = .67$) and GA 20 ($r = .68$). No classification accuracy information was reported because the DSM-IV-J was used as the criterion to test the classification accuracy of the SOGS-RA and GA 20; however, there was a fairly high degree of agreement between the instruments.

Jacques and Ladouceur (43) examined the confusion regarding the scoring of the DSM-IV-J. The nine DSM-IV-J criteria are measured by 12 items and some investigators have made the error of computing the cut score from all 12 items rather than from the nine criteria. This error can make a difference in the reported prevalence rate and therefore investigators are urged to follow the scoring instructions for nine criteria.

Olason, Sigurdardottir and Smari (34) compared the DSM-IV-MR-J with the SOGS-RA in a prevalence survey of 750 adolescents in Iceland. The authors computed a Principal Components Analysis and reported a one-factor solution accounting for 41% of the variance and a coefficient alpha of .78. The correlation between the DSM-IV-MR-J and SOGS-RA was $r = .79$. They reported that the DSM-IV-MR-J identified 2% with problem gambling, which was slightly less than the 2.7% identified by the SOGS-RA and a concordance rate of kappa = .62.

9.4 Massachusetts Gambling Screen (MAGS)

Shaffer et al. (9) developed the Massachusetts Gambling Screen (MAGS), a seven-item screening instrument designed to measure the gambling problems of excessive gamblers and to obtain an estimate of the prevalence of problem gambling. The MAGS was developed in 1993 on a sample of 589 Boston high school students who had gambled in the past year. The MAGS was not developed exclusively for adolescents, but because the development sample comprised high school students and also because the "A" in the acronym MAGS has oftentimes mistakenly been referred to as Adolescent (rather than MA for Massachusetts), the MAGS is erroneously referred to as an adolescent instrument. Nevertheless, Shaffer and colleagues indicate that the instrument was developed for both adolescents and adults. The MAGS inquires about behavior during the past year. The MAGS includes 14 items adapted from the Short Michigan Alcoholism Screening Test (SMAST), an alcoholism screen developed by Selzer, Vonokur, and van Rooijen (10). Of these 14 items, 7 were selected as the best discriminators in a discriminant function analysis, and the MAGS comprises these 7 items. In the MAGS development study, a measure of DSM-IV diagnostic criteria for PG was also developed, consisting of 12 items, which served as the criterion. Each item is assigned a 0 for a "no" response and a 1 for a "yes" response. Scoring is based on item weights that are multiplied by each item score and summed, along with a constant. The MAGS classifies respondents into three categories: (a) nonpathological gambling, (b) transitional gambling, or (c) pathological gambling. Cut scores are based on a weighted scoring equation derived from a discriminant function analysis. The seven-item MAGS scale had an internal consistency reliability coefficient alpha of .83. In terms of validity, the MAGS total discriminant score obtained a high correlation ($r = .76$) with total DSM-IV score.

The brevity of the MAGS is one of its strong points. However, one concern is the use of item weights for scoring that were derived from the development sample of a limited number of high school students. Though item weights may have provided excellent classification accuracy in the development sample, it is unlikely that this same level of accuracy will be maintained when administered to other samples. Item weights can be unique to a given sample and therefore may not generalize to other samples. This issue requires further research.

The MAGS was compared with the SOGS-RA by Langhinrichsen-Rohling et al. (32) in a survey of high school students. The MAGS and SOGS-RA were found to have little concordance in their classifications and the MAGS yielded much more conservative estimates than the SOGS-RA. Of the 1,395 high school students who had gambled in the past year, the MAGS only classified 26 as probable pathological gamblers whereas the SOGS-RA classified 80 as problem gamblers. The authors concluded that the prevalence estimates of adolescent problem gambling vary as a function of the instrument used. This study exhibited some limitations, including the use of different time frames for SOGS-RA (past 12 months) versus the MAGS (lifetime), however, the MAGS development article used a past 12 months time frame (9). As noted previously, though the authors report that the MAGS item "arrested for gambling" was the best item for discriminating the "probable pathological gamblers from all the other groups," but how many high school students get arrested for gambling?

9.5 Canadian Adolescent Gambling Inventory (CAGI)

The most recent adolescent instrument to be developed is the Canadian Adolescent Gambling Inventory (CAGI) (11, 12, 13). This adolescent instrument is not the typical adaptation of an adult instrument. The goal of the CAGI was to develop a scale specifically for adolescents. The intent was to develop a scale that represents a continuum of gambling problem severity from low to high, rather than items that tap into high problem severity alone, as is done with adult scales that have been adapted for youth, such as the DSM-IV-J. The CAGI moves beyond a single, simple scale to the measurement of more complex, multiple domains of gambling problem severity. The CAGI measures the two main elements of youth gambling, gambling behavior itself, and gambling problem severity, including preoccupation and negative consequences. The development of the CAGI included defining the behaviors of interest, creating an item pool, pilot testing items with adolescent focus groups, psychometric analyses of items and scales, and procedures to obtain estimates of reliability, validity, and classification accuracy.

The CAGI has a past three months time frame and measures five areas: (a) types of gambling activities played, (b) frequency of participation for each gambling activity, (c) time spent gambling for each activity, (d) money spent gambling, and (e) gambling problem severity. The CAGI is available in both English and French language versions. The gambling activities section includes a fake gambling item to test for validity of self-report. The gambling problem severity items have four-point response options. Though it is still under development, there is a working draft of the instrument and preliminary psychometric estimates.

Temporal stability was measured with a test-retest procedure 7–14 days apart and test-retest correlations ranged from acceptable ($r = .60$) to excellent ($r = .91$). Internal consistency measured with Cronbach's alpha ranged from .74 to .88. The CAGI includes a 9-item Gambling Problem Severity Subscale (GPSS). CAGI items use four-point response options of "Never", "Sometimes", "Most of the times" and "Almost always", scored 0, 1, 2 and 3, respectively. The nine items are summed and a threshold of 6 or more was found to be the best cut score for classification accuracy. Using DSM-IV as the gold standard criterion, the GPSS yielded a sensitivity of .96, a specificity of .89, and a Youden Index of .85. In terms of convergent validity, the CAGI scales were correlated with gambling frequency ($r = .58$), time spent gambling in a typical week ($r = .67$), and sum of money lost gambling ($r = .51$).

9.6 Conclusions

In response to the need for instruments to measure problem gambling among adolescents, a small number of instruments have been developed. Most of these instruments have adapted adult instruments for adolescents, and this is a questionable practice given that problem gambling among adolescents is believed to have somewhat different characteristics than among adults. Developers who have adapted adult scales for adolescents have also tended to use a lower cut score to indicate problem gambling in adolescents than is used to indicate problem gambling for adults. For example, the cut score on the SOGS is 5, but the cut score on the SOGS-RA is 4; and the cut score on the DSM-IV is 5 and the cut score on the DSM-IV-MR-J is 4.

Large differences have been reported in prevalence rates in epidemiological studies of adolescent problem gambling, from as low as 0.3% to as high as 10% (14, 23, 45), and at least part of this discrepancy is likely attributable to imprecision in existing adolescent assessment tools. As this review has shown, these instruments have little information on their psychometric properties and in particular, there has been a lack of rigorous research on the classification accuracy of these instruments. This may, in part, explain the wide range of prevalence estimates reported in gambling surveys. The adult instruments from which the adolescent instruments were adapted were developed for clinical purposes but have often been used for other purposes and populations. The psychometric properties of an instrument must be investigated for the different settings and the populations for which it is applied. The classification accuracy of an instrument is affected by the base rate of the disorder within the population to which it is being applied, and therefore an instrument developed to measure PG in a clinical sample where the base rate is fairly high will have weaker classification accuracy when applied to the general population where the base rate is extremely low. The current state of adolescent problem gambling assessment makes it difficult for a clinician or researcher to select a psychometrically sound instrument that will measure problem gambling in a population of interest. A number of steps must be taken to address these issues.

First, existing instruments have to be put to rigorous psychometric evaluation, and this research will build a body of evidence for (or against) the reliability, validity, and classification accuracy of existing adolescent problem gambling instruments. Research on the psychometric properties of these instruments has to be conducted for the settings and populations in which they are used, such as students in a school setting. This research will justify the continued use of those instruments found to exhibit satisfactory reliability, validity, and classification accuracy, and will serve to encourage the revision and refinement of those instruments found lacking.

Second, for the assessment of adolescent problem gambling, new instruments must be developed that take into account the developmental issues of youth at different ages. This effort should include refining the definition of problem gambling for youth with a focus on describing the phenomenon of problem gambling among youth. Is adolescent problem gambling the same as or different from adult problem gambling? Is youth problem gambling the same or different at varying ages and developmental stages? Gambling is exhibited by 8- and 9-year-old children as well as young adults. How does problem gambling display itself in youth of varying ages and developmental stages? Can the same instrument be used for youth of varying ages and developmental stages? Can the same cut score be used for youth of varying ages and developmental stages?

Third, investigators must use scientific standards for test development. It is recommended that investigators and test users follow the standards for testing set forth by the American Educational Research Association, the American Psychological Association, and the National Council on Measurement in Education (45). These guidelines describe technical standards for test construction and evaluation, including reliability and validity. The use of these guidelines will facilitate the development of psychometrically sound instruments that will be recognized as standards in the field.

Fourth, DSM-IV diagnostic criteria for PG are used to make clinical, scientific, and public policy decisions. The DSM-IV diagnostic criteria are the accepted standard for the identification of PG, but some (or all) of the criteria may not be relevant for youth. Debate continues about the adequacy of definitions and diagnostic criteria of pathological gambling, particularly as it applies to youth (11, 12, 14, 45). Therefore, one of the most pressing questions in the field of adolescent problem gambling is: What criteria should be used to diagnose adolescent PG?

Psychometric research on measures of adolescent PG will lead to refinement of measurement tools and greater precision, which is the mark of good science. After a body of research has been generated, the goal of a "gold standard" instrument(s) to measure adolescent PG, or at least one that receives favorable consensus, will be achieved.

References

1. Lesieur HR, Blume SB. The South Oaks Gambling Screen (SOGS): A new instrument for the identification of pathological gamblers. Am J Psychiatry 1987;144:1184–8.
2. Lesieur HR, Blume SB. Revising the South Oaks Gambling Screen in different settings. J Gambl Stud 1993;9:213–23.
3. Stinchfield R. Reliability, validity, and classification accuracy of the South Oaks Gambling Screen (SOGS). Addict Behav 2001;27:1–19.
4. Winters KC, Stinchfield R, Fulkerson J. Towards the development of an adolescent gambling problem severity scale. J Gambl Stud 1993;9:63–84.
5. Winters KC, Stinchfield R, Fulkerson J. Patterns and characteristics of adolescent gambling. J Gambl Stud 1993;9:371–86.
6. American Psychiatric Association. Diagnostic and statistical manual of Mental Disorders. 4th ed. Washington, DC: Autho;, 1994.
7. Fisher SE. Measuring pathological gambling in children: The case of fruit machines in the UK. J Gambl Stud 1992;8:263–85.

8. Fisher S. Developing the DSM-IV-MR-J criteria to identify adolescent problem gambling in non-clinical populations. J Gambl Stud 2000;16:253–73.

9. Shaffer HJ, LaBrie R, Scanlon KM, Cummings TN. Pathological gambling among adolescents: Massachusetts Gambling Screen (MAGS). J Gambl Stud 1994;10:339–62.

10. Selzer ML, Vonokur A, van Rooijen L. A self-administered short Michigan alcoholism screening test (SMAST). J Stud Alcohol 1975;36:117–26.

11. Wiebe, J., Wynne, H., Stinchfield, R., & Tremblay, J., (2005). *Measuring problem gambling in adolescent populations: Phase I Report*. Canadian Centre on Substance Abuse. Download from HYPERLINK "http://www.ccsa.org/"www.ccsa.org/2008 CCSA Documents2/Cagi phase 1 report.pdf.

12. Wiebe, J., Wynne, H., Stinchfield, R., & Tremblay, J., (2008). *Canadian Adolescent Gambling Inventory (CAGI): Phase II Final Report*. Canadian Centre on Substance Abuse. Download from HYPERLINK "http://www.ccsa.org/2008 CCSA Documents2/CAGI_Phase_2_Report-English.pdf"www.ccsa.org/2008 CCSA Documents2/CAGI_Phase_2_Report-English.pdf

13. Tremblay, J., Stinchfield, R., Wiebe, J., & Wynne, H. (2010). *Canadian Adolescent Gambling Inventory (CAGI): Phase III Final Report*. Canadian Centre on Substance Abuse. Download from HYPERLINK "http://www.ccsa.org/"www.ccsa.org/2010 CCSA Documents/CAGI_Phase_III_Report_e.pdf

14. National Research Council. Pathological gambling: A critical review. Washington, DC: Natl Acad Press; 1999.

15. Allen MJ, Yen WM. Introduction to measurement theory. Monterey, CA: Brooks/Cole, 1979.

16. Nunnally JC. Psychometric theory. 2nd ed. New York: McGraw-Hill; 1978.

17. Cronbach L. Coefficient alpha and the internal structure of tests. Psycho-metrika 1951; 16:297–334.

18. Cicchetti DV. Guidelines, criteria, and rules of thumb for evaluating normed and standardized assessment instruments in psychology. Psychol Assess 1994;6:284–90.

19. Baldessarini RJ, Finklestein S, Arana GW. The predictive power of diagnostic tests and the effect of prevalence of illness. Arch Gen Psychiatry 1983;40: 569–73.

20. Fleiss JL. Statistical methods for rates and proportions. 2nd ed. New York: Wiley; 1981.

21. Jacobs DF. Illegal and undocumented: A review of teenage gamblers in America. In: Shaffer HJ, Stein SA, Gambino B, Cummings TN, eds. Compulsive gambling: Theory, research and practice. Lexington, MA: Lexington Books; 1989:249–92.

22. Lesieur HR, Klein R. Pathological gambling among high school students. Addict Behav 1987;12:129–35.

23. Shaffer HJ, Hall MN. Estimating the prevalence of adolescent gambling disorders: A quantitative synthesis and guide toward standard gambling nomenclature. J Gambl Stud 1996;12 (2):193–214.

24. Winters KC, Stinchfield R Kim L. Monitoring adolescent gambling in Minnesota. J Gambl Stud 1995;11:165–83.

25. Govoni R, Rupcich N, Frisch GR. Gambling behavior of adolescent gamblers. J Gambl Stud 1996;12:305–17.

26. Derevensky JL, Gupta R. Prevalence estimates of adolescent gambling: A comparison of the SOGS-RA, DSM-IV-J, and the GA 20 questions. J Gambl Stud 2000;16:227–51.

27. Ladouceur R, Bouchard C, Rheaume N, Jacques C, Ferland F, Leblond J, Walker M. Is the SOGS an accurate measure of pathological gambling among children, adolescents and adults? J Gambl Stud 2000;16:1–24.

28. Derevensky JL, Gupta R, Winters K. Prevalence rates of youth gambling problems: Are the current rates inflated? J Gambl Stud 2003;19(4):405–25.

29. Wiebe J, Cox BJ, Mehmel BG. The South Oaks Gambling Screen Revised for Adolescents (SOGS-RA): Further psychometric findings from a community sample. J Gambl Stud 2000;16:275–88.

30. Poulin C. Problem gambling among adolescent students in the Atlantic provinces of Canada. J Gambl Stud 2000;16:53–78.
31. Poulin C. An assessment of the validity and reliability of the SOGS-RA. J Gambl Stud 2002; 18 (1):67–93.
32. Langhinrichsen-Rohling J, Rohling ML, Rohde P, Seeley JR. The SOGS-RA vs. the MAGS-7: Prevalence estimates and classification congruence. J Gambl Stud 2004;20(3): 259–81.
33. Ladouceur R, Ferland F, Poulin C, Vitaro F, Wiebe J. Concordance between the SOGS-RA and the DSM-IV criteria for pathological gambling among youth. Psychol Addict Behav 2005;19(3):271–6.
34. Olason DT, Sigurdardottir KJ, Smari J. Prevalence estimates of gambling participation and problem gambling among 16–18 year old students in Iceland: A comparison of the SOGS-RA and DSM-IV-MR-J. J Gambl Stud 2006;22(1):23–39.
35. Boudreau B, Poulin C. The South Oaks Gambling Screen-revised Adolescent (SOGS-RA) revisited: A cut-point analysis. J Gambl Stud 2007;23:299–308.
36. Welte JW, Barnes GM, Tidwell MO, Hoffman JH. The prevalence of problem gambling among U.S. adolescents and young adults: Results from a national survey. J Gambl Stud 2008;24:119–33.
37. Fisher SE. Gambling and pathological gambling in adolescents. J Gambl Stud 1993;9:277–87.
38. Fisher SE. The amusement arcade as a social space for adolescents. J Adolesc 1995;18:71–86.
39. Fisher SE. A prevalence study of gambling and problem gambling in British adolescents. Addict Res 1999;7:509–38.
40. Wood RTA, Griffiths MD. The acquisition, development and maintenance of lottery and scratchcard gambling in adolescence. J Adolesc 1998;21:265–73.
41. Becona E. Pathological gambling in Spanish children and adolescents: An emerging problem. Psychol Rep 1997; 81:275–87.
42. Gupta R, Derevensky J. Adolescent gambling behaviour: A prevalence study and examination of the correlates associated with excessive gambling. J Gambl Stud 1998; 14:319–45.
43. Jacques C, Ladouceur R. DSM-IV-J criteria: A scoring error that may be modifying the estimates of pathological gambling among youths. J Gambl Stud 2003;19(4):427–31.
44. Lesieur HR, Rosenthal RJ. Pathological gambling: A review of the literature (Prepared for the American Psychiatric Association Task Force on DSM-IV Committee on Disorders of Impulse Control Not Elsewhere Classified). J Gambl Stud 1991;7:5–39.
45. Shaffer HJ, Hall MN, Vander Bilt J. Estimating the prevalence of disordered gambling behavior in the United States and Canada: A meta-analysis. Boston: Harvard Med School, Div Addict; 1997.
46. American Educational Research Association, American Psychological Association and National Council on Measurement in Education. Standards for educational and psychological testing. Washington, DC: Am Psychol Assoc; 1985.

Treating youth problem gamblers

10 Treatment of adolescent gambling problems: More art than science?

Jeffrey L. Derevensky, Caroline Temcheff, and Rina Gupta

Despite the relatively high prevalence rates of adolescent problem gambling, most individuals go untreated. Estimates are that only 10% of adults with gambling problems and even fewer adolescents seek help for a gambling problem. Adolescents do not present in the same manner as adults; they do not lose their wives, husbands, or children (they are generally unmarried); they do not lose a home (they typically live with their parents); they have not lost a job (most often they are students); and their accumulated debts, though impactful for them, tend not to be at the same level as those of adults. Yet the negative social, psychological, familial, mental health, and often legal consequences resulting from their excessive gambling can be pervasive. This chapter explores the possibility of different treatment approaches for adolescent problem gamblers and presents the model employed at the International Centre for Youth Gambling Problems and High-Risk Behaviors as a model for helping these youth.

10.1 Introduction

The fact there have been no universal empirically validated treatment programs established for problem gamblers has not deterred clinicians from employing a wide diversity of treatment approaches. These paradigms, explained more fully by Gupta and Derevensky (1), Petry (2), National Research Council (3), McCown and Howatt (4), and Shaffer and LaPlante (5), suggest that most clinicians adopt one or more of the following approaches in treating adult pathological gamblers; psychoanalytic/psychodynamic, behavioral, cognitive, cognitive-behavioral, psychopharmacological, physiological, self-help, or addiction-based models. Several of these approaches have specific time frames and more or less standardized approaches and goals for each session (these are typically the cognitive or behavioral interventions); others are more dependent on the individuals' concomitant psychological or mental health problems as assessed by the therapist; others advocate for self-help strategies (these can be accomplished through tutorials, workbooks, or support group meetings). A number of these models are more fully explained throughout this book.

There has been abundant research conducted during the past 30 years clearly suggesting that problem gamblers are not a homogenous group. They not only differ on the basis of their gender, age, types of gambling activities preferred, length of proposed treatment plan, but on critical bio-psycho-social individual aspects. This conceptualization and understanding has suggested that rather than incorporating a rather restrictive approach suitable for all pathological gamblers, a more tailored approach has merit. This is not to suggest that one's theoretical ordination must be altered but rather that the therapist must be cognizant of the individual's underlying problems, cognitive distortions, co-occurring mental health disorders, gambling availability and accessibility, triggers prompting one to gamble, one's support system, as well as the individual's gambling habits, preferences, and associated gambling-related problems.

The mechanism of addiction involves not only direct physiological effects but a cascade of events, cognitions, and consequences that lead to short-term pleasurable and rewarding experiences, but both short and long-term harm. Precipitating events or emotions, erroneous beliefs, cognitive distortions, and intermittent reinforcement schedules work together to make gambling a potentially highly addictive activity for some individuals. Given this, psychological treatment and intervention for individuals with a gambling addiction must address all steps of the mechanism underlying the addiction in order to achieve meaningful and lasting change.

Given the paucity of research examining the efficacy of treatment programs and outcomes in general, and for adolescents in particular, with respect to problem and pathological gambling, it is not surprising that there currently exists no best practices. This is likely a result of the lack of systematic examination, the diversity of approaches, the heterogeneity of individuals seeking help, the small numbers of youth seen in treatment programs, and the limited research community examining this issue. Walker, Schellink, and Anjoul (6) highlight the notion that human gambling is an enigma. How to best understand motivation for gambling where individuals are willing to wager on the outcome of unpredictable events when the expected return is less than the initial stake, may be difficult to explain if the central premise of gambling focuses on the notion of winning money. If, however, one assumes that other concomitant reasons for engaging in this behavior include enjoyment, excitement, as well as social aspects, winning money then becomes only one of a number of important reasons for engaging in this behavior. If one further assumes that the major motivation is the need to relieve some form of mental issue/disorder or dysregulation, coupled with erroneous beliefs and cognitions, then it is possible to better understand why some individuals continue to gamble in spite of repeated losses and their desire to stop. Do cognitions become distorted and erroneous beliefs overtake common sense? Does the need for an exhilarating experience, a desire for an adrenaline rush, or the impulse to satisfy a craving trump rational thought? Understanding the underlying reasons why individuals gamble and develop excessive gambling problems will undoubtedly help in the treatment of problem gamblers.

There is clear evidence that most adults and adolescents learn from their mistakes and though they sometimes exceed their preset gambling limits, both in terms of time and/or money, and may suffer some short-term consequences, most eventually refrain from excessive gambling. Some may stop and others may retake control of their wagering behavior. Yet for some individuals, their physiological needs, perceived skill, and erroneous cognitions, and/or need for escape from daily stressors lead them to increase the frequency and intensity of their gambling in spite of the fact that they realize that their odds of winning are indeed limited. Where else can one find large numbers of intelligent people who leave their intelligence outside the door when they enter a casino? Can it be that most individuals think they are smarter than the owners of casinos who have invested hundreds of millions and billions of dollars?

Adolescents in many ways are in fact no different than adults when it comes to the underlying reasons for their gambling, although it has been argued that brain maturation is not completed until approximately age 24. Yet, the developmental period of adolescence is marked by distinct beliefs, physiological and psychological changes, concerns, and challenges. As such, most therapists typically would agree that an understanding of the psychology of adolescence would be extremely important in the treatment of most disorders.

Although there is no empirically validated treatment protocol specifically designed for adolescents with a gambling disorder, a limited number of treatment studies have been reported in the psychological and psychiatric literature. These studies, however, have typically been predicated on very small samples of treatment-seeking adolescents (7) and have been criticized for not upholding rigorous scientific standards (3, 8–10). For a description and overview of the adult studies the reader is referred to Petry (2), Shaffer and LaPlante (5), Toneatto and Ladouceur (11), and Zangeneh, Blaszczynski, and Turner (12). The limitations of these studies, in particular for adolescents, are illustrated in a study by Ladouceur and his colleagues (7), which provided one of the earliest studies examining a cognitive-behavioral approach in treating four adolescent male pathological gamblers. Their treatment paradigm included five components: (a) general information about gambling, (b) cognitive interventions and strategies, (c) problem-solving training, (d) relapse prevention, and (e) social skills training. Cognitive therapy was provided individually to these youth for approximately 3 months (a mean number of 17 sessions). Ladouceur and his colleagues (7) reported clinically significant gains resulting from treatment, with three of the four adolescents remaining abstinent between 3 and 6 months following treatment. They further concluded that the treatment duration necessary for adolescents with severe gambling problems was relatively short compared to that required for adults, and that cognitive therapy represents a promising new paradigm for treatment of adolescent pathological gamblers. Although treatment effects based on this study were promising, the limited sample (four adolescents) is not sufficiently representative to draw firm conclusions. It is also important to note that these adolescents reportedly had no co-occurring mental health or addictive disorders. Understanding erroneous cognitions and beliefs remained a central focus. Their premise was that adolescents, like their adult counterparts, will continue to gamble in spite of repeated losses as they maintain the unrealistic perception and belief that ultimately they are able to recoup their losses (chasing behavior). Ladouceur and his colleagues (7) contend that it is the desire to recoup losses and win money that provides the primary motivation to gamble. In a number of studies we have found that for most adolescent gamblers the primary reasons for gambling are for the enjoyment and excitement, as well as to make money, with 50% of all adolescents problem gamblers reporting doing so as a means of escaping stressors in their lives, be they academic, social, familial, interpersonal, legal, and so on (13). The desire to recoup losses, though important, is typically not the underlying reason driving their gambling behavior. Yet, when discussing this issue with adolescent problem gamblers it is frequently reported that all they want to do is "get even" and recoup previous losses given their excessive debts. Having adolescents realize the underlying reason motivating their gambling behavior becomes central to long-term changes and has become the focus of our treatment paradigm. As previously noted in the chapters within this book by Gupta and Derevensky (14), and Shead, Derevensky, and Gupta (15), understanding the etiology and risk factors for the individual remain central to developing an effective treatment strategy.

10.2 Treating youth: The McGill treatment approach

It is important to preface the section describing the McGill treatment program by acknowledging that, like many other addictive behaviors, there is evidence that a number of individuals with gambling disorders have likely modified their behaviors without formal psychotherapeutic or psychopharmacological treatment (5, 16), with a number of individuals electing self-help or support group recovery programs. Shaffer and LaPlante (5) have argued that if gambling disorders are similar to substance abuse disorders, it is plausible that many individuals experience a process of natural recovery at a similar rate to other addictive disorders (17). Given that very few adolescents present for treatment (adolescents tend not to present themselves for counseling or therapy for most psychological disorders), and the general prevalence rates for disordered gambling among adults are significantly less than for adolescents, it would appear that most teens go through a process of natural recovery sometime during these transitional years. However, it is essential to note that there remain long-term, sometimes life-altering, negative consequences resulting from their pathological gambling (personal, interpersonal, familial, school, legal, and financial).

For the past 15 years, we have been providing treatment for youth (adolescents and young adults) experiencing gambling and gambling-related problems. The treatment facility is housed within McGill University's International Centre for Youth Gambling and High Risk Behaviors. Our understanding of risk and protective factors associated with youth experiencing gambling problems during this period has grown exponentially. At the same time, we have witnessed a distinct shift in the gambling activities in which young people engage. Although sports wagering is still commonplace, many young people are now becoming excessively involved in poker (Texas Hold'em being the game of choice) and Internet wagering (poker playing, sports wagering, and casino games are also quite popular). Much of this poker playing has been instigated by the pop up messages and advertisements received by adolescents on their personal computers, the heavy advertising on television, radio, and in the print media, and the phenomenal success of televised poker tournaments (strongly endorsed by multiple Internet gambling sites) (18, 19). The fact that a number of celebrities, well known by these young people, and past winners of the World Series of Poker have been quite young (early 20s), winning millions of dollars, has strengthened its appeal. Still further, a recent study conducted by McBride and Derevensky (20) among college students found that a primary reason for Internet wagering was to relieve boredom. As also noted by Griffiths, Parke, and Derevensky in this volume (21), a growing number of adolescents and young adults are using Internet wagering as their preferred venue due to its convenience, easy accessibility, and less restrictive and lax enforcement of age requirements.

Though no formal evaluation of the treatment outcome has occurred due to the diversity of our clientele and the need to individualize and match clients with our clinical intervention, a great deal of knowledge and information has been acquired into the strategies that promote gambling abstinence, techniques to help youths' overall improvement of their psychological well-being, and the importance of relapse prevention. There is some controversy among clinicians and academics concerning whether abstinence or controlled gambling is acceptable for adults with severe gambling problems (22–26). Our clinical experience with adolescents and young adults suggests that abstinence remains a desired goal given that this age group of individuals has difficulty not in setting time and/or money goals but rather in maintaining and adhering to these limits. In spite of the large percentage of adolescents and young adults preferring a controlled gambling approach ("Just teach me to gamble in moderation so I can enjoy myself"), our research and clinical experience suggest that controlled gambling can be an interim goal, but abstinence is necessary to prevent increased levels of gambling and relapse. Ultimately our goal is to have these youth resume a healthy lifestyle, ensure that no other risky behavior replaces their gambling, and achieve abstinence.

Similar to adolescents with other mental health issues, adolescents with gambling problems typically do not to present themselves for treatment in the absence of some type of outside (typically parental or peer) pressure or influence. A number of reasons have been suggested, including (a) fear of being identified, (b) the belief that they can control or stop their gambling without support, (c) self-perceptions of invincibility and invulnerability to future negative consequences, (d) negative views of therapy, (e) guilt associated with their gambling problems, (f) a lack of recognition and acceptance that they have a gambling problem despite scoring high on gambling severity screens or associated gambling problems, (g) they are not ready to stop their gambling in spite of the negative consequences, and (h) an inherent belief in natural recovery and self-control (for a more detailed explanation see Derevensky, and Gupta, Derevensky, and Gupta and Winters [27, 28]). DiClemente, Story, and Murray (29), adopting the basic elements of the process of intentional behavior change model originally outlined in the Stages of Change from the Transtheoretical Model (30), have argued that the motivational aspects for change are indeed crucial. Thus, while "strongly encouraged" to seek help, the individual must in fact desire to ultimately change his/her behavior. Movement from the precontemplation stage (not considering initiating or lack of real desire to change the behavior) to preparation (commitment and planning) to action (engaged in actual behavioral change) and finally to maintenance (sustaining behavioral changes) stage sets an optimal framework for working with youth who are either unmotivated to change or possibly who have modified their behavior but are concerned about relapse (a number of adolescents and young adults have entered our treatment program already being abstinent but concerned about relapse).

Referrals from parents, friends, teachers, the court system, and the local Help/Referral Line are the primary sources through which we acquire our treatment population. As part of our outreach prevention/intervention program, posters and brochures are distributed to schools, media exposure and media campaigns are frequent, and workshops are provided for school psychologists, guidance counselors, social workers, teachers, and directly to children and adolescents to raise awareness about issues related to youth gambling. As a result of this outreach program, we receive calls from a number of adolescents and family members directly requesting assistance. The Centre's Internet site has also generated several inquiries for online help and assistance.

Research and our clinical experience suggest that adolescent problem gamblers develop a social network consisting of other peers with gambling problems (13, 31). This results in clients recommending their friends for treatment. Once the adolescent accepts and realizes that he/she has a serious gambling problem, awareness of gambling problems among their friends typically becomes acute. Eventually, some successfully convince their peers to seek help as well.

Because adolescents with gambling problems have limited access to discretionary funds and many initially seek treatment without parental knowledge, treatment is provided without cost. This is obviously not practical for treatment providers in independent practice. However, state, provincial, and/or national funding (or support by insurance providers where available) is crucial for the establishment and maintenance of treatment centers for adolescents with a gambling addiction.

The location of the treatment facility plays an important role in successfully working with young gamblers. Concerns about being seen entering an addiction treatment facility, mental health center, or hospital may discourage some youth from seeking treatment. Accessibility by public transportation is essential as most young clients do not own cars or have money for taxi fare. Although our clinic is adjacent to a university counseling center, it operates as a self-contained facility exclusively for work with youth experiencing gambling problems. The Centre is located centrally in a large urban setting.

The treatment approach has been developed and is predicated on recent research findings and our clinical work with adolescents and young adult problem gamblers. It is important to reiterate that the treatment philosophy is based on the assumption that sustained abstinence is ultimately necessary for youth to recover from gambling and gambling-related problems and to reduce the likelihood of relapse, and that many life areas and mental health issues must be concomitantly addressed (e.g., social networks, coping skills, cognitive distortions, attention deficit hyperactive disorders, depression). We have observed a large percentage of youth in treatment whose initial goal is "controlled gambling." There has been some debate among clinicians about whether complete abstinence or controlled use should be the final goal for addictions therapy among adults. Our clinical work suggests that although controlled gambling (ability to respect self-imposed limits) can be an interim goal for adolescents, abstinence is eventually necessary. Accepting that adolescents set initial goals to decrease their gambling (controlled gambling) instead of becoming abstinent, allows us time to develop strong working alliances with clients before introducing the need for sustained abstinence. It is our clinical judgment that if we initially encouraged adolescents toward total abstinence as a prerequisite for treatment, we would risk losing a large number of adolescents due to their sense of failure or disconnect between their objective and that of the treatment provider.

In our clinic, attempts are made to closely monitor these youth for at least one year post treatment, with long-term follow-up often being difficult. Several youth call periodically beyond the one-year follow-up period to report their progress, but we remain acutely aware that youth who may have relapsed may be unwilling to contact the treatment center again unless they are prepared to re-enter treatment. There is also some evidence with adults that pathological gamblers who have successfully completed treatment and who have relapsed often fail to return to the same treatment center for assistance, but are more likely to seek treatment elsewhere given their belief that they do not want to disappoint their original therapists (32).

10.3 Steps of treatment

10.3.1 Intake interviews

Intake interviews typically take place over several sessions. The primary goals of the intake sessions include diagnosis of gambling severity, identification of mental health issues, completion of a functional assessment, understanding of the individual's motivation and readiness for change, establishment of a good working alliance marked by mutual respect, and preliminary work on fostering motivation if the client's motivation appears tenuous. Each of these goals is discussed separately below.

Diagnosis

The intake procedure includes a semi-structured interview using the DSM-IV-MR-J or DSM-IV criteria (depending on the individual's age) for pathological gambling as well as the identification of relevant gambling behaviors (e.g., preferred activities, frequency, wagering patterns, history of gambling, accumulated losses, financial and legal issues, etc.). It must be underlined that although the diagnostic instruments have utility in research settings, within the clinical setting, adopting a dichotomous view of a gambling addiction can be too simplistic. The trained and specialized clinician should feel comfortable with incorporating clinical judgment when diagnosing presence and particularly severity of gambling problems. The fact that the individual has presented himself/herself for treatment of a gambling problem is in itself strong evidence of a gambling disorder. As previously noted, a number of youth enter our treatment program having already abstained from gambling but seeking assistance concerning maintenance and acutely aware of relapse. Many of these youth have had gambling-free periods but have eventually relapsed.

Functional assessment

The functional assessment is a vital component when planning any therapeutic intervention. The functional assessment includes information gathering in a number of areas including triggers for problematic gambling, cognitions, behaviors, emotions before and during gambling episodes, and consequences following gambling episodes. Triggers can include specific places (casinos, bars with electronic gambling machines, Internet pop-up messages, televised or radio advertisements, poker parties, etc.), people (socializing with friends who gamble), activities (going to a party, excessive consumption of alcohol), or dysregulation of emotional states (e.g., anxiety, loneliness, sense of loss, depression). Although initially many individuals are unaware of their specific triggers, they can be identified through discussions of prior experiences or by examining the client's written journals (a component within the therapeutic process). Cognitions and cognitive distortions that follow from exposure to triggers must also be identified and made explicit (e.g., "If I gamble now, I will be more relaxed for the party tonight and I will have a better time"), as well as emotions that might follow from the cognitions or interpretations of events. Finally, consequences following excessive, out-of-control, or binging gambling episodes should be explored.

Assessing and fostering motivation for change

It has been suggested that those individuals who present themselves for treatment are distinct, representing a minority of young pathological gamblers. It is important to note that though those individuals seeking help voluntarily come for treatment, a number may be less than motivated to initially participate. A considerable number attend as a result of parental pressure, mandatory referrals from the judicial system, or strong encouragement by significant others (i.e., boyfriends, girlfriends) and comply for fear of losing relationships. One youth who was brought in by his parents commented on the DSM-IV list of items on a poster in our waiting room. He reported that he endorsed every item on the gambling screen but he did not have a gambling problem in spite of the fact that his parents, relatives, friends, and girlfriend thought he had a gambling problem.

Any type of psychological therapy for addiction is a very arduous process that demands significant effort and focus on the part of the client. For this reason, before beginning therapy, it is important to assess the client's readiness for change as well as motivation for change and work to foster motivation as needed (29). Client motivation can be encouraged by several techniques and practices that are incorporated into the motivational interviewing style of therapy (see Miller and Rollnick [33] and Hodgins and Diskin [34]). The general tenets of this approach include the belief that motivation to change must come from the client (i.e., cannot be imposed by others), that though the therapist can be directive, it is ultimately the client's task to articulate and resolve ambivalence, and that the therapeutic relationship is a collaborative partnership. Further, Miller and Rollnick (33) contend that motivation is not a stable client trait, but rather may fluctuate throughout treatment. Some important therapeutic elements included in motivational interviewing with individuals experiencing gambling problems include (a) providing personalized and specific feedback relevant to the individual's situation (reality check), (b) shifting responsibility for treatment to the client, (c) allowing clients to engage in a "decisional balance" exercise in which they can weigh the hypothetical costs and benefits of continuing versus quitting gambling, (d) providing several options and objective advice, (e) and the encouragement of the client's self-efficacy. Of course, the provision of a safe place to share experiences and challenges as well as empathic listening are key components of the therapeutic alliance and should be given special attention when trying to foster client motivation. The use of these techniques with adult problem gamblers has been shown to have a positive impact (34, 35). It is likely that such techniques would also greatly benefit adolescent problem gamblers.

Allowing individuals to receive help with the primary notion of controlled gambling is essential while working toward an abstinence approach. For many of these individuals, gambling becomes the ultimate form of escape from problems, a way of coping with depressive symptomatology, an exhilarating activity that gives them much pleasure. Over time, they come to realize the short-term and long-term harms associated with their excessive gambling. For many, stopping gambling is analogous to losing their best friend. Therapists have a tendency to focus solely on the negative aspects and consequences associated with gambling without addressing the positive aspects. Both perspectives need to be addressed.

10.3.2 Therapy

General therapeutic environment. A staff psychologist provides individual therapy at the Centre. It should be noted that on occasion, peers with similar gambling problems, family members, and/or significant others are often requested to participate. Our past experience is that group therapy has been extremely difficult to coordinate due to multiple clients' differing timetables. Therapy is typically provided weekly, however if the therapist deems more frequent sessions are required, appropriate accommodations are made on a short-term basis. The overall number of sessions varies significantly based on the level of motivation, degree, and length of gambling severity, and severity of co-morbid disorders. Typically, treatment lasts between 20 and 50 sessions.

For adolescents experiencing gambling problems, total honesty during therapy is emphasized and a nonjudgmental relationship is provided. This is fundamental in terms of creating an environment in which the adolescent does not fear reactions of disappointment or condemnation if weekly personal goals are not successfully achieved.

Mutual respect is a top priority and adolescents are held to a high standard of personal responsibility in this area. Treatment is provided at no cost, but clients are required to respect the therapist's time. This involves calling ahead to cancel and reschedule appointments, punctual attendance at sessions, and a commitment to complete assignments between sessions.

Goal setting

Overarching goals for therapy are set at the beginning of treatment and are revised several times during the therapeutic process. Smaller objective and measurable weekly goals are also a crucial part of creating a space in which clients can feel supported and motivated and can track progress through their healing process. It is important that goals be tailored to the client's priorities, gambling severity, and comorbid disorders. For example, a client with comorbid personality or anxiety disorder is not approached in the same way as a client with gambling addiction without depressive symptomatology. In most cases, multiple therapeutic goals are addressed simultaneously over many sessions, while tailoring the time allocated to each goal to the needs of the client.

Environmental changes and triggers

Once triggers are identified as part of the functional assessment, it becomes possible to proactively address them during the therapeutic process. For example, one of the most common triggers for gamblers is the handling of large sums of money. In this case, adolescents would be helped to adopt strategies to minimize carrying large sums of money and limit their access to cash withdrawals from bank machines. In one case, a parent who was financially supporting his son made daily deposits into his account rather than weekly deposits. Other examples of triggers include gambling advertisements or landmarks, personal anxiety or depressed feelings, interpersonal difficulties, enticement of peers, stressful academic or work-related situations, and the need to acquire money quickly. Sometimes, merely having the awareness of one's triggers provides the individual with a better ability to deal with gambling urges. Individuals with a machine gambling addiction (e.g., slots, VLTs, Pokies) are urged not to spend time in establishments housing these machines. Though it is likely not possible to eliminate all triggers (e.g., pop-up messages, lottery tickets on checkout counters in convenience stores, etc.), it is possible to help individuals understand the importance of triggers in prompting them to gamble. Additional research is needed to better understand the relationship between triggers and mechanisms of self-control.

Understanding motivations for gambling

Adolescents experiencing serious gambling problems frequently continue gambling in the face of repeated losses and serious negative consequences as result of their need to dissociate and escape from daily stressors. Many youth with gambling problems report that when they are gambling they enter a "different world," a world without problems and stresses. They report that while gambling, they feel invigorated and alive, they are admired and respected, that time passes quickly, and all their problems are forgotten – be they psychological, financial, social, familial, academic, work-related, or legal. As such, for a large number of youth experiencing gambling problems, their gambling becomes the ultimate escape, albeit for a short period of time. From their perspective, a good day for these youth is when their gambling money lasts all day; a bad day is when their money runs out in an hour.

Adolescents are asked to write a short essay on why it is they feel the need to gamble – "What gambling does for me." Writing about what gambling provides for the adolescent is important for several reasons. First, it enables the therapist to have a better understanding of the individual's perceptions of the reasons underlying why they are gambling excessively. Second, and more importantly, it enables the individual to articulate and understand the underlying reasons for gambling. Gambling can be both positively and negatively reinforcing to players; providing intermittent pleasurable feelings or escape from negative situations or emotions. This is at least partly responsible for the fact that adolescents with gambling problems continue playing despite potentially serious negative longer-term consequences. A recent study by Gillespie, Derevensky, and Gupta (36) revealed that most adolescent problem gamblers perceive both the risks and benefits associated with gambling. What appears to differentiate problem gamblers from their nonproblem gambling peers is that problem gamblers view the risks and negative consequences associated with excessive gambling to occur at a much later time and by then they believe they will have stopped gambling.

The following are excerpts from several clients' writings. The first highlights difficulties with interpersonal relationships and poor coping/adaptive skills, the second illustrates an individual's gambling to alleviate a depressed state and psychological escape.

> I always had trouble making friends, and never had a girlfriend. Gambling has now become my best friend and my one true love. I can turn to her in good times and bad and she'll always be there for me. (Male, age 18)

> Gambling, well, it's strange to talk about the positive side because of how upside down it has turned my life, but I guess the pull of it is how it makes me feel so alive, so happy, and so much like I belong, but only when I am gambling. The low I feel after I realize what I did, and how much I have lost, is worse than anything I can explain. I guess I just need to feel good from time to time, it lets me escape the black hole that is my life. (Male, age 17)

Analysis of gambling episodes

Gaining awareness and achieving acceptance of gambling triggers, psychological, emotional, and behavioral reactions to those triggers, and the consequences that follow from this sequence is important. This type of understanding and critical analysis can have an empowering impact on adolescents and can encourage them to make long-term changes in their behaviors. It is essential that the individual does not attribute the repeated losses to an external event (e.g., bad luck, or as one client noted "my parents are on my back all the time and I was unable to concentrate and review all the statistics needed to pick the winning team"). Problem gamblers are in some ways like alcoholics.

Many alcoholics have a favorite drink but if one removes their favorite drink they will switch to another. One youth who was an excessive gambler at the casino playing blackjack had told us that individuals who played the electronic gambling machines were "stupid" as there was no skill involved. After we managed to keep him out of the casino he became a machine gambler until eventually he stopped gambling.

The importance of identifying and dealing with triggers has already been discussed in this chapter. However, it is also important to understand the times in a client's day when he/she does not seem to have the urge to gamble. Identifying the circumstances, time of day, emotional state, activity levels, physical proximity to gambling venues, etc. is essential. Understanding the circumstances under which the urge to gamble is lower or absent helps provide a set of guidelines by which the therapist can help re-create similar situations at other times in the day. For example, we have noted that many of the young gamblers undergoing treatment often report that when actively engaged in playing sports with friends, bicycling, other physical activity (e.g., gym, skiing) they feel better and their minds clear of their gambling desires both during and after the activity. As a result, for these youth, when helping them to structure and organize their week, attempts are made to include similar types of activities on a daily basis.

Establishing a baseline of gambling behavior and encouraging a decrease in gambling

Once the motivations for gambling are understood and an analysis of gambling patterns has been made, efforts are focused on making changes to the adolescent's gambling behavior. In order to set goals and measure improvements, we find it useful and important to initially establish a baseline of gambling behavior. Adolescents are required to record their gambling behaviors in terms of frequency, duration, time of day, type of gambling activity, amount of money spent, losses and wins. When establishing goals for a decrease in gambling participation, adolescents are guided to establish reasonable goals for themselves. Some elect to target multiple indices such as frequency, duration, and amount spent simultaneously, whereas others may focus on one aspect of gambling (e.g., frequency or duration). For these individuals, we encourage a decrease in frequency or duration of each gambling episode versus initially focusing on amount wagered. Some meet their goals immediately at which point we generally support decisions to maintain this decrease for a short period before establishing new goals. Others struggle to meet their goals, at which point goals can be modified and amended.

Cognitive therapy and cognitive distortions

It has been well established that individuals with gambling problems experience multiple cognitive distortions (37, 38). They are prone to have an illusion of control, perceive that they can control the outcome of random events, underestimate the amount of money lost and overestimate the amount won, fail to utilize their knowledge of the laws of independence of events, and believe that if they persist at gambling they will likely regain all money lost. Addressing these cognitive distortions remains an important treatment goal. In particular, male adolescents externalize their losses (e.g., bad luck, bad dealer) whereas females internalize their behavior (e.g., "I should have known the odds, I made a poor decision"). Furthermore, an analysis of their gambling behavior typically reveals the rationalizations they make to justify their gambling behavior. These rationalizations need to be directly addressed, as they too represent distortions of reality. One such example is, "By gambling now, the urge will be out of my system and I'll be more able to focus on studying for my exam." The overarching goal is to ensure that the individual comprehends that the gambling episode will likely result in a bad mood if they lose money, and an inability to focus on studying for an exam. Ultimately, the goal of addressing many of the cognitive distortions is to highlight how one's thinking can be self-deceptive, to provide examples and pertinent information about randomness, to encourage a realization that gamblers are incapable of controlling outcomes of random events and games, payout rates, etc.

In addition to examining constructs such as the illusion of control, laws of independence of events, and randomness, we have tried to incorporate specific examples for both sports gamblers and poker players. For sports gamblers, we discuss the results of several large studies conducted by the National Collegiate Athletic Association in the United States (approximately 20,000 college athletes in each study) (39, 40). The results of these studies suggest that there is a small but identifiable number of college athletes who try to manipulate the outcome of games as a result of their personal gambling. We challenge adolescents' perceptions of selecting winning teams, in spite of their extensive knowledge about the sport, if the outcome of the game may be altered by a player.

The identification of specific cognitive distortions particular to each client forms a critical component of therapy. Erroneous cognitions are addressed throughout the therapeutic process. There is evidence that such erroneous cognitions and beliefs can be altered and modified (41).

Establishing the underlying causes of stress, anxiety, depression, and other mental health disorders

In light of empirical research (13, 42–44) and clinical findings it becomes essential to identify and address any underlying problems that result in increased stress, anxiety, and depression. For some, the financial losses and delinquent behaviors associated with their excessive gambling result in increased anxiety, stress, and/or depression. Yet for others these mental health issues are the reason for gambling. As most winnings and losses are intermittent, individuals experience both benefits and consequences associated with their playing behavior. Our clients have presented with a wide diversity of mental health issues: poor self-image, depression, anxiety disorders, attention deficit disorders, conduct disorders, oppositional defiant disorders, suicide ideation, and social and interpersonal issues. As well, it is not uncommon for them to be experiencing academic, work-related, and/or legal issues. Psychopharmacological treatment in conjunction with traditional forms of therapy is provided in collaboration with consulting psychiatrists when necessary.

Evaluating and improving coping abilities

Once underlying anxieties or affective states that contribute to the adolescent's desire to gamble have been identified, another therapeutic goal is to assist the adolescent in the acquisition of new positive and prosocial coping strategies. Recent research has pointed to the importance of resilience as a protective factor in helping individuals refrain from excessive gambling (45). Problematic and excessive gambling as a need to escape one's problems usually occurs more frequently among individuals who have poor coping and adaptive skills (46). Using gambling or other addictive activities to deal with daily stressors, anxiety, or depression represents a form of maladaptive coping. Recent research efforts have confirmed these clinical observations, where adolescents who meet the criteria for pathological gambling demonstrated poor coping skills and depression compared to same-age peers without a gambling problem (47, 48).

Given this information, building and expanding the individual's repertoire of coping abilities remains important in enabling adolescents to be resilient in light of adversity. As adolescents begin to acquire more sophisticated adaptive strategies and their repertoire of coping responses expands, they are more apt to apply these skills in their daily lives. Examples of healthy coping skills include effective communication with others, enhanced social support seeking behavior, and the ability to differentially respond to situations based on risks and benefits. Also included in the discussions and role-playing exercises are ways to improve social skills (e.g., learning to communicate with peers, developing healthy friendships, being considerate of others, and developing trust).

Rebuilding healthy interpersonal relationships

A common consequence of a serious gambling problem involves impaired and damaged relationships with friends, peers, and family members. Helping adolescents rebuild these crucial relationships constitutes an important therapeutic goal. Because of lies, manipulative, and antisocial behaviors stemming from the gambling problem, friends and family members become alienated, leaving unresolved negative feelings and disrupted relationships. Once a youth has been identified as being a liar or thief, it becomes difficult to regain the trust of others and to resume healthy relationships. This becomes one of the more difficult situations faced by the problem gambler. They have typically lied numerous times about having quit gambling, but once they actually do stop their gambling they want to be trusted almost immediately. Although on a cognitive level they understand the lack of trust by significant others, they have great difficulty being repeatedly questioned as to their daily activities. We often remind youth that it took quite some time to destroy the trust and will likely take even longer to rebuild it. One parent asked his son to bring receipts for all expenses to help account for his money. This proved both embarrassing and difficult, having to ask friends for receipts when purchasing coffee. This type of situation requires some intervention by the therapist on behalf of the adolescent. One needs to explain to family members and friends that these deceptive actions are part of the constellation of problematic behaviors exhibited by individuals who cannot control their gambling. Consequently, once the gambling is under control, family members and friends can anticipate being treated with honesty and respect.

Family members, peers, and significant others become important support personnel to help ensure abstinence and can take an active role in relapse prevention. Youth with gambling problems are likely to be happier and more apt to abstain from gambling if they feel they belong to a peer group and are supported by family and friends. As a result, the periodic inclusion of family members and friends in therapy sessions has proven to be very beneficial. Nevertheless, the process of rebuilding relationships can be long and arduous. and is often met with only partial success. In some circumstances, some friends or family members may not be willing to forgive the problem gambler or re-establish contact.

Restructuring free time

Adolescents struggling to overcome a gambling problem experience more positive outcomes when not faced with large amounts of unstructured time. Some adolescents in treatment are still in school and/or have a job, and as such their free time consists mainly of evenings and weekends. Others have dropped out of school and may have a part-time job, and others are not working. For these youth, structuring their time becomes paramount as they initially find it exceedingly difficult to resist urges to gamble when they are bored. We frequently ask adolescents to carry a notepad to keep track of their daily schedule. Spending time with friends, family, school- or work-related activities are beneficial. Other suggested activities involve participating in organized sports activities, engaging in a hobby, watching movies, and performing volunteer work. The success of their week is evaluated on how they well they achieve the weekly goals agreed upon, with their gambling-related goals (reduction or abstinence) being one part of the program. Thus, if an individual fails to meet their goals surrounding their gambling behavior, they still may achieve success in other areas. This approach tends to keep the clients from being discouraged, and motivates them to attain a balanced lifestyle and to continue treatment.

Fostering effective money management skills

These skills are typically lacking in adolescents who have a gambling problem. Therapeutic goals involve educating them as to the value of money (as they tend to lose perspective after gambling large sums), building money management skills, and helping them develop and maintain a reasonable debt repayment plan. Interestingly, problem gamblers often view purchases in line with their gambling behaviors. When asked how one teenager travelled to the casino, he replied "half a hand." He went on further to explain that he typically wagered $25 per hand on blackjack and taxi fare to the casino was only $13. Having youth carry less money, in small denominations (large bills enhance their stature and self image as the "big shot") is also important.

10.3.3 Preparation for cessation of treatment and relapse prevention

As previously noted, our clinical work suggests that abstinence from gambling is the optimal goal. Abstinence among our clinical sample has improved the likelihood of relapse of gambling problems. It should be noted that small, occasional relapses (we tend to refer to them as "slips" with our clients) throughout the treatment process are to be expected. However, once gambling has ceased for an extended period of time (i.e., 6 months), an effective relapse prevention program should help these individuals remain free of gambling.

Given that gambling treatment usually goes on over an extended period of time, it is important to phase therapy out gradually. This allows the adolescent to get accustomed to having longer stretches without therapeutic support during which he/she must take control of maintenance of therapeutic gains autonomously. Difficulties encountered during this phasing-out process provide useful information and can be dealt with while the adolescent is still actively engaged in therapy.

Relapse prevention post termination includes continued access to the primary therapist for "booster" sessions, the existence of a good social support network, engagement in either school or work, the practice of a healthy lifestyle, and avoidance of powerful triggers. Youth are contacted periodically via telephone, text messages, or email for one year post treatment to ensure they are maintaining their abstinence and doing well in general. Additional support is offered when required.

10.4 Enhancing a social responsibility perspective

A major part of the Centre's mission is to promote a social responsibility perspective to policymakers, parents, and youth. For most adolescents as well as adults, gambling is generally done in moderation without enduring serious social, economic, and personal costs. Yet, the fact that many youth, parents, and educators remain unaware of the negative consequences associated with adolescent gambling is problematic. Gambling has become glamorized and normalized in our society. We take the widespread popularity of poker playing among adolescents as one prime example.

As previously noted, there are a growing number of adolescents and young adults whose gambling problems are related to their poker playing. This increase is likely due to widespread advertising, Internet gambling opportunities, televised tournaments, celebrity endorsements, its normalization, and the changing face of tournament winners. No longer is the winner the elderly gentleman from Texas wearing the large "10 gallon" hat but rather the young person, with a pierced ear, baseball cap turned backward, and wrap around sunglasses. These new champions of the World Series of Poker allow the adolescent to more closely identify with the tournament winners. As a result, we often share an excerpt of an e-mail sent to us from a professional poker player in response to an editorial that appeared in multiple newspapers warning youth not to think of themselves as the next winner:

> I am a very, solid player and have finished 97th place out of over 3000 players at a WSOP [World Series of Poker] event and do well especially at limit poker. I've ranked at one point in the top 300 of over one million online players. But I have been taught by people that are exceptional players prior to playing money games and have read many books to the point where I know my hands odds at any point during the betting process as if it were like breathing and most importantly what my opponent will do most of the time prior to betting.
>
> Without the top calibre tutelage and in-depth study of the game prior to playing, I would have lost a lot of money. But I and especially a select few like Jonathan Duhamel [the 2010 winner of the Wold Series of Poker] and minute others are probably the exception as we learn that bank roll management skills amongst other rules is above and beyond the most important rule. . . . which most players lack. I never ever play house casino games such as blackjack, roulette etc.
>
> But even after all this accumulated skill and knowledge it is still VERY, VERY difficult to make an income at it and I can't even imagine how someone starting out could do it without going bankrupt first.
>
> After reading the article, I would have to conclude your findings, theories and hypothesis as being absolutely correct. Over 99.5% of the players do not have the discipline, focus, patience and skill to become "professional". I see this over and over again at the table, how emotion not logic causes many to lose their money by the end of the night. I know who will win and who will lose it within 20 minutes and I also know they will not walk away until they lose it all. Very sad really as it happens to many players especially within certain ethnic groups. I would not over exaggerate by saying that gambling is a "disease".

It is probably the only "sport" where someone honestly thinks that overnight after winning a small tournament they consider themselves a "professional poker player", just because I score a goal against a great goalie doesn't mean I can play in the National Hockey League.

I know of top online poker world professionals that have won over $500,000 in online tournaments in one year and lose $130,000 in 2 months playing almost all the events and some cash games during the WSOP. It is not for the faint of heart.

There has also been an online discussion on how many online poker sites have their tournament games "random number generators" programmed for a high rate of set up hands (AA vs KK or KK vs QQ etc) to finish a tournament quickly so that the poker site saves money on Internet bandwidth costs. For example, a popular poker site refuses to have their random number generator reviewed by a third party for fairness.

There are other things to consider such as online team collusion, bots and advanced poker software and of course those many notorious online bad beats that creates this fuel of rage, and now someone will spend whatever it takes to win the money back only to lose it all. It is like a old record player that gets stuck on repeat, it will not change without outside help. People are creatures of habits and in poker and other gambling its bad habits.

My strongest advice is that if people *have* to play I think it should be mandatory at the very minimum especially online to set a low maximum deposit limit for the week or month. . . . . The game can be fun if you set a reasonable timeframe and budget.

10.5 Concluding comments

This treatment program's efficacy has not been empirically validated using the standards necessary for a rigorous, scientifically controlled study (i.e., no random assignments to a control group matching for severity of gambling problems and other mental health disorders, controlling for age, gender, SES, frequency and type of gambling activity preferred, etc.). As such, more clinical research is necessary before definitive conclusions can be drawn. Nevertheless, based on clinical criteria established for success (i.e., abstinence for six months post treatment, return to school or work, no longer meeting the DSM criteria for pathological gambling, improved peer and family relationships, improved coping skills, and no marked signs of depressive symptomatology, delinquent behavior, or excessive use of alcohol or drugs), the McGill University treatment program appears to have reached its objectives in successfully working with youth suffering from serious gambling problems.

The description of our treatment philosophy and approach in this chapter hopes to provide clinicians and treatment providers with a better understanding of the different components deemed necessary when working with young problem gamblers. Treating youth with severe gambling problems requires clinical skills, a knowledge of adolescent development, an understanding of the risk factors associated with problem gambling, and a thorough grounding in the empirical work concerning the correlates and risk factors associated with gambling problems. By no means should this chapter substitute for proper training.

Although we did not elaborate upon how to treat youth with multiple addictions in this chapter, it is clear that gamblers with concomitant substance abuse problems pose a greater challenge for treatment (49). Youth with clinical levels of depression, high levels of impulsivity, and anxiety disorders are often referred to psychiatry to simultaneously undergo pharmacological treatment while undergoing our therapy. The use of serotonin re-uptake inhibitors can be effective in helping these youth manage their depression and anxiety, and preliminary research suggests that they may be useful in lowering levels of impulsivity that often underlie pathological gambling behavior (Grant and Potenza, in this volume [50], and Grant, Kim, and Potenza [51]).

Though the incidence of severe gambling problems among youth remains relatively small, the devastating short-term and long-term consequences to the individual, their families, and friends are significant. One adolescent, when discussing the severity of his gambling problem, responded, "It's an all-encompassing problem that invades every facet of my life. I wouldn't wish this problem on my worst enemy, for it's way too harsh a punishment."

The vast majority of the youth seen in our clinic have a wide array of problems. Merely treating the gambling problem without examining the individual's overall mental health functioning will likely result in less than optimal results. The following is a text written by a young pathological gambler from our treatment program, one year post-treatment:

> Gambling is an extremely addictive activity which can get unbelievably out of control. It can lead to a very horrible reality, one in which just getting out of bed can seem unthinkable. Unfortunately, I have lived this reality. I was eighteen when I began to fight for my life back. My future did not look very good. I was severely depressed, anxious and overweight, I wanted to disappear. Thankfully, with the support of an amazing team I have managed to overcome my addiction, lose thirty pounds and continue my schooling. I feel like I am relearning how to live. This continues to be a very long and emotionally painful process, however it does get easier with time. My memories of the gambling, the lies and unhappiness are slowly fading away. . . becoming part of the past. However I will never forget my struggle or how easy it was to lose control. In my gambling years I have seen and experienced first hand an incredible amount of heartache. I hope to never witness such avoidable pain again. Now at twenty years old, I am beginning a journey which holds an endless amount of opportunity. My dream to be a health-care professional seems closer than ever. Please let my story be a source of hope for anyone in a similar situation. I understand how bad life can seem, I've been there, believe me. You are not alone. Get the help you need, be true to yourself and start your own journey.

Although it appears as though some adolescents who gamble problematically appear to resolve their gambling problems without traditional therapeutic intervention or support groups, providing support for those in need remains essential. Our governments, private corporations, and charitable organizations, recipients of the revenues generated from gambling, need to help address this issue by providing appropriate funding for the establishment of treatment centers and training of professionals. Problem gambling, for adults and adolescents, can have devastating short- and long-term consequences.

In spite of gains in knowledge concerning the correlates and risk factors associated with severe gambling problems among youth during the past fifteen years, a general lack of public and parental awareness exists (52). The fact that the prevalence rates for youth with severe gambling problems remain higher than those for adults is of significant concern. Whether maturation will result in individuals stopping their excessive gambling behavior by the time they become adults with additional responsibilities still remains an unanswered question. As we have argued elsewhere, independent of whether or not individuals with severe gambling during adolescence become more responsible 'social gamblers' as adults, the personal costs and consequences incurred along the way often are severe and remain with them.

Gambling problems among youth will continue to raise important public health and social policy issues in the 21st century. Greater emphasis on outreach, awareness, and prevention programs remains essential. The search for best practices in the treatment of adolescent gambling problems is only beginning. Our governments must help fund more basic and applied research and be responsible for supporting and developing effective and scientifically validated prevention and treatment programs. The treatment of young problem gamblers is a complex, multidimensional process. Though such an approach can take months or longer, the long-term benefits to the individual and society outweigh the immediate costs of funding such programs.

References

1. Gupta R, Derevensky J. A treatment approach for adolescents with gambling problems. In: Zangeneh M, Blaszczynski A, Turner N, eds. In the pursuit of winning. New York: Springer; 2008.
2. Petry N. Pathologiocal gambling: etiology, comorbidity, and treatment. Washington: American Psychological Association; 2004.
3. National Research Council. Pathological gambling: A critical review. Washington, DC: National Academy Press; 1999.
4. McCown W, Howatt W. Treating gambling problems. New Jersey: John Wiley; 2007.
5. Shaffer HJ, LaPlante D. Treatment of gambling disorders. In: Marlatt G, Donovan D, eds. Relapse prevention: Maintenance strategies in the treatment of addictive behaviors. New York: Guilford; 2008.
6. Walker M, Schellink T, Anjoul F. Explaining why people gamble. In: Zangeneh M, Blaszczynski A, Turner N, eds. In the pursuit of winning. New York: Springer; 2008.
7. Ladouceur R, Boisvert J, Dumont JM. Cognitive-behavioral treatment for adolescent pathological gambling. Behav Modif 1994;18:230–42.
8. Blaszczynski AP, Silove D. Cognitive and behavioural therapies for pathological gambling. J Gambl Stud 1995;11(2):195–220.
9. National Gambling Impact Study Commission. Chicago, IL: National Opinion Research Center; 1999.
10. Nathan P. Best practices for the treatment of gambling disorders: Too soon? Paper presented at the annual Harvard-National Center for Responsible Gambling Conference Las Vegas. 2001.
11. Toneatto T, Ladouceur R. Treatment of pathological gambling: A critical review of the literature. Psychol Addict Behav 2003;17(4):284–92.
12. Zangeneh M, Blaszczynsky A, Turner N, eds. In the pursuit of winning: Problem gambling theory, research, and treatment. New York: Springer; 2008.
13. Derevensky J. Gambling behaviors and adolescent substance use disorders. In: Kaminer Y, Buckstein OG, eds. Adolescent substance abuse: Psychiatric comorbidity and high risk behaviors. New York: Haworth; 2008:403–33.
14. Gupta R, Derevensky J. Defining and assessing binge gambling. In: Derevensky J, Shek D, Merrick J, eds. Youth gambling problems: The hidden addiction. Berlin: De Gruyter; in press.
15. Shead NW, Derevensky J, Gupta R. Youth problem gambling: Our current knowledge of risk and protective factors. In: Derevensky J, Shek D, Merrick J, eds. Youth gambling problems: The hidden addiction. Berlin: De Gruyter; in press.
16. Hodgins D, Wynne H, Makarchuk K. Pathways to recovery from gambling problems: Follow-up from a general population survey. J Gambl Stud 1999;15(2):93–104.
17. Wisdom J, Cavaleri M, Gogel L, Nacht M. Barriers and facilitators to adoelscent drug treatment: Youth, family and staff reports. Addict Res Theory 2011;19:179–89.

18. Sklar A, Derevensky J, Way to play: Analyzing gambling ads for their appeal to underage youth. Can J Commun 2010;35(4):533–54.
19. Derevensky J, Sklar A, Gupta R, Messerlian C. An empirical study examining the impact of gambling advertisements on adolescent gambling attitudes and behaviors. IJMA 2010;8:21–34.
20. McBride J, Derevensky J. Internet gambling behaviour in a sample of online gamblers. IJMA 2009;7:149–67.
21. Griffiths M, Parke J, Derevensky J. Remote gambling in adolescence. In: Derevensky J, Shek D, Merrick J, eds. Youth gambling problems: The hidden addiction. Berlin: De Gruyter; in press.
22. Blaszcynski AP, McConaghy N, Frankova A. Control versus adstinence in the treatment of pathological gambling: A two to nine year follow-up. Br J Addict 1991;86:299–306.
23. Dowling N, Smith D, Thomas T. A comparison of individual and group cognitive-behavioral treatment for female pathological gambling. Behav Res Ther 2007;45(9):2192–202.
24. Ladouceur R, Lachance S, Fournier P-M. Is control a viable goal in the treatment of pathological gambling? Behav Res Ther 2009;47(3):189–97.
25. Ladouceur R. Controlled gambling for pathological gamblers. J Gambl Stud 2005;21:51–9.
26. Slutske WS, Piasecki T, Blaszczynski A, Martin NG. Pathological gambling recovery in the absence of abstinence. Addiction 2010;105:2169–75.
27. Derevensky J, Gupta R, Winters K. Prevalence rates of youth gambling problems: Are the current rates inflated? J Gambl Stud 2003;19(4):405–25.
28. Derevensky J, Gupta R. Adolescents with gambling problems: A review of our current knowledge. e-Gambling 2004;10:119–40.
29. DiClemente CC, Story M, Murray K. On a roll: The process of initiation and cessation of problem gambling among adolescents. J Gambl Stud 2000;16:289–313.
30. DiClemente CC, Prochaska JO. Self-change and therapy change of smoking behavior: A comparison of processes of change in cessation and maintenance. Addict Behav 1982;7(2):133–42.
31. Wynne H, Smith G, Jacobs DF. Adolescent gambling and problem gambling in Alberta. Prepared for the Alberta Alcohol and Drug Abuse Commission, Edmonton; 1996.
32. Chevalier S, Geoffrion C, Audet C, Papineau É, Kimpton M-A. Évaluation du programme expérimental sur le jeu pathologique. Rapport 8-Le point de vue des usagers. Montreal: Institut nationale de sante publique du Québec; 2003.
33. Miller W, Rollnick S. Motivational interviewing: Preparing people to change addictive behavior. New York: Guilford; 1991.
34. Hodgins D, Diskin K. Motivational interviewing in the treatment of problem and pathological gambling. In: Arkowitz H, Westra W, Rollnick S, eds. Motivational interviewing in the treatment of psychological problems. New York: Guilford; 2008.
35. Arkowitz H, Westra H, Miller W, Rollnick S, eds. Motivational interviewing in the treatment of psychological problems. New York: Guilford; 2008.
36. Gillespie M, Derevensky J, Gupta R. The utility of outcome expectancies in the prediction of adolescent gambling behaviour. JGI 2007;19:69–85.
37. Ladouceur R, Walker M. Cognitive approach to understanding and treating pathological gambling. In: Bellack AS, Hersen M, eds. Comprehensive clinical psychology. New York: Pergamon; 1998.
38. Langer EJ. The illusion of control. J Pers Soc Psychol 1975;32(2):311–28.
39. Huang J-H, Jacobs DF, Derevensky J, Gupta R, Paskus T, Petr T. Pathological gambling amongst college athletes. J Am Coll Health 2007;56(2):93–9.
40. Shead NW, Derevensky J, Paskus T. Trends in gambling behavior among college student-athletes: A comparison of 2004 and 2008 NCAA survey data. Unpublished manuscript.
41. Derevensky J, Gupta R, Baboushkin H. Underlying cognitions in children's gambling behaviour: Can they be modified? IGS 2007;7(3):281–98.
42. Dickson L, Derevensky J, Gupta R. Youth gambling problems: An examination of risk and protective factors. IGS 2008;8(1):25–47.

43. Shead NW, Derevensky J, Gupta R. Risk and protective factors associated with gambling. Int J Adolesc Med Health 2010;22:39–58.
44. Ste-Marie C, Gupta R, Derevensky J. Anxiety and social stress related to adolescent gambling behavior and substance use. J Child Adolesc Subst Abuse 2006;16(4):55–74.
45. Lussier I, Derevensky J, Gupta R, Bergevin T, Ellenbogen S. Youth gambling behaviors: An examination of the role of resilience. Psychol Addict Behav 2007;21:165–73.
46. Gupta R, Derevensky J. Adolescent gambling behavior: A prevalence study and examination of the correlates associated with problem gambling. J Gambl Stud 1998;14:319–45.
47. Gupta R, Derevensky J, Marget N. Coping strategies employed by adolescents with gambling problems. Child Adolesc Ment Health 2004;9(3):115–20.
48. Nower L, Gupta R, Blaszczynski AP, Derevensky J. Suicidality and depression among youth gamblers: A preliminary examination of three studies. IGS 2004;4(1):70–80.
49. Ladd G, Petry N. A comparison of pathological gamblers with and without substance abuse treatment histories. Exp Clin Psychopharmacol 2003;11:202–9.
50. Grant J, Potenza M. Adolescent problem gambling: Pharmacological treatment options. In: Derevensky J, Shek D, Merrick J, eds. Youth gambling problems: The hidden addiction. Berlin: De Gruyter; in press.
51. Grant JE, Kim SW, Potenza MN. Advances in the pharmacological treatment of pathological gambling. J Gambl Stud 2003;19:85–109.
52. Campbell C, Derevensky J, Meerkamper E, Cutajar J. Parents' perceptions of adolescent gambling: A Canadian national study. JGI; in press.

11 Seeking help online: A new approach for youth-specific gambling interventions

Sally Gainsbury

A substantial proportion of adolescents and young adults gamble and rates of problem gambling among youth appear to be significantly higher than in adult populations. Despite this, few youth seek treatment, suggesting that traditional services are failing to help this vulnerable population. Youth are progressively active online and use the Internet for social networking, education, recreation, and increasingly, to look for help for health and mental health issues where they would not be comfortable seeking traditional forms of professional help. In recognition of this, Internet-based therapy and self-guided interventions have been launched specifically for adolescents and young adults in an attempt to reduce high-risk behaviors and increase program utilization. Research demonstrates that online therapeutic support is perceived to be acceptable and useful by youth. Furthermore, online interventions have demonstrated success in reducing smoking and heavy drinking among this typically hard-to-reach population. Given the success of similar programs, online problem gambling services are predicted to be effective in increasing youth awareness of their potentially problematic gambling behavior and in assisting adolescents and young adults in retaining control and minimizing and reducing gambling-related problems.

11.1 Introduction

Although typically seen as an adult pursuit, increasing numbers of adolescents and young adults are engaging in gambling and experiencing gambling-related problems. Studies from Australia, Canada, the United States, and the United Kingdom that have assessed the rate of problem gambling among adolescents (aged 12–17 years) report rates of problem gambling typically 2–3 times that found in adults (1–4). Young adults aged 18–24 also appear to have significantly more gambling-related problems than any other adult age cohort (5–7). Gambling among youth is particularly disconcerting as young gamblers are more likely to engage in alcohol and drug use and abuse/dependence, and to develop significant psychiatric problems including pathological gambling, substance use, and mood disorders (8).

Despite the high rates of problem gambling among youth, this age group rarely acknowledges their problems or seeks treatment. One reason for this is that young gamblers do not typically suffer life-changing experiences, such as losing one's house, job, or spouse, that are often associated with problem gambling as they do not have these things to lose. However, youth gamblers may still experience significant psychosocial problems including financial losses, anxiety, guilt or depression, disruption and neglect of work, school, and relationships, lost opportunities, and engagement in illegal activities (9).

Reluctance to seek help is not limited to young problem gamblers; however, young people have specific barriers when it comes to accessing mental health services (10). These include both structural barriers including time, costs, and travel, and personal barriers such as being overwhelmed by unfamiliar issues, lack of confidence in seeking help, or not recognizing the extent of their problem. Further, adolescents often prefer to seek help from nonprofessional resources, such as family and friends, rather than from formal professional support including school counselors and mental health professionals (11). The reluctance to seek help may be particularly significant among boys. A survey of young male callers to the Australian Kids Help Line found that although nearly half (49%) wanted to discuss their emotional experiences, they were concerned that people would react negatively, and that they would be seen as weak or judged as "crazy" or "uncool"(12).

Reflecting the apparent failure of traditional treatment programs to recruit clients in need of help, a survey of international experts and attendees at a U.S. problem gambling conference ranked "treatment issues" as being the most important area for future research to address (13). Within this priority area, improving treatment attendance and service utilization and developing manualized treatments were identified as the most important research topics. Subsequently, it is important that new interventions be developed that are accessible to adolescents and young adults and utilized by this population.

Interest in online therapeutic interventions has gained momentum with the emergence of increasing research that online programs for health and mental health problems, including addictions, have efficacy equal to or better than traditional programs including face-to-face therapy and brief interventions and educational and self-help options, particularly for motivated individuals and those with moderate or less severe difficulties (14–19). The current chapter discusses the feasibility of utilizing online therapeutic support for helping young people experiencing gambling issues. There are currently a number of youth-focused informational Web sites aimed at preventing gambling-related harms (e.g., www.friends4friends.ca and www.wannabet.org). However, there are currently no active interventions specifically dealing with gambling for youth that involve interactive self-help programs including personalized feedback or Internet-based interactions with therapists or peers through e-mail, chat, or discussion forums. Subsequently, evidence from the fields of alcohol and tobacco cessation is examined to inform the development of such programs.

11.2 Internet use

Results from the Pew Internet and American Life Project show that in 2007–2008, 93% of American teenagers between the ages of 12 and 17 reported using the Internet, an increase from 73% in 2001, and in 2010, 95% of those aged 18 to 29 years reported using the Internet (20–22). Thirty-seven percent of the respondents indicated that they used e-mail, instant messaging, and/or chat rooms to discuss subject matter that they would not have discussed with someone in person (22). Similar access rates have been found worldwide, with a survey of adolescents in 13 countries observing that 100% of 12–14-year-olds reported having Internet access in the United Kingdom, followed by 98% in the Czech Republic, 96% in Macau, and 95% in Canada (23). Even in countries with the least Internet access, usage was still common, with 70% of adolescents in

Hungary and Singapore reporting regular Internet use. In a similar study of 9- to 19-year-olds in the United Kingdom, 47% of adolescents used e-mail, chat, or instant messaging and users indicated that talking to people online was the same or more satisfying as talking to people in real life (24), demonstrating the high comfort levels that adolescents have with Internet use.

The Internet is rapidly becoming a major source of health information for adolescents and young adults (25–26). Youth regard the Internet as appealing, as it is an accessible and anonymous method of seeking help (25, 27). For example, a study by Mission Australia (28) found that young people aged 11–19 years rated the Internet as the fourth most important source of advice and support after friends, parents, and relatives/family friends. Furthermore, Kids Help Line client data reveals that compared to telephone support, young people are five times more likely to seek help for mental health concerns, three times more likely to seek help about suicide and eating behavior issues, and twice as likely to seek help for self image, sexual orientation, and sexual assault online (29). Similarly, among older teenagers (15–17 years old), 21% reported searching the Internet for information on sensitive subjects, which they found difficult to talk about face-to-face (30).

11.3 Rationale for Internet therapy and online interventions

High rates of Internet use among adolescents, young adults, and college students (31) have prompted trials of online interventions for smoking and alcohol use. There are several reasons that make online interventions potentially advantageous in seeking to treat high-risk behaviors among youth. Firstly, the confidentiality and nonjudgmental quality of the Internet may increase the potential for youth to divulge personally relevant information, which may facilitate knowledge, attitude, or behavioral changes (32). Compared with paper-and-pencil questionnaires, computerized programs for young people increase self-disclosure in sensitive areas, such as risky sexual behavior, excessive alcohol use, marijuana use, and family problems (33–34). The anonymity and accessibility of the Internet may allay young people's concerns about seeking help, especially their fears about being personally identifiable (35–36), which is particularly important for interventions for illegal activities such as underage gambling.

A further advantage of online interventions is the ability to assess a large and vulnerable population in a cost-effective and confidential manner and to provide relevant resources to those in need. For those without Internet access in their homes, Web sites can be easily accessed from computers in schools, colleges, libraries, and Internet cafes. Adolescents and young adults can complete online screening questionnaires in private and at their convenience and receive automatic and personalized feedback to determine their need for further intervention and be directed to relevant resources. There is evidence that brief online feedback that sets an individuals' gambling behavior against social norms is perceived as being useful for nonproblem and problem gamblers and may encourage behavioral change (37). Although youth may be skeptical about discussing high-risk and illegal behaviors with a health practitioner, parent, or other adult, they are nevertheless interested in how their behavior compares with that of their peers (38). Online feedback interventions appeal to this curiosity while reducing apprehension associated with face-to-face discussions with a professional. Furthermore, research indicates that youth respond better to electronic feedback than to in-person feedback regarding high-risk behaviors such as drinking (39–41). Studies also report that adolescents find it easier to write than talk about severe and complex and emotional problems and that the anonymity offered by online interventions makes communication easier and facilitates greater expression of emotions and interpersonal issues (42–43).

Internet interventions can be tailored to be made more relevant for the individual accessing it, providing customized information, exercises, and support based on their reported problems, age, gender, stage of readiness, and needs. This is particularly useful for problem gambling interventions given the variety of forms (e.g., electronic gaming machines, sports wagering, online gambling) and reasons for gambling (e.g., risk-taking, excitement, boredom, social pressure, emotional escape). Tailored program content is more likely to be read, remembered, and viewed as personally relevant (44–45), which may ultimately increase program utilization and effectiveness.

Internet-based interventions also enable users to control their learning environment, move at their own pace, and receive information on demand (46). This may encourage youth to access the interventions at a time convenient to them and when they are at the appropriate stage of readiness for change. The convenience of online programs allows youth to access therapeutic support from professionals or peers at any time if they need advice, counseling, or have questions. There is also less stigmatism associated with online counseling, as no one knows that the individual is seeking help, in contrast to meetings with school counselors or other professionals. Online programs overcome barriers to traditional treatment including geographical isolation, inability to attend individual or group sessions due to timing, transportation, or conflicting commitments, fears of stigmatization, and/or privacy concerns.

11.4 Internet therapy and online interventions for adolescents

Interventions for adolescents concerning high-risk behaviors are very important as this is a critical developmental period in which behavioral experimentation occurs, peer pressure is high, and maladaptive behavioral patterns can be formed. Although research is still emerging, there is increasing evidence to support the use of online interventions for youth during this difficult period of emerging adulthood. In one large-scale study, 17,000 year 10 students from South Australia were surveyed about their use of the Internet to seek counseling and advice for personal problems (47). The results revealed that the adolescents surveyed were seeking help from the Internet at the same rate they sought help from other mental health professionals such as school counselors, psychiatrists, and psychologists. The authors commented on the particular benefit of Internet therapy for teenage boys, who used the Internet as much as females, but are much less likely to seek help in person. This hypothesis is supported by further research demonstrating that about one in three adolescents were more able to self-disclose online than offline (48).

Kids Help Line (www.kidshelp.com.au) is a free confidential 24-hour online counseling service (provided in real-time, chat-based text exchange) specifically for Australians aged between 5 and 18 (typically used by adolescents). Online focus groups reported that the online environment was less confronting than traditional forms of counseling, with responses indicating that it was less "intimidating" and "scary," that counselors would not think they were "weird" and could not see if they cried (11). Additional advantages included privacy issues, particularly that they would not be overheard, and being able to take time in writing replies, which increased feelings of control and comfort with the counseling process. Participants indicated that they were comfortable with text communication and felt online counselors were more supportive than telephone counselors. A study of Kids Help Line (49) directly compared one online counseling session with one telephone counseling session. Significant pre-existing differences were found between the groups as the online counseling group contained significantly more females, was older, and reported high pre-counseling distress compared with the telephone counseling group. The higher distress levels were consistent with reported internal findings that young people using online counseling are more likely to be coded with mental health problems, suicidality, and sexual abuse than youth seeking telephone support. Although both interventions had a substantial positive overall effect on distress levels, telephone counseling had a much more substantial impact than online counseling. Telephone counseling also generated greater therapeutic alliance, lower resistance, and higher collaboration as compared to online counseling. However, these variables did not predict counseling outcomes. The authors hypothesized that while the duration of the telephone and online sessions were equivalent, due to the time involved with composing and typing messages, youth using the telephone were able to address their problems more effectively because of the greater speed and efficiency of communication. The authors argue that increasing the duration of online sessions would likely enhance the impact of this form of intervention.

Internet interventions may act as an adjunct to existing programs for adolescents to reduce risky behaviors. A trial of a Web-based high school smoking cessation program included a specially designed Web site for adolescents, along with proactive phone calls from the group facilitator to the participant (50). Significant positive effects were found for the online intervention, with 57% of participants reporting visiting the Web site, which was rated positively on several dimensions. Most importantly, Web site utilization was associated with positive smoking cessation outcomes. In contrast, proactive phone calls failed to increase cessation rates or abstinence, which may have occurred because it was difficult to reach the adolescents and engage them in conversation at the time of the call, and in their home where they may be overheard.

An important component of online interventions can include tailored e-mails that provide personalized feedback, relevant cognitive and behavioral strategies, and promote self-efficacy. Classroom-based Web-assisted tobacco interventions found high school student smokers who participated in an interactive smoking cessation online program and received tailored e-mails were significantly more likely to reduce their intentions to smoke and were more resistant to cigarette use at 6-month follow-up than those in a control condition (51). The intervention also significantly reduced the likelihood of cigarette use by non-smokers. Similarly, promising outcomes have been demonstrated with a "virtual world chat room" for adolescent smoking cessation. The Internet therapy program allows young smokers to interact with a trained cessation counselor and other teen smokers in a real-time "virtual world." In a randomized controlled trial, smokers participated in 45-minute sessions weekly for seven weeks (52). Those who participated in the online program were significantly more likely than controls to report weekly abstinence, reduced smoking, and higher quit rates at the conclusion of the program. Only the number of times quit was statistically significant at the one-year follow-up, suggesting booster sessions may be necessary to increase program effectiveness. Participants rated the intervention positively in terms of its ease of use, appeal, and usefulness; however, only 9% logged on to receive all seven sessions, with most participants receiving three online sessions.

Less promising results were found for a home-based self-guided online smoking cessation program for adolescents, which resulted in no difference in abstinence rates when compared to four brief face-to-face therapy sessions (53). Adolescents were randomly allocated to conditions, regardless of their intention to quit, and although attendance rates were high for the brief office interventions, there was relatively low utilization of the Web site, indicating that it did not keep teenagers sufficiently engaged. The program attempted to use a non-directive, impersonal, patient-education approach, without professional guidance or prompting. The failure of this program suggests that online interventions may be more effective as an adjunct to face-to-face or online therapy, should be coupled with reminders and prompts to use the site, and offer should personalized, directive and interactive content and feedback to engage teenage smokers. Adolescents who used the online site made greater progress in reducing the number of days smoked compared to the face-to-face condition, suggesting that the self-help site may be used as a self-management tool for those not ready to quit.

11.5 Internet therapy and online interventions for young adults

As with adolescent Internet interventions, research is at early stages, but positive effects have been found for Internet-based programs for high-risk behaviors including smoking and alcohol consumption (54–56). Online interventions appear to be more appealing to young adults than traditional programs. In an online survey of 1,564 university students, Kypri and colleagues (39) found significantly greater support (82%) among hazardous drinkers for online interventions than for health education seminars (40%) or practitioner-delivered interventions (58%). Similar positive results were found in an evaluation of an online smoking cessation program for young adults (57) and Internet-based counseling services for general mental health issues among college students (58), indicating Internet-based therapy programs may reach a wider population of those in need of assistance, who would not seek traditional services.

A trial of an Internet-based smoking cessation program among young adults found participants were more engaged in the program activities, rated their treatment more favorably, and had quit for more consecutive days at 3- and 6-month follow-ups compared to participants who received an in-person counseling session and traditional print-based self-help materials (54). The online intervention was introduced in an in-person session and consisted of a self-help kit, but was augmented by 10–12 counseling e-mails tailored to the individual. Participants were encouraged to reply by e-mail to their counselors with questions and comments, and to update their counselors on their cessation progress. E-mails were sent weekly for the first month and then monthly for the following five months. Additional e-mails were sent around the participant's cessation date. Although all participants received the same cognitive and behavioral techniques from the self-help guide and in-person session, those in the online condition were more likely to have adopted these and to have made a quit attempt. The majority of participants (92%) read "most" or "all" or their e-mails, indicating that this may be an appropriate medium for communicating with young adults. Another online smoking cessation program incorporated content of general interest to young adults, weekly reminder e-mails, interactive quizzes with tailored feedback, behavioral monitoring, peer-support via weekly e-mails from peer coaches, and weekly incentives ($10 gift card) (55). Compared to a control group, participants had increased short-term abstinence rates. Although long-term cessation rates were not found, given that this study included participants who had no immediate plans to quit, an emphasis on taking breaks from smoking may encourage quitting attempts in the future.

Given the increasing availability and popularity of Internet-enabled mobile phones and the high use of texting among young adults, this technology has been utilized to disseminate information and implement smoking cessation interventions in young adult and college-aged smokers (16). Smoking interventions delivered via the Internet, mobile-enabled videos, and mobile phone text messages have resulted in 43% of participants making at least one 24-hour attempt to stop smoking and 22–42% abstinence rates at 6-week follow-up (59–61). Participants that continued smoking reported significantly reduced smoking rates and dependence (59). The amount of and timing of Internet- and mobile-based contacts appears to be an important factor for intervention efficacy (62).

Online interventions have also been shown to be effective in reducing hazardous drinking and improving attitudes on drinking among college students (32, 56, 58). Trials demonstrate that self-administered Internet-based CBT interventions that include personalized feedback with tailored motivational information about high-risk drinking are more effective in modifying attitudes and behavior post-treatment and at 3- and 6-month follow-ups compared to assessment only, educational Web sites, and interactive online interventions that do not include tailored feedback (32, 38, 56, 63–65). Of significant note, these effects have also been shown for subgroups of heavy drinkers including women, persistent heavy drinkers, those who intend to drink heavily for a particular occasion (e.g., 21st birthday), and those with low motivation to change (32, 65), demonstrating the usefulness of an online approach among a typically hard-to-reach population.

Importantly, brief online interventions have also been found effective for reducing high-risk behaviors among young adults (38). A trial of an Internet alcohol reduction intervention for college students found that students who completed a brief online screener for problem drinking and received personalized feedback found it easy to use, personally relevant, and would recommend it to friends (66). The intervention prompted help-seeking behavior, with 30% of participants accessing additional information on support services through the Web site. These results must be interpreted with caution due to the lack of information on corresponding behaviors. Westrup et al. (67) found that despite positive interest in a self-help alcohol Internet site with personalized feedback, most participants did not report any changes in alcohol use, stress, or coping, regardless of the extent of feedback they received.

Although some online self-administered programs for problematic and risky behaviors appear to have promising results, this new mode of intervention requires further development. A brief self-administered Web-based program with personalized feedback delivered to college students led to less drinking at 6-week follow-up, but was not significantly different from printed material at a 6-month follow-up (68). Similarly, no differences were found in binge drinking behavior 30 days following college students receiving a newsletter by e-mail or post mail (69).

A systematic review of the published literature on computerized treatments for drug and alcohol abuse and dependence and smoking addiction found that the majority of studies examined incorporated self-administrated methods with therapist contact for assessment at most (16). These methods included interactive, multi-component Web sites, and personalized feedback and analysis of studies demonstrated mixed results regarding efficacy of treatments. In comparison to programs with ongoing therapist assistance, the interventions with minimal therapist contact appeared to be more efficacious with gains maintained over time, suggesting that therapist contact may not be necessary to modify alcohol-use behavior and related attitudes.

11.6 Internet therapy and online interventions for problem gambling

Although Internet interventions are being increasingly implemented and evaluated to reduce some high-risk behaviors among youth, there is little empirical evidence supporting the use of online interventions for gambling-related problems for youth. Based on the evidence presented previously, it is reasonable to conclude that Internet interventions may likely be an acceptable form of treatment for gambling-related issues and preferred to traditional face-to-face or self-help alternatives. Internet therapy has been introduced to treat adults with gambling problems in Australia, Canada, Finland, New Zealand, Sweden, Norway, Germany, and the United Kingdom. Although evidence is preliminary, positive results have been found, indicating that Internet therapy, using self-guided interactive exercises combined with therapeutic support via telephone or e-mail, is effective compared to wait-list controls, reaches individuals who would not otherwise present for treatment, and is viewed positively by clients (70–75).

Gambling Help Online is an Internet-based counseling service available in Australia offering live chat-based counseling (24 hours a day, 7 days a week) and short-term (approximately 6 weeks) e-mail therapy, branded as support. The site includes self-assessment pages for gambling-related problems and faulty cognitions, educational content, self-help information and strategies, in addition to the therapeutic services offered. Analysis of the first 12 months of the online intervention found that first contacts were generally crisis-driven, and clients also sought help for relapse prevention, as an adjunct to treatment, to seek strategies and information, or to discuss another person's gambling problems (76). Although the program is not intended as a youth intervention, the highest proportion of clients using the chat services was under the age of 30. Further analysis indicates an age by gender interaction as the chat clients under 30 years of age were significantly more likely to be male, whereas those aged over 40 or 50 were significantly more likely to be female. For example, 85% of males with sports betting concerns were under the age of 30. Although young males were generally problem gamblers, they appeared to have significantly lower problem-gambling severity scores than older males. Analysis of clients seeking e-mail support again found that males were more likely to be under the age of 30.

Problem gambling has a significant impact beyond the negative consequences experienced by the problem gambler. Families and friends also face significant negative consequences and require help and support. Approximately 16% of individuals seeking assistance from Gambling Help Online were family and friends of gamblers (76). In the first 12 months of operation, 47% of these were under the age of 30 and 19% reported being the son or daughter of a problem gambler. The high usage of Internet-based services by young adults, despite the availability of telephone and face-to-face support, indicates that online interventions are preferable to this population for help-seeking. This is further demonstrated by results from an evaluation of gamblers seeking help through Victoria's problem gambling counseling services between 1995 and 2000 (77). This study reported that clients were typically over the age of 30 and despite being the most likely to experience problem gambling, the under-25 age group was the least represented in treatment services.

There do not currently appear to be any online services specifically aimed at youth with gambling problems. However, a pilot project, conducted in Canada by the International Centre for Youth Gambling Problems and High-Risk Behaviors at McGill University, aimed to provide online help for adolescents and young adults with gambling problems. An online platform offered individual and group chats with various topics focusing on gambling and problems associated with gambling. Separate teen and young adult sites were widely promoted throughout Canadian high schools, universities, healthcare providers, and in popular media. From January through June 2007 the site had 2,161 different visitors, 4,102 visits, and 1,031,893 hits. In total, from inception (November 2005) through the end of June 2007 the site received almost 2 million hits. Although the Web site received a large number of visitors, and strong endorsement from the clinical and educational community, the number of adolescents and young adults who engaged in this service was minimal. Upon completion of the pilot project funding was not continued and the Web sites are no longer operational.

Although the pilot project described above was not successful in attracting large numbers of adolescents with gambling problems, those who did respond viewed the information and help as invaluable. Lessons from the development of online smoking cessation and hazardous drinking sites aimed at adolescents and young adults may aid in the development of a more effective youth-oriented online problem gambling intervention. Components of online interventions with some success include tailored feedback directing clients to relevant information and resources, interactive exercises and quizzes with automatic feedback, e-mail reminders and prompts, e-mail communication with therapists, and content and formatting relevant to a youth audience (whether adolescent or young adult). Due to the apparent reluctance of youth to recognize the seriousness of their gambling-related problems, an important component of an online gambling treatment for youth may be an Internet-based assessment with automatic, personalized normative feedback. Receiving feedback on how their own gambling behavior compares with their peers may encourage adolescents and young adults to consider taking steps to modify their gambling involvement. Furthermore, recruitment strategies can be used to encourage all youth to complete online assessments, and these can be actively encouraged or mandated within schools and universities and by health care providers.

The absence of youth from traditional gambling treatment services suggests both the perceived inaccessibility of existing services for youth and the reluctance to recognize gambling-related problems (78). To overcome these barriers to help-seeking, online support services may be used in educational settings whereby youth use the services as part of structured school or college class activities. In educational terms, the Internet is being increasingly used as a media for progressive learning that appears to have some advantages over traditional teaching methods. For example, groups of online learners can motivate and support each others' learning experiences. Such an approach can communicate gambling prevention information to youth, as well as information on how to spot the signs of a gambling problem and how/where to seek help.

Given the limited evidence on the utility of providing online support for youth gambling problems it is premature to determine whether such a program would be effective. However, based on the successful implementation of online interventions for other high-risk behaviors, this treatment option deserves further consideration and research, particularly given the success of this approach with adults.

11.7 Conclusions

Online therapeutic support services appear to have a great deal of potential to assist youth in dealing with gambling-related problems, given their access to and familiarity with the media and the anonymous capabilities of such services. This is evidenced in their use of online therapeutic support for other health-related issues and high-risk behaviors. In particular, this type of support may be one way that could potentially help to bridge the gap between the few youth that seek help and the much larger number identified as experiencing problems overall. Certainly, existing evidence suggests that Internet-based interventions do already appear to help youth reduce smoking and heavy drinking. Furthermore, adult problem gamblers, who are often otherwise reluctant to seek support, have experienced positive effects of online gambling therapy. The key challenge lies in designing appropriate online services and communication strategies that will appeal to and be accessible by youth while at the same time ensuring that youth are aware of both the problems they may face in relation to their gambling behavior and the availability of such online services to assist them. Important design elements include ease of access (e.g., via e-mailed hyperlinks to a target population, hyperlinks on other highly accessed Web sites, or easily searchable), reduced length, ease of navigation, nonjudgmental language, brief assessments with personalized normative feedback, and tailored content where appropriate and links to other services. Programs should emphasize the anonymity and privacy of users by encouraging nonidentifiable user names and anonymous e-mails to be used. Only careful attempts at engaging youth in this way will ultimately demonstrate the utility of online therapeutic support for helping youth overcome gambling problems, paired with evaluation studies to help further shape what does and does not work in this emerging branch of therapeutic support.

References

1. Delfabbro P, Thrupp L. The social determinants of youth gambling in South Australian adolescents. J Adolesc 2003;26:313–30.
2. Derevensky J, Gupta R. Gambling problems in youth: Theoretical and applied perspectives. New York: Kluwer Acad/Plenum; 2004
3. Ipsos MORI. British survey of children, the national lottery and gambling 2008–09. London: Ipsos MORI; 2009.
4. Shaffer H, Hall M. Updating and refining prevalence estimates of disordered gambling behaviour in the United States and Canada. Can J Public Health 2001;92:168–72.
5. Delfabbro P. Australasian gambling review, 3rd ed. Adelaide: Independent Gambling Authority South Aust; 2008

6. Derevensky J. Foreword. In: Meyer G, Hayer T, Griffiths M, eds. Problem gambling in Europe. New York: Springer; 2009:xv–xviii.

7. Welte J, Barnes G, Wieczorek W, Tidwell M, Parker J. Alcohol and gambling pathology among U.S. adults: Prevalence, demographic patterns and comorbidity. J Stud Alcohol 2001;62:706–13.

8. Lynch WJ, Maciejewski PK, Potenza MN. Psychiatric correlates of gambling in adolescents and young adults grouped by age at gambling onset. Arch Gen Psychiatry 2004;611:1116–22.

9. Shaffer HJ, Hall MN, Walsh JS, Vanderbilt J. The psychosocial consequences of gambling. In Tannenwald R, ed. Casino development: How would casinos affect New England's economy. Special report No.2. Boston: Federal Reserve Bank of Boston; 1995:130–41.

10. Owens PL, Hoagwood K, Horwitz SM, Leaf PJ, Poduska JM, Kellan SG, et al.,. Barriers to children's mental health services. J Am Acad Child Adolesc Psychiatry 2002;41:731–8.

11. King R, Bambling M, Lloyd C, Gomurra R, Smith S, Reid W, et al. Online counselling: The motives and experiences of young people who choose the Internet instead of face to face or telephone counselling. Counselling and Psychotherapy Research 2006;6:169–74.

12. Kids Help Line. Visual counselling 'tools' revolutionise online service. Newsletter August 1-2, 2003.

13. Nower L. National priorities for problem gambling research: Future directions. Washington, DC: National Council on Problem Gambling; 2009.

14. Gainsbury S, Blaszczynski A. A systematic review of Internet-based therapy for the treatment of addictions. Clin Psychol Rev 2010;doi:10.1016/j.cpr.2010.11.007.

15. Newman MG, Szkodny LE, Llera SJ, Przeworski A. A review of technology-assisted self-help and minimal contact therapies for anxiety and depression: Is human contact necessary for therapeutic efficacy? Clin Psychol Rev 2011;3;89–103.

16. Newman MG, Szkodny LE, Llera SJ, Przeworski A. A review of technology-assisted self-help and minimal contact therapies for drug and alcohol abuse and smoking addiction: Is human contact necessary for therapeutic efficacy? Clin Psychol Rev 2011;31:178–86.

17. Barak A, Hen L, Boniel-Nissim M, Shapira N. A comprehensive review and a meta-analysis of the effectiveness of internet based psychotherapeutic interventions. J Technol Hum Serv 2008;26:109–60.

18. Bennett GC, Glasgow RE. The delivery of public health interventions via the internet: Actualizing their potential. Annu Rev Public Health 2009;30:273–92.

19. Cuijpers P, van Straten A, Andersson G. Internet-administered cognitive behavior therapy for health problems: A systematic review. J Behav Med 2008;31:169–77.

20. Pew Internet & American life Project. Demographics of Internet users. http://ww.pewinternet.org/. Accessed December 14, 2010.

21. Pew Internet & American Life Project. Teenage life online: The rise of the instant-message generation and the internet's impact on friendships and family relationship. 2001. http://www.pewinternet.org/. Accessed February 18, 2009.

22. Pew Internet & American Life Project. Generations online in 2009. http://www. pewinternet.org/. Accessed February 18, 2009.

23. Centre for the Digital Future. World Internet Project: International Report 2008. http://www.digitalcenter.org/pages/site_content.asp?intGlobalId=42

24. Livingston S, Bober M. UK children go online. London School of Economics and Political Science, London. 2004. http://www.lse.ac.uk/collections/children-go-online/. Accessed April 7, 2009.

25. Gray LA, Klein JD, Noyce PS, Sesselberg T, Cantrill JA. Health information-seeking behaviour in adolescence: the place of the Internet. Soc Sci Med 2005;60:1467–78.

26. Kaiser Family Foundation. Generation Rx.com: How young people use the internet for health information 2001. http://www.kff.org/entmedia/loader.cfm?url=/commonspot/security/getfile.cfm&PageID=13719.

27. Nicholas J, Oliver K, Lee K, O'Brien M. Help-seeking behaviour and the internet: An investigation among Australian adolescents. Australian e-Journal for the Advancement of Mental Health 2004;3:1–8. http://auseinet.flinders.edu.au/journal/
28. Mission Australia. National survey of young Australians. Melbourne: Mission Australia; 2007.
29. Kids Help Line. Online Counselling. Kids Helpline Infosheet 2000;27. www.kidshelp.com.au
30. Borzekowski DLG, Rickert VI. Adolescent cybersurfing for health information: A new resource that crosses barriers. Arch Pediatr Adolesc Med 2001;155:813–7.
31. Pew Internet and American Life Project. The internet goes to college, 2002. http://www.pewinternet.org/pdfs/PIP_College_Report.pdf.. Accessed August 26, 2009.
32. Chiauzzi E, Green TC, Lord S, Thum C, Goldstein M. My student body: A high-risk drinking prevention web site for college students. J Am Coll Health 2005;3:263–73.
33. Paperny DM, Ayono JY, Lehman RM, Hammar SL, Risser J. Computer–assisted detection and intervention in adolescent high-risk health behaviors. J Pediatr 1990;116:456–62.
34. Turner CF, Ku L, Rogers SM, Lindbergh LD, Pleck JH, Sonenstein FL. Adolescent sexual behavior, drug use, and violence. Science 1998;280:867–73.
35. Gould MS, Munfakh JLH, Lubell K, Kleinman M, Parker S. Seeking help from the internet during adolescence. J Am Acad Child Adolesc Psychiatry 2002;41:1182–9.
36. Skinner H, Biscope S, Poland B. Quality of internet access: Barrier behind internet use statistics. Soc Sci Med 2003; 57:875–80.
37. Wood R, Williams R. Internet gambling: Prevalence, patterns, problems and policy options. Final report prepared for the Ontario Problem Gambling Research Centre, Guelph, Ontario, 2009.
38. Doumas DM, McKinley LL, Book P. Evaluation of two web-based alcohol interventions for mandated college students. J Subst Abuse Treat 2009;36:65–74.
39. Kypri K, Saunders JB, Gallagher SJ. Acceptability of various brief intervention approaches for hazardous drinking among university students. Alcohol Alcohol 2003;38:626–8.
40. Larimer ME, Cronce JM. Identification, prevention, and treatment revisited: Individual-focused college drinking prevention strategies 1999–2006. Addict Behav 2007;32:2439–68.
41. Saunders JB, Kypri K, Walters ST, Laforge RG, Larimer ME. Approaches to brief intervention for hazardous drinking in young people. Alcohol Clin Exp Res 2004;28:322–9.
42. Glasheen KJ, Campbell MA. Are you keeping up with the kids? In Connections 2006; 23;3: 2–7, Queensland Guidance and Counselling Association Inc.
43. Zimmerman DP. A psychosocial comparison of computer-mediated and face-to-face language use among severely disturbed adolescents. Adolescence 1987;22:827–40.
44. Brug J, Campbell M, van Assema P. The application and impact of computer generated personalized nutrition education: a review of the literature. Patient Educ Couns 1999;36: 145–56.
45. Dijkstra A, De Vries H. The development of computer-generated tailored interventions. Patient Educ Couns 1999;36:193–203.
46. Cheiten S, Walters M. Comprehensive school health education and interactive multimedia. In Harris LM, ed. Health and the new media: Technologies transforming personal and public health. Mahwah, NJ: Erlbaum; 1995: 145–62.
47. Oliver K, Nicholas J. The use of the internet to seek help among Australian adolescents. Combined Abstracts of the 2005 Australian Psychology Conferences. Innes M, Katsikitis M. The Australian Psychological Society Ltd. Melbourne, 239, 2005.
48. Schouten AP, Valkenburg PM, Peter J. Precursors and underlying processes of adolescents' online self-disclosure: Developing and testing an "Internet-attribute-perception" model. Media Psychol 2007;10:292–314.
49. King R, Bambling M, Reid W, Thomas I. Telephone and online counselling for young people: A naturalistic comparison of session outcome, session impact and therapeutic alliance. Counselling & Psychotherapy Research 2006b;6:175–81.

50. Mermelstein R, Turner L. Web-based support as an adjunct to group-based smoking cessation for adolescents. Nicotine Tob Res 2006;8:S69-S76.

51. Norman CD, Maley O, Li X, Skinner H. Using the Internet to assist smoking prevention and cessation in schools: A randomized, controlled trial. Health Psychol 2008;27:799–810.

52. Woodruff SI, Conway TL, Edwards CC, Elliott SP, Crittenden J. Evaluation of an internet virtual world chat room for adolescent smoking cessation. Addict Behav 2007;32:1769–86.

53. Patten CA, Croghan IT, Meis TM, Decker PA, Pingree S, Colligan, RC, et al. Randomized clinical trial of internet-based versus brief office intervention for adolescent smoking cessation. Patient Education & Counselling 2006;64:249–58.

54. Abroms LC, Windsor R, Simons-Morton B. Getting young adults to quit smoking: A formative evaluation of the X-Pack Program. Nicotine Tob Res 2008;10:27–33.

55. An LC, Klatt C, Perry CL, Lein EB, Hannrikus DJ, Pallonen UE, et al. The RealU online cessation intervention for college smokers: A randomized controlled trial. Prev Med 2008;47:194–99.

56. Walters ST, Hester RK, Chiauzzi E, Miller E. Demon rum: Hightech solutions to an age-old problem. Alcohol Clin Exp Res 2005;29:270–7.

57. Escoffrey C, McCormick L, Bateman K. Development and process evaluation of a Web-based smoking cessation program for college smokers: Innovative tool for education. Patient Educ Couns 2004;53:217–25.

58. Lintvedt OK, Sørensen K, Østvik AR, Verplanken B, Wang CE. The need for web-based cognitive behavior therapy among university students, J Technol Hum Serv 2008;26:239–58

59. Obermayer JL, Riley WT, Asif O, Jean-Mary J. College smoking-cessation using cell phone text messaging. J Am Coll Health 2004;53:718.

60. Riley W, Obermayer J, Jean-Mary J. Internet and mobile phone text messaging intervention for college smokers. J Am Coll Health 2008;57:245–8.

61. Whittaker R, Maddison R, McRobbie H, Bullen C, Denny S, Dorey E, et al. A multimedia mobile phone-based youth smoking cessation intervention: Findings from content development and piloting studies. J Med Internet Res 2008;10: e49

62. Rodgers A, Corbett T, Bramley D, Riddell T, Wills M, Lin RB, et al. Do u smoke after txt? Results of a randomised trial of smoking cessation using mobile phone text messaging. Tob Control 2005;14:255–61.

63. Neighbors C, Larimer ME, Lewis MA. Targeting misperceptions of descriptive drinking norms: Efficacy of a computer-delivered personalized normative feedback intervention. J Consult Clin Psychol 2004;72:434–47.

64. Neighbors C, Lewis MA, Bergstrom RL, Larimer ME. Being controlled by normative influences: Self-determination as a moderator of a normative feedback alcohol intervention. Health Psychol 2006;25:571–9.

65. Neighbors C, Lee CM, Lewis MA, Fossos N, Walter T. Internet-based personalized feedback to reduce 21st-birthday drinking: A randomized controlled trial of an event-specific prevention intervention. J Consult Clin Psychol 2009;77:51–63.

66. Hallett J, Maycock B, Kypri K, Howat P, McManus A. Development of a web-based alcohol intervention for university students: Processes and challenges. Drug Alcohol Rev 2009;28:31–9.

67. Westrup D, Futa KT, Whitsell SD, Mussman L, Wanat SF, Koopman C, et al. Employees' reactions to an interactive website assessing alcohol use and risk for alcohol dependence, stress level and coping. J Subst Use 2003;8:104–11.

68. Kypri K, Saunders JB, Williams SM, McGee RO, Langley JD, Cashell-Smith ML, et al. Web-based screening and brief intervention for hazardous drinking: A double-blind randomized controlled trial. Addiction 2004;99:1410–17.

69. Moore MJ, Soderquist J, Werch C. Feasibility and efficacy of a binge drinking prevention intervention for college students delivered via the Internet versus postal mail. J Am Coll Health 2005;54:38–44.

70. Carlbring P. Internet-based self-help for pathological gambling. Presentation given at the 6th European Conference on Gambling Studies and Policy Issues. Malmo, Sweden, 2005.
71. Carlbring P, Smit F. Randomised trial of internet-delivered self help with telephone support for pathological gamblers. J Consult Clin Psychol 2008;76:1090–4.
72. Eidem M. Distance based therapy for problem gamblers in Norway. Paper presented at the 7th European Conference on Gambling Studies and Policy Issues. Nova Gorica, Slovenia, July 2008. http://www.assissa.eu/easg/wednesday/1400-ses4/eidem_magnus.pdf.
73. Eidem M. Distance based therapy for problem gamblers in Norway. Paper presented at the 14th International Conference on Gambling & Risk Taking, Lake Tahoe, NV, 2009.
74. Farrel-Roberts K. Problem gambling: www.gamblingtherapy.org: an online advice and counselling helpline. Presentation given at the 6th European Conference on Gambling Studies and Policy Issues. Malmo, Sweden, 2005.
75. Peltoniemi T, Bothas H. Virtual prevention and treatment in Finland: Some addictions-related examples. Paper presented at the *Media Seminar.* Haarlem, October 4–6, 2007. http://www.a-klinikka.fi/ajankohtaista/paihdetiedotusseminaari07/Peltoniemi%20Bothas_Virtual%20prevention%20and%20treatment%20in%20Finland.pdf. Accessed April 27, 2009.
76. Rodda S. Gambling Help Online: Program Engagement and Client Characteristics. Paper presented at the National Association for Gambling Studies 20th annual conference. Gold Coast, December 1–3, 2010.
77. Jackson AC, Thomas SA, Holt TA, Thomason N. Change and continuity in a help-seeking problem gambling population: A five-year record. Journal of Gambling Issues 2005. http://www.camh.net/egambling/issue13/jgi_13_jackson.html
78. Hardoon K, Derevensky J, Gupta, R. Empirical vs. perceived measures of gambling severity: Why adolescents don't present themselves for treatment. Addict Behav 2003;28:933–46.

12 Adolescent problem gambling: Pharmacological treatment options

Jon E. Grant and Marc N. Potenza

Randomized controlled studies in adults with pathological gambling suggest that pharmacotherapy may offer significant promise in reducing gambling symptoms. No studies, however, have directly investigated the safety and efficacy of pharmacological treatments for pathological gambling in adolescents. Given the rates of adolescent problem gambling and its impact on affected individuals and their families, effective treatments are needed. Pharmacotherapy may be a useful adjunct in a treatment plan for adolescent problem gambling, but patients, parents, and guardians should understand the risks and potential benefits of pharmacotherapy and other treatment options. This chapter briefly reviews the literature on effective treatments in adults and describes safety data for the use of these drugs in adolescents.

12.1 Introduction

Problem gambling among adolescents can be conceptualized as belonging to a larger constellation of "developmental addictions." Data support a relationship between "behavioral" and drug addictions in adolescents (1, 2) and gambling, substance use, and other impulsive behaviors frequently co-occur in adolescents (3–6). The co-aggregation of impulsive behaviors appears particularly frequent in adolescent males (7). Arguably the most consistent and robust finding across youth gambling studies is that boys are more involved in gambling than girls and have higher rates of problem gambling than do girls (8–11).

Research on developmental biology suggests that the adolescent brain is a changing organ and this has several important correlates. First, it suggests that treatments for adults might not work in the same manner in adolescents. Second, it suggests that treatments within adolescent groups might differ according to brain maturational stage (12), and that within subjects the effectiveness of specific treatments might vary over time. Third, treatments during specific developmental epochs in adolescence may have an enduring impact on the presence or manifestation of adult psychiatric syndromes. These points highlight the importance of directly studying the efficacies and tolerabilites of specific treatments in adolescents.

Adolescents as a group appear to constitute a high-risk population for gambling problems. Although most adolescents gamble occasionally and do so responsibly, approximately 3–8% have been found to have a significant gambling problem (13–15). Given the rates of adolescent problem gambling and its impact on affected individuals and their families, effective treatments are important (16). There are, however, no pharmacological treatments for pathological gambling in children, adolescents, or adults that are currently approved by the U.S. Food and Drug Administration (FDA).

Thus, it is important for patients, parents, and guardians to understand that any use of medications for pathological gambling is off-label, and a review of the benefits and risks of pharmacotherapies and other treatment options is warranted in order to devise an appropriate treatment plan. No studies have directly investigated the safeties and efficacies of pharmacological treatments for pathological gambling in adolescents. Therefore, we will review briefly the literature on effective treatments in adults, describe safety data for the use of these drugs in adolescents, and provide a rationale for future studies to investigate the efficacies and tolerabilites of pharmacotherapies for pathological gambling in adolescents.

12.2 Pharmacotherapy

The peer-reviewed literature indicates that pharmacological treatments have only been examined using randomized clinical trial methodologies in adults with pathological gambling, and, therefore, there is no direct evidence of either safety or efficacy of any pharmacotherapy in adolescent pathological gambling. Developmental issues are important to consider when prescribing medication for adolescents. Because adolescents may metabolize medications more rapidly than do adults, some adolescents may require higher doses relative to body weight compared to adults. On the other hand, because adolescents may have less adipose tissue than adults, there may be more bioactive drug available and therefore a greater likelihood of adverse events or a need for lower doses. Differences in central nervous system functioning and hormonal changes may further influence adolescents' responses to various medications. Additionally, although other medications have shown some promise for pathological gambling in adults (for example, valproate, topiramate, memantine) (17–19), we include only those medications that have been examined in double-blind, placebo-controlled studies.

12.2.1 Opioid antagonists

Given their ability to modulate dopaminergic transmission in the mesolimbic pathway, opioid receptor antagonists have been investigated in the treatment of pathological gambling. There is evidence suggesting that naltrexone, a mu-opioid receptor antagonist, is effective in reducing gambling and gambling urges in adults with pathological gambling. An initial double-blind study suggested the efficacy of naltrexone, an FDA-approved treatment for alcohol dependence and opioid dependence, in reducing the intensity of urges to gamble, gambling thoughts, and gambling behavior (20). In an 11-week, double-blind, placebo-controlled study of 45 subjects with pathological gambling, significant improvement was seen in 75% of naltrexone-treated subjects (mean dose 188 mg/day) compared to 24% of those treated with placebo. In particular, individuals reporting higher intensity gambling urges responded preferentially to treatment (20).

Although an 11-week study comparing naltrexone to placebo in 52 adults with co-occurring gambling and alcohol dependence failed to demonstrate any differences when medication was combined with cognitive behavioral therapy (21), the initial naltrexone study findings (20) were replicated in a larger, longer study of 77 subjects randomized to either naltrexone or placebo over an 18-week period. Subjects assigned to naltrexone had significantly greater reductions in gambling urges and gambling behavior compared to those receiving placebo. Subjects assigned to naltrexone also had greater improvement in psychosocial functioning. By study endpoint, 39.7% of those on naltrexone were able to abstain from all gambling for at least one month, whereas only 10.5% of those subjects receiving placebo attained complete abstinence for the same time period (22).

Another opioid antagonist, nalmefene, has also shown promise in the treatment of pathological gambling. Nalmefene is currently not available in oral form in the United States. In a large, multi-center trial, using a double-blind, placebo-controlled, flexible-dose design, 207 subjects were assigned to receive either nalmefene at varying doses or placebo. At the end of the 16-week study, 59% of those assigned to nalmefene showed significant reductions in gambling urges, thoughts, and behavior compared to only 34% receiving placebo (23). A second study using lower doses of nalmefene, however, failed to find a positive response in the intent-to-treat analysis, compared to placebo (24).

Using data from nalmefene and naltrexone trials described above, analyses were performed to identify factors associated with a positive treatment outcome (25). Consistent with the influence of opiate antagonists on alcohol consumption, a familial history of alcoholism was associated with a positive treatment response, as were strong gambling urges at treatment onset. In placebo-treated patients, younger age was the factor most closely associated with a positive placebo response. This finding, in conjunction with high placebo response rates observed in clinical trials involving adults with pathological gambling, suggests that placebo responses in adolescents with pathological gambling warrant consideration and that the findings from open-label trials be considered cautiously.

Naltrexone has been used in the treatment of opioid dependence, alcohol use disorders, and autism in adolescents and appears to be well tolerated in young patients (26–29). Although naltrexone has demonstrated some efficacy in adolescents with autism, opiate dependence, and alcohol use disorders when used at 50 mg/day, the safety of naltrexone at the higher doses used in the adult gambling studies (up to 200 mg/day) has not been examined in an adolescent population. Doses of naltrexone greater than 50 mg/day have warranted a "black box" warning due to the medication's propensity for hepatotoxicity, particularly at higher doses (30). Therefore, more research on both the efficacy and safety of naltrexone in adolescent pathological gambling is needed to inform prescribing guidelines.

12.2.2 Antidepressants

Clomipramine

Serotonin reuptake inhibitors (SRIs) block the action of the serotonin transporter and thus increase synaptic availability of serotonin. These medications have been used with varying degrees of success in treating adults with pathological gambling. Clomipramine, a relatively non-selective SRI, was administered in a double-blind, placebo-controlled trial of one female subject who reported a 90% improvement in gambling symptoms when treated with 125 mg of clomipramine (31). Gambling behavior remitted at week three of the trial and improvement was maintained for the next 7 weeks of the trial.

Clomipramine is currently FDA-approved for the treatment of obsessive-compulsive disorder (OCD) in adolescents. Three studies have found the medication safe and efficacious in treating adolescent OCD (32–34). The most common adverse effects observed in adolescents, including dry mouth, somnolence, and dizziness, are comparable to those seen in adults. Adverse cardiac effects are possible and patients should be followed with blood levels and EKGs for safety purposes.

Fluvoxamine

Fluvoxamine, a selective SRI (SSRI), has demonstrated mixed results in two placebo-controlled, double-blind studies of adults with pathological gambling, with one 16-week, crossover study supporting its efficacy at an average end-of-study dose of 207 mg/day (35), and a second six-month parallel-arm study with high rates of drop-out finding no significant difference in response to active or placebo drug (36). Fluvoxamine was the first SSRI to gain FDA approval for the treatment of adolescent OCD. Two studies have demonstrated that fluvoxamine at doses ranging from 50 to 300 mg/day is effective and generally safe in the treatment of adolescents with OCD (37, 38)

Paroxetine

Two studies examining paroxetine in the treatment of adults with pathological gambling have been conducted, but the results have been mixed. The first 8-week study demonstrated significantly greater improvement for those individuals assigned to paroxetine compared to placebo (39), but a 16-week, multi-center study of paroxetine failed to find a statistically significant difference between active drug and placebo, perhaps in part due to the high placebo response rate (48% to placebo, 59% to active drug) (40).

Although never formally tested in adolescents with pathological gambling, paroxetine has been studied in adolescents suffering from major depressive disorder and OCD (41, 42). Some research has found paroxetine treatment in adolescents to be associated positively with suicidality (42), and due to these findings, as well as the mixed results in adults with pathological gambling, the off-label use of paroxetine in the treatment of adolescent pathological gambling should take these considerations into account.

Sertraline

In a double-blind, 6-month, placebo-controlled trial evaluating sertraline for pathological gambling in adults, a mean dosage of 95 mg/day demonstrated no statistical advantage over placebo in a group of 60 pathological gamblers (43). Sertraline is FDA-approved for OCD in children and adolescents age 6–17 years, but has not been studied in adolescents with pathological gambling. Data suggest that sertraline appears generally safe when examined in adolescents (44), but the FDA black-box warning for potential suicidality applies to all antidepressants (45).

Escitalopram

Escitalopram was used in a 12-week, open-label trial with an 8-week double-blind discontinuation phase for responders in 13 subjects with pathological gambling and co-occurring anxiety disorders (46). At the end of the open-label phase (mean dose 25.4 mg/

day), six subjects were considered responders, with concurrent decreases in gambling and anxiety severity observed. Improvements in gambling and anxiety were maintained for those randomized to continue receiving active escitalopram, while assignment to placebo was associated with a resumption of gambling and anxiety symptoms.

The FDA recently granted approval to escitalopram for the treatment of adolescent depression. Two double-blind studies found it safe and more efficacious than placebo in treating depression in adolescents aged 12–17 years (47).

Bupropion

A recent study used bupropion in a 12-week, double-blind, placebo-controlled design in 39 adults with pathological gambling. Analyses demonstrated that 36% of bupropion subjects and 47% of placebo subjects were classified as responders. However, high treatment discontinuation rates of nearly 44% were observed in this study, thus rendering definitive statements difficult to make regarding the efficacy of bupropion in the treatment of adult pathological gambling (48).

Response of adult gambling symptomatology to medications approved for depression and anxiety, particularly in the placebo-controlled trials of SSRIs, usually involves decreased thoughts about gambling, reductions in gambling, and improvement in social and educational or occupational functioning. Patients may initially report feeling less preoccupied with gambling and feeling less anxious about having thoughts of gambling. As these studies have often excluded individuals with significant depressive or anxious symptoms and changes in gambling behaviors and overall clinical status occur independently from changes in depression or anxiety, the data suggest that modulation of serotonin function in adults with pathological gambling may mediate improvement in symptoms specifically related to gambling.

Data supporting the efficacy of SRIs in the treatment of adult pathological gambling, albeit mixed, suggest that some of these medications may be beneficial in adolescents with pathological gambling. However, given changes during adolescence in serotonergic neuronal structure and function in such brain regions as the prefrontal cortex, direct investigation of the efficacies and tolerabilities of specific SRIs in adolescents with pathological gambling is warranted. The use of these medications in adolescents suffering from mood disorders or OCD suggests that many of these medications may be safe in adolescents with pathological gambling. These medications, however, carry a warning about the possible increase in suicidality in young people, and therefore should be used cautiously.

12.2.3 Glutamatergic agents

Because improving glutamatergic tone in the nucleus accumbens has been implicated in reducing reward-seeking behavior in addictions (49), N-acetyl cysteine (NAC), a glutamate modulating agent, was administered to 27 adults with pathological gambling over an 8-week period with responders randomized to receive an additional 6-week double-blind trial of NAC or placebo. Fifty-nine percent of subjects in the open-label phase experienced significant reductions in pathological gambling symptoms and were classified as responders. At the end of the double-blind phase, 83% of those assigned to receive NAC were still classified as responders compared to only

28.6% of those assigned to placebo (50). The only reported side effects included mild nausea or flatulence. In studies of marijuana dependence and autism in children and adolescents, similar doses of NAC have been examined with side effect profiles similar to those in adults. Given its safety profile, NAC may be a promising treatment option for adolescents with problem gambling.

12.2.4 Mood stabilizers

Lithium

Sustained-release lithium carbonate was used in a 10-week, double-blind, placebo-controlled study of 40 adults with bipolar spectrum disorders and pathological gambling. Lithium (mean level 0.87 meq/liter) was superior to placebo in reducing the thoughts and urges associated with pathological gambling. Lithium was also superior to placebo in reducing manic symptoms, and these improvements paralleled the changes in gambling thoughts and urges. No significant differences between groups were found in the episodes of gambling per week, time spent per gambling episode, or the amount of money lost (51).

Lithium has been FDA-approved for the treatment of bipolar disorder in adolescents and has demonstrated safety in this population (52). Common adverse effects of lithium appear similar to those in adults: nausea, polyuria, tremor, and acne. Long-term use, however, can result in problems with thyroid and kidney functioning. Lithium may be a potentially useful treatment for adolescent pathological gambling, but studies of efficacy and safety are needed.

12.2.5 Atypical antipsychotics

Atypical antipsychotics, including drugs such as risperidone, olanzapine, and ziprasidone, generally share the ability to antogonize serotonin $5HT_2$ and dopamine D_2-like (D_2, D_3, and D_4) receptors (53). These drugs have been explored as monotherapies and augmenting agents in the treatment of non-psychotic disorders and behaviors, including pathological gambling. Two recent studies have examined the use of olanzapine as monotherapy in the treatment of pathological gambling.

In a 12-week, double-blind, placebo-controlled trial of 42 adults with pathological gambling, olanzapine (mean dose 8.9 [5.2] mg) resulted in a 35% or greater reduction in gambling symptoms in 66.7% of the olanzapine group. However, 66.7% of the placebo group had the same reduction in symptoms. No statistically significant treatment effect was noted for olanzapine (54).

In another study using olanzapine, Fong and colleagues (55) tested 21 adults with pathological gambling in a 7-week, double-blind, placebo-controlled trial. All subjects reported their primary form of gambling as video poker. Reductions in cravings to gamble and gambling behavior were noted in both the olanzapine and placebo groups but no statistically significant differences were observed.

Currently several atypical antipsychotics are FDA-approved for use in adolescents (e.g., schizophrenia, bipolar disorder, or autism). Although atypical antipsychotic drugs have been found to be well-tolerated in short-term trials involving adolescents (56), increasing concerns have been raised regarding their adverse effect profile, particularly regarding their propensity for impaired glucose control and weight gain in adults and adolescents (56). As such, emerging data regarding the long-term risk-benefit ratio may influence the decision to use these drugs in adolescents in general. Given the lack of support for the use of atypical antipsychotics in treating adults with pathological gambling and the potential risks of using these drugs with regard to such adverse effects as weight gain and impaired glucose regulation, their use in adolescents with pathological gambling would need to be well justified and carefully monitored over time.

12.3 Conclusions

Despite the high prevalence of pathological gambling in adolescents, research on this disorder, particularly with respect to pharmacological therapies, is in its relative infancy. Our understanding of neurodevelopmental changes that occur during adolescence, and their influence on adolescent behaviors, is at an early stage. Longitudinal studies involving neuroimaging, genetics, and behavioral assessments should help advance our understanding of adolescents, and with this understanding should come advances in prevention and treatment strategies for problems frequently experienced by adolescents, including risk behaviors such as pathological gambling.

Available data on pathological gambling in adults suggest several possible pharmacological interventions. At present, arguably the best evidence suggests the use of naltrexone and lithium in treating pathological gambling in adults. However, no data exist directly evaluating the efficacy and safety of pharmacological treatments for pathological gambling in adolescents. Pharmacological treatment of other disorders in adolescents suggests that certain medications – SRIs, mood stabilizers, naltrexone – appear safe and effective at certain doses and for certain indications. Although the data suggest potentially promising pharmacological treatments for adolescent pathological gambling, definitive treatment recommendations await completion of controlled treatment studies in this population. As the combination of behavioral and drug therapies has been demonstrated in other addictive disorders to be superior to either treatment alone (57), future investigations in the treatment of pathological gambling in adolescents and adults should consider empirically validating such combined treatment approaches.

Acknowledgements

This work was supported by an American Recovery and Reinvestment Act (ARRA) Grant from the National Institute on Drug Abuse (1RC1DA028279-01) to Dr. Grant and grants from the National Center for Responsible Gaming and its Institute of Research on Gambling Disorders to Drs. Grant and Potenza. Its contents are solely the responsibility of the authors and do not necessarily represent the official views of any of the funding agencies. Dr. Grant has received research grants from Forest Pharmaceuticals and GlaxoSmithKline. Dr. Grant has received compensation as a consultant for law offices on issues related to impulse control disorders. Dr. Potenza has received financial support or compensation for the following: consulting for and advising Boehringer Ingelheim; consulting for and financial interests in Somaxon; research support from Mohegan Sun

Casino, Forest Laboratories, Ortho-McNeil, Oy-Control/Biotie, and Glaxo-SmithKline pharmaceuticals; and consulting for law offices and the federal public defender's office on issues related to impulse control disorders.

References

1. Wagner FA, Anthony JC. From first drug use to drug dependence: Developmental periods of risk for dependence upon marijuana, cocaine, and alcohol. Neuropsychopharmacology 2002;26:479–88.
2. Chambers RA, Potenza MN. Neurodevelopment, impulsivity, and adolescent gambling. J Gambl Stud 2003;19:53–84.
3. Proimos J, DuRant RH, Pierce JD, Goodman E. Gambling and other risk behaviors among 8th- to 12th-grade students. J Pediatr 1998;102:e23.
4. Romer D, ed. Reducing adolescent risk: Toward an integrated approach. Thousand Oaks, CA: Sage; 2003.
5. Tsitsika A, Critselis E, Janikian M, Kormas G, Kafetzis DA. Association between internet gambling and problematic internet use among adolescents. J Gambl Stud 2010 Oct 16. Epub ahead of print.
6. Brezing C, Derevensky JL, Potenza MN. Non-substance-addictive behaviors in youth: Pathological gambling and problematic internet use. Child Adolesc Psychiatr Clin North Am 2010;19:625–41.
7. Villella C, Martinotti G, Di Nicola M, et al. Behavioural addictions in adolescents and young adults: Results from a prevalence study. J Gambl Stud 2010 Jun 18. Epub ahead of print
8. Wallisch L. Gambling in Texas: 1992 Texas survey of adolescent gambling behavior. Austin, TX: Texas Commission Alcohol Drug Abuse; 1993.
9. Wynne Resources Ltd. Adolescent gambling and problem gambling in Alberta. Edmonton, Alberta: Alberta Alcohol Drug Abuse Commission; 1996.
10. Gupta R, Derevensky JL. Adolescent gambling behavior: A prevalence study and examination of the correlates associated with problem gambling. J Gambl Stud 1998;14:319–45.
11. Stinchfield R. A comparison of gambling among Minnesota public school students in 1992, 1995 and 1998. J Gambl Stud 2001;17:273–96.
12. Burnett S, Sebastian C, Cohen Kadosh K, Blakemore S-J. The social brain in adolescence: Evidence from functional magnetic resonance imaging and behavioral studies. Neurosci Biobehav Rev 2010;doi: 10.1016/j.neubiorev.2010.10.011.
13. Shaffer HJ, Hall MN. Estimating the prevalence of adolescent gambling disorders: A quantitative synthesis and guide toward standard gambling nomenclature. J Gambl Stud 1996;12:193–214.
14. Dervensky JL, Gupta R. Prevalence estimates of adolescent gambling: A comparison of the SOGS-RA, DSM-IV-J, and the GA 20 Questions. J Gamb Stud 2000;16:227–51.
15. Splevins K, Mireskandari S, Clayton K, Blaszczynski A. Prevalence of adolescent problem gambling, related harms and help-seeking behaviors among an Australian population. J Gambl Stud 2010;26:189–204.
16. Nastally DL, Dixon MR. Adolescent gambling: Current trends in treatment and future direction. Int J Adolesc Med Health 2010;22:95–111.
17. Pallanti S, Quercioli L, Sood E, et al. Lithium and valproate treatment of pathological gambling: A randomized single-blind study. J Clin Psych 2002;63:559–564.
18. Dannon PN, Lowengrub K, Gonopolski Y, et al. Topiramate versus fluvoxamine in the treatment of pathological gambling: A randomized, blind-rater comparison study. Clin Neuropharmacol 2005;28:6–10.
19. Grant JE, Chamberlain SR, Odlaug BL, et al. Memantine shows promise in reducing gambling severity and cognitive inflexibility in pathological gambling: A pilot study. Psychopharmacology (Berl) 2010;212:603–12.

20. Kim SW, Grant JE, Adson DE, et al. Double-blind naltrexone and placebo comparison study in the treatment of pathological gambling. Biol Psychiatry 2001;49:914–21.
21. Toneatto T, Brands B, Selby P. A randomized, double-blind, placebo-controlled trial of naltrexone in the treatment of concurrent alcohol use disorder and pathological gambling. Am J Addict 2009;18:219–25.
22. Grant JE, Kim SW, Hartman BK. A double-blind, placebo-controlled study of the opiate antagonist naltrexone in the treatment of pathological gambling urges. J Clin Psychiatry 2008;69:783–9.
23. Grant JE, Potenza MN, Hollander E, et al. Multicenter investigation of the opioid antagonist nalmefene in the treatment of pathological gambling. Am J Psychiatry 2006;163:303–12.
24. Grant JE, Odlaug BL, Potenza MN, et al. Nalmefene in the treatment of pathological gambling: Multicentre, double-blind, placebo-controlled study. Br J Psychiatry 2010;197:330–1.
25. Grant JE, Kim SW, Hollander E, et al. Predicting response to opiate antagonists and placebo in the treatment of pathological gambling. Psychopharmacology 2008;200:521–7.
26. Campbell M, Anderson LT, Small AM, et al. Naltrexone in autistic children: Behavioral symptoms and attentional learning. J Am Acad Child Adolesc Psychiatry 1993;32:1283–91.
27. Kolmen BK, Feldman HM, Handen BL, et al. Naltrexone in young autistic children: A double-blind, placebo-controlled crossover study. J Am Acad Child Adolesc Psychiatry 1995;34:223–31.
28. Lifrak PD, Alterman AI, O'Brien CP, et al. Naltrexone for alcoholic adolescents. Am J Psychiatry 1997;154:439–41.
29. Fishman MJ, Winstanely EL, Curran E, et al. Treatment of opioid dependence in adolescents and young adults with extended release naltrexone: Preliminary case-series and feasibility. Addiction 2010;105:1669–76.
30. Physician's Desk Reference, 57th ed, Thompson PDR, Montvale, NJ; 2003.
31. Hollander E, Frenkel M, Decaria C, et al. Treatment of pathological gambling with clomipramine. Am J Psychiatry 1992;149:710–1.
32. Flament MF, Rapoport JL, Berg CJ, et al. Clomipramine treatment of childhood obsessive-compulsive disorder: a double-blind controlled study. Arch Gen Psychiatry 1985;42:977–83.
33. Leonard HL, Swedo SE, Rapoport JL, et al. Treatment of obsessive-compulsive disorder with clomipramine and desipramine in children and adolescents: A double-blind crossover comparison. Arch Gen Psychiatry 1989;46:1088–92.
34. DeVeaugh-Geiss J, Moroz G, Biederman J, et al. Clomipramine hydrochloride in childhood and adolescent obsessive-compulsive disorder: A multicenter trial. J Am Acad Child Adolesc Psychiatry 1992;31:45–9.
35. Hollander E, DeCaria CM, Finkell JN, et al. A randomized double-blind fluvoxamine/placebo crossover trial in pathological gambling. Biol Psychiatry 2000;47:813–17.
36. Blanco C, Petkova E, Ibanez A, et al. A pilot placebo-controlled study of fluvoxamine for pathological gambling. Ann Clin Psychiatry 2002;14:9–15.
37. Apter A, Ratzoni G, King RA, et al. Fluvoxamine open-label treatment of adolescent inpatients with obsessive-compulsive disorder or depression. J Am Acad Child Adolesc Psychiatry 1994;33:342–8.
38. Riddle MA, Reeve EA, Yaryura-Tobias JA, et al. Fluvoxamine for children and adolescents with obsessive-compulsive disorder: A randomized, controlled, multicenter trial. J Am Acad Child Adol Psychiatry 2001;40:222–9.
39. Kim SW, Grant JE, Adson DE, et al. A double-blind placebo-controlled study of the efficacy and safety of paroxetine in the treatment of pathological gambling. J Clin Psychiatry 2002;63:501–7.
40. Grant JE, Kim SW, Potenza MN, et al. Paroxetine treatment of pathological gambling: A multicenter randomized controlled trial. Int Clin Psychopharmacol 2003;18:243–9.
41. Keller MB, Ryan ND, Strober M, et al. Efficacy of paroxetine in the treatment of adolescent major depression: A randomized controlled trial. J Am Acad Child Adolesc Psychiatry 2001;40:762–72.

42. Abbott A. British panel bans use of antidepressant to treat children. Nature, 2003;423:792.
43. Sáiz-Ruiz J, Blanco C, Ibanez A, et al. Sertraline treatment of pathological gambling: A pilot study. J Clin Psych 2005;66:28–33.
44. Robb AS, Cueva JE, Spron J, et al. Sertraline treatment of children and adolescents with post-traumatic stress disorder: A double-blind, placebo-controlled trial. J Child Adolesc Psycho-pharmacol 2010;20:463–71.
45. Schneeweiss S, Patrick AR, Solomon DH, et al. Variation in the risk of suicide attempts and completed suicides by antidepressant agent in adults: A propensity score-adjusted analysis of 9 years' data. Arch Gen Psych 2010;67:497–506.
46. Grant JE, Potenza MN. Escitalopram treatment of pathological gambling with co-occuring anxiety: An open-label pilot study with double-blind discontinuation. Int Clin Psychopharma-col 2006;21:203–9.
47. Yang LP, Scott LJ. Escitalopram in the treatment of major depressive disorder in adolescent patients: Profile report. CNS Drugs 2010;24:621–3.
48. Black DW, Arndt S, William WH, et al. Bupropion in the treatment of pathological gambling: A randomized, double-blind, placebo-controlled, flexible-dose study. J Clin Psychopharmcol 2007;27:143–50.
49. Kalivas PW, Peters J, Knackstedt L. Animal models and brain circuits in drug addiction. Mol Interv 2006;6:339–44.
50. Grant JE, Kim SW, Odlaug BL. N-acetyl cysteine: A glutamate-modulating agent in the treat-ment of pathological gambling: a pilot study. Biol Psychiatry 2007;62:652–7.
51. Hollander E, Pallanti S, Allen A, et al. Does sustained-release lithium reduce impulsive gam-bling and affective instability versus placebo in pathological gamblers with bipolar spectrum disorders? Am J Psychiatry 2005;162:137–45.
52. Geller B, Cooper TB, Sun K, et al. Double-blind and placebo-controlled study of lithium for adolescent bipolar disorders with secondary substance dependency. J Am Acad Child Adolesc Psychiatry 1998;37:171–8.
53. Potenza MN, McDougle CJ. The potential of atypical antipsychotics in the treatment of non-psychotic disorders. CNS Drugs 1998;9:213–32.
54. McElroy SL, Nelson EB, Welge JA, et al. Olanzapine in the treatment of pathological gambling: A negative randomized placebo-controlled trial. J Clin Psychol 2008;69:433–40.
55. Fong T, Kalechstein A, Bernhard B, et al. A double-blind, placebo-controlled trial of olan-zapine for the treatment of video poker pathological gamblers. Pharmacol Biochem Behav 2008;89:298–303.
56. Stigler KA, Posey D, Potenza MN, et al. Bodyweight gain associated with atypical antipsychotic use in children and adolescents: Prevalence, clinical relevance and management. Pediatric Drugs 2004;33–44.
57. Carroll KM. Integrating psychotherapy and pharmacotherapy to improve drug abuse treatment outcome. Addict Behav 1997;22:233–45.

Prevention initiatives

13 Youth gambling prevention initiatives: A decade of research

Jeffrey L. Derevensky and Rina Gupta

In this chapter we will attempt to illustrate the importance of using a conceptual model as the foundation for prevention efforts and will argue that research, development of prevention programs, and their acceptability into school-based curriculum and community programs are all important. There is a growing empirical base indicating that well-designed, appropriately implemented school-based prevention can positively impact multiple social, heath, and academic outcomes. Despite our limited knowledge of the role of protective factors in gambling problems, there is ample research to suggest that direct and moderator effects of protective factors can be used to guide the development of future prevention and intervention efforts to help minimize risk behaviors. There is a strong belief that competence and health-promotion programs are best initiated before youth are pressured to experiment with risky behaviors. Early intervention prevention programs that follow adolescents through high school will likely result in fewer youth with gambling problems. Socio-cultural factors also remain crucial in developing effective programs. Prevention programming will need to account for the changing forms and opportunities for gambling. Ultimately, school-based initiatives may have to examine the commonalities among multiple risky behaviors before educators become inundated with the implementation of prevention programs for risky behaviors and have little time for the educational curriculum. Greater parental, teacher, and school administrators' awareness of youth gambling problems will similarly be fundamental before real changes are realized.

13.1 Introduction

There is little doubt that today's youth live in an environment where gambling has become normalized and is a socially acceptable form of entertainment. Most jurisdictions around the world have some form of gambling, be it a lottery, electronic gambling machines, sports wagering, horse tracks, keno, land-based casinos, or Internet gambling. Such regulated forms of gambling are accompanied by unregulated interpersonal wagering among youth themselves. Prevalence studies conducted in the United States, Canada, Europe, Asia, and Australasia point to the popularity of wagering for money by children and adolescents as well as adults. Early reviews of the scientific literature (1–2) noted a trend toward the increasing proliferation of gambling venues, increased expenditures, and the seriousness of the adverse consequences for those individuals with a gambling problem. Though the prevalence rates of youth gambling for both adolescents and young adults vary between jurisdictions, there is ample evidence that they are gambling at high rates and some are experiencing multiple gambling-related problems. In fact, most prevalence studies suggest that adolescent problem gambling rates are approximately 2–4 times those of adults (1, 3). Still further, when examining the adult prevalence rates of problem gambling, the research suggests that individuals between 18 and 25 have the highest adult problem gambling rates (3–4). Although the prevalence rates of problem gambling have not dramatically risen in spite of greater availability, accessibility, and increased venues, concerns still exist. It is also noteworthy that the overall U.S. population in the past decade rose 9.7%. As a result, though the prevalence rates of problem gambling may not have risen, the overall number of individuals suffering from problem gambling has increased. Of significant concern is the changing landscape of gambling, with an increased use of technologically based venues being particularly attractive to youth (5–6). These new forms of gambling, Internet and mobile gambling, capitalize on youth's perceived skill and knowledge.

In spite of our increased knowledge about risk and protective factors, correlates associated with youth gambling, and the deleterious impact of problem gambling for adolescents, there have been few systematic attempts at educating youth about the risks and warning signs associated with excessive gambling. The normalization of gambling has presented gambling as a benign form of entertainment. Most individuals actually gamble in a responsible manner, setting and generally maintaining both time and money limits, but a number of youth go on to have quite severe gambling-related problems. Yet current attempts at primary prevention of gambling problems have been limited at best. Reducing the prevalence and risks associated with gambling problems remains an important goal from a public health framework.

Primary prevention programs can be conceptualized for individuals of any age, but the vast majority of primary prevention programs intended to prevent gambling problems have focused on youth, with others starting to target particularly high-risk and vulnerable groups (e.g., elderly/seniors, minorities, individuals with low income, and those experiencing other impulse and addictive disorders). (The Massachusetts Council on Compulsive Gambling has an excellent resource of prevention programs.) This chapter summarizes the current literature on the prevention of gambling problems and harm minimization, highlights our current knowledge gaps, identifies issues of concern, presents a viable model for the development and evaluation of prevention programs, and provides recommendations for future directions. Though our conceptual knowledge and understanding concerning adolescent gambling behavior in general, and problematic gambling specifically, has grown considerably in the past two decades, its social impact continues to lag far behind. This lack of scientific knowledge is compounded by a lack of youth and parental awareness about the risks and hazards associated with gambling. A number of studies have reported that youth do not think that their gambling behavior is of significant concern (7–8). These reports have recently been confirmed by parents. In a national Canadian study, when asked to identify potential problematic adolescent behaviors, more than 50% of parents identified multiple potentially risky behaviors as a concern (drug use [87%], alcohol use [82%], drinking and driving [81%], unsafe sexual activity [81%], violence in schools and bullying [75%], smoking [73%], obesity and eating disorders [66%], excessive online Internet use [66%], negative body image [64%], excessive video game playing [64%], and depression [60%]. The only exception was gambling where 40% of parents expressed concern (9).

13.2 Prevention programs

Most existing primary prevention programs are universal, focusing on the entire population versus only high-risk groups. These programs are designed to minimize and/or prevent multiple mental health disorders, antisocial, and risk-taking behaviors. Recent analyses have suggested that today's youth are at high risk for engaging in a multitude of risky behaviors including substance use, tobacco use, teen pregnancy, unprotected sex, eating disorders, violence, school dropout, as well as conduct and antisocial disorders (10–12). More recently, a number of clinical researchers have begun to develop and examine the impact of gambling prevention programs (13–19).

Understanding the severity of the consequences associated with youth problem gambling can be difficult in light of the generally accepted perception that youth have little readily available access to money, that accessibility to gambling venues is limited, and the widespread belief that few adolescents have significant gambling or gambling-related problems. Volberg and her colleagues (3), in an excellent review of adolescent gambling prevalence studies, suggest that youth often begin gambling at an early age. Data from the Australian Productivity Commission (2) has suggested that adult pathological gamblers report beginning during their childhood, often as young as 9 years of age. Independent of sanctions and legal prohibitions and restrictions youth appear to have managed to gamble on most forms of legalized and state sanctioned gambling activities (1, 7, 20–24).

Adolescent prevalence rates of problem gambling have been consistently reported to be between 3 and 8% (two to four times that of adults) (1, 3, 25–28), with another 10–15% of youth being at-risk for the development of a serious gambling problem (1, 3, 21, 25, 27, 29). The relatively rapid movement from social gambler to problem gambler (7) and the induction of gambling as the new rite of initiation into adulthood (30) attest to adolescents' desire to participate in a wide diversity of gambling activities, and to their vulnerability. Given that this behavior can easily go undetected for long periods of time, it has often been referred to as a "hidden addiction."

Similar to adults, our current understanding of youth problem gambling includes a profile that reflects its serious nature (31). Increased efforts to understand the economic, social, familial, and psychological costs of gambling, and the recognition of the adolescent population as being particularly at risk for developing problem behaviors (11, 32–33) and gambling-related problems (25, 34) amplifies the necessity for effective prevention initiatives (1, 17).

Within the past two decades there has been increased interest in the prevention of high-risk behaviors (35). This research, converging with the examination of etiologies and remedies for psychological disorders, to become prevention science, has formed the basis of many school-based prevention efforts (36–37). Though our current knowledge of the efficacy of prevention of youth gambling problems is limited, and a clear need for more intensive and extensive efforts has been acknowledged (16), few empirical studies have been undertaken to assess the usefulness of such programs, nor do most of the programs have any theoretical underpinnings.

There is a growing body and substantial literature on prevention of adolescent alcohol and substance abuse. Substance abuse prevention has a rich history of research, program development/implementation, and evaluation, which can help to shape future directions for the prevention of gambling problems (18). As both a mental and a public health issue, the conceptualization of problem gambling as another form of risk-taking behavior, and its adverse consequences, substantiates the need for effective prevention initiatives (38).

In spite of the importance of developing such programs, most existing programs have not been shown to be successful in altering behaviors because of their short duration, lack of intensity, atheoretical nature, and ineffective administration. Still further, there has been a general lack of follow-up due to insufficient funding to provide long-term behavioral evaluations. In general, efforts to address adolescent risky behaviors have typically been streamed into prevention programs aimed toward non-users (primary prevention), screening for potential problems (secondary prevention), and treatment (tertiary prevention) for those who have developed problems (e.g., alcohol use and abuse, substance abuse, smoking). In terms of primary prevention, the bulk of resources have been allocated toward initiatives with the goal of preventing or postponing the initial use of substances or activities including gambling. This is also predicated on research suggesting that pathological gambling adolescents and adults both begin initiating at an early age (2, 25, 34). Although the authors in principle would advocate for youth abstinence, the reality remains that an abstinence approach would likely not be successful. The traditional approach of promoting non-use/experimentation as a means of preventing problems has been challenged (18, 39–44), especially in the field of alcohol consumption and gambling (45).

Though relatively few reduction prevention initiatives currently exist specifically targeting problem gambling, the increasing widespread use of the harm-reduction approach in the field of alcohol and substance abuse necessitates an examination of the validity of a harm-reduction approach for gambling. It has recently been advocated that initiatives move toward designing prevention strategies that target multiple risk behaviors based on theoretical and empirical evidence of common risk and protective factors across adolescent risky behaviors (11, 46–50) including problem gambling (17, 26, 45, 51). Ample research points to the serious consequences of problem gambling. Such negative consequences have short-term and far-reaching negative consequences. In light of the proliferation and expansion of gambling venues, the normalization of gambling, and the relative ease of accessibility by underage minors (52), the importance of primary prevention takes center stage in addressing this issue. Though prevention efforts are critical in protecting vulnerable populations, no current best practices or standards have been empirically established.

13.3 Abstinence versus harm reduction approach

There are two global paradigms under which specific prevention approaches can be classified, either abstinence or harm-reduction (the terms harm-reduction and harm minimization have often been used interchangeably). These two approaches are not completely mutually exclusive, but they are predicated on different short-term goals and processes. Abolitionists and gambling critics would argue for an abstinence approach, whereas others have suggested that the normalization of gambling within society would preclude such an approach.

Harm-reduction strategies (policy, programs, intervention) primarily seek to help individuals without demanding abstinence (53–54). Included in such an approach would be secondary prevention strategies, based on the assumption that individuals cannot be prevented from engaging in particular risky behaviors (32, 55); tertiary prevention strategies (56); and a "health movement" perspective (38, 57–59).

Though the negative consequences resulting from excessive gambling are evident (e.g., financial difficulties, depression, suicide ideation and attempts, health problems, academic problems, criminal and antisocial behavior, familial disruptions, peer difficulties, interpersonal problems, etc.) (48, 60), it remains unclear as to whether the social costs associated with legalized gambling outweigh the benefits. Social cost/benefit studies are limited in number and their methodological approaches have been criticized. As gambling expansion increases, governments seem to have adopted by default a harm-minimization approach, whereby policy efforts (where applicable) are aimed at reducing or minimizing the negative impact of gambling while not limiting access for the general public. Such policies may not be explicit but rather implicit. The change in governmental and industry advocates in the past twenty years has been remarkable. Both groups now readily acknowledge some of the potential harms associated with excessive gambling and some have taken proactive measures in trying to minimize these harms. Corporate Social Responsibility (CSR) is now becoming firmly accepted in the gaming/gambling industry.

Almost universally, underage youth are prohibited access to government-regulated forms of gambling and venues. (It should be noted that different jurisdictions have different regulations as to the age permitted to gamble and/or gamble on certain types of activities.) Though these laws are necessary, research also indicates that early gambling experiences mostly occur with nonregulated forms of gambling (e.g., playing cards for money among peers, placing informal bets on sports events, wagering on games of skill, or parents gambling for/and with their children) (3, 9, 22, 25). The fact that parents are aware of their children's gambling both within and outside the home and fail to address this issue represents tacit approval (9). This highlights both the paradox and the confusion as to which primary prevention approach to promote; abstinence or harm-reduction. If one were to advocate an abstinence approach, is it realistic to expect youth to stop gambling when between 70 and 80% of children and adolescents report having gambled during the past 12 months? Similar to their adult counterparts, one could argue that it would be unrealistic to expect youth to stop gambling completely, especially because it is exceedingly difficult to regulate access to gambling activities organized among themselves (e.g., card betting, sports betting, wagering on personal games of skill, etc.) as well as their reports that they often receive lottery scratch tickets as gifts (61). Other proponents of a harm-minimization approach would argue that in spite of legal restrictions, most youth gamble without developing any significant negative consequences.

Ample research highlights the age of onset of gambling behavior as a significant risk factor associated with problem gambling, with a younger age of initiation being correlated with the development of gambling-related problems (1–3, 22, 25, 34, 45). Thus, delaying the age of onset of gambling experiences would be one strategy in a successful prevention paradigm. Though this argument would support an abstinence approach, other mitigating factors would suggest its limitations.

We have long argued that a harm-reduction approach makes intuitive sense on other levels. As gambling has been historically part of our culture (62–63), it has become strongly endorsed by government, and most adults remain unaware of the potential negative consequences for underage youth. As such, a harm-minimization approach seems a reasonable alternative. This is not to suggest that we are advocating for underage minors to gamble. Rather, we are suggesting that the pressures and accessibility to do so negates a total abstinence approach. Included under the principles of harm-minimization is the promotion of responsible behavior, teaching and informing youth about the facts and risks associated with gambling, changing erroneous cognitions, misperceptions, and beliefs, along with enhancing skills needed to maintain control when gambling. If these skills are encouraged and reinforced for youth through their formative years, it is plausible that they may be less vulnerable to the risks of a gambling problem once gaining legal access to gambling forums (48). The authors recognize that the harm-minimization approach is not without criticism. However, given that there are a number of socially and widely acceptable risk behaviors (e.g., alcohol consumption and gambling) where involvement in such activities can be viewed as a continuum ranging from no problems to significant psychological, social, physical, and financial harm to one's self and others, the utility of the harm-reduction approach as a means to prevent problem behavior remains promising.

13.4 Gambling as a socially acceptable activity

There is ample reason to believe that individual involvement in potentially risky behaviors may be approached in a responsible manner. For example, the majority of youth who drink alcohol or gamble do not do so excessively nor do they develop significant problems. Rather, their behaviors are done in a moderate manner, setting and adhering to acceptable limits although these limits may be intermittently disrespected. Research on the patterns of use and personal and social control mechanisms of various substance use points to the possibility of achieving controlled involvement in risky behaviors, free from problematic involvement (64–65). There is also evidence from studies using adults that substance users do in fact make rational choices, weighing the perceived positive gains versus risks of drug or alcohol use, and utilize informal control mechanisms of social networks (66–68). Interestingly, adolescent problem gamblers were able to discern both the benefits and risks associated with problem gambling. However, it appears that problem gamblers either do not recognize themselves as problem gamblers and/or that they see the risks coming much later (assuming they will "stop" their gambling when the consequences become problematic) (69).

Research on risk and protective factors offers an important reminder that the cause of such variance results from the interaction of present risk and protective factors operating within complex person-environment-situation interactions. Thus, it can be argued that the continuum of harm is associated with a number of different risk profiles and that harm-reduction is a useful means to prevent normal adolescent gambling behavior from becoming increasingly problematic (69).

13.5 Harm-reduction prevention programs

The strategies of harm-reduction prevention have the potential for reducing the prevalence of problem gambling and are consistent with a public health framework (38). As an example, school-based drug education programs and media campaigns are common strategies used regardless of prevention orientation (e.g., abstinence, harm-reduction). To date, universal harm-reduction programs have generally been primarily integrated in the form of school-based drug, alcohol, and smoking awareness, education and prevention programs. A greater variety of strategies are employed when considering selective prevention, given the variety of at-risk populations that selective programs may target (e.g., street youth at high risk for drug and alcohol abuse, individuals with antisocial conduct, delinquent and/or behavioral disorders, or entire schools at high risk for a multiplicity of problems due to sociocultural factors).

Such universal harm-reduction prevention programs are intended to modify inappropriate attitudes toward risky behaviors, enhance positive decision making, educate youth about both short-term and long-term risks associated with excessive use, and facilitate their understanding of tolerance. A basic premise underlying such an approach is that once the individual's awareness and knowledge increase about potentially risky activities and they have developed proficient decision-making skills, they can then make appropriate decisions about whether they need to avoid substances (e.g., alcohol, tobacco, and illegal drugs), and/or monitor their use carefully (39).

13.6 Resilience

A long history of research suggests that resilient youth typically have adequate or competent problem-solving skills (the ability to think abstractly, and to generate and implement solutions to cognitive and social problems), social competence (encompassing the qualities of flexibility, communication skills, concern for others, and pro-social behaviors), autonomy (self-efficacy and self control), and a sense of purpose and future (exhibited in success orientation, motivation, and optimism) (70). The field of prevention, in particular work by SAMSHA, has moved our understanding from a risk-prevention framework to one that includes both risk-prevention and the promotion of protective factors. Masten, Best, and Garmezy (71) have suggested that protective factors can serve to mediate or buffer the effects of individual vulnerabilities or environmental adversity so that the adaptational trajectory is more positive than if the protective factors are not at work. Protective factors, in and of themselves, do not necessarily promote resiliency. If the strength or number of risk factors outweigh the impact of protective factors, the chance that poor outcomes will ensue increases.

Multiple studies have examined the impact of a large number of risk and protective factors associated with excessive alcohol and substance abuse (72–73). Such risk and protective factors can be grouped into a number of domains. In their conceptual model, Bournstein, Zweig, and Gardner (74) suggest an interactive effect between each of these domains and the individual, who processes, interprets, and responds to various factors, based on unique characteristics brought to the situation. The Centre for Substance Abuse Prevention model, modified by Dickson et al. (73) (see Fig. 13.1), provides a conceptual framework for targeting high-risk groups and their potential outcomes. This model remains widely used in the development of prevention programs.

Protective and risk factors have been shown to interact such that protective factors reduce the strength of the relation of the stressor and its outcomes. There are numerous examples as to how protective factors influence positive outcomes. For example, the

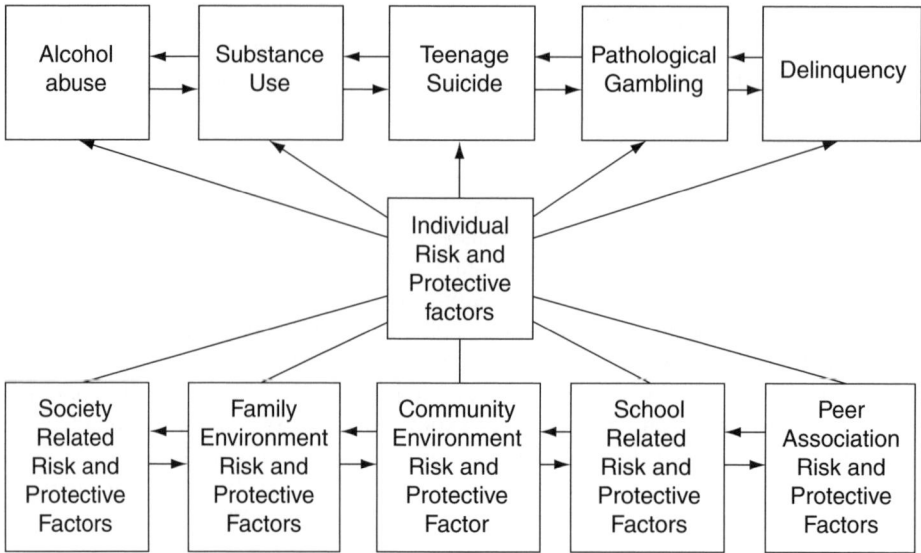

Fig. 13.1: A conceptual model for understanding the domains of risk and protective factors that influence an individual's behavior. Adapted from Understanding Substance Abuse Prevention: Toward 21st Century Primer on Effective Programs (73). Centre for Substance Abuse Prevention (CSAP) and Substance Abuse and Mental Health Services Administration (SAMHSA). Modified by Dickson and her colleagues.

effects of positive school experiences have been shown to moderate the effects of family conflict, which in turn decreases the association between family conflict and several adolescent problem behaviors (e.g., pathological gambling, alcohol and substance abuse, suicide, and delinquency) (75).

In an attempt to conceptualize our current state of knowledge concerning the risk factors associated with problem gambling, a similar paradigm was developed based on the existing knowledge of youth with severe gambling problems (17). Within the individual domain, poor impulse control, high sensation-seeking, unconventionality, poor psychological functioning, low self-esteem, early and persistent problem behaviors, and early initiation are commonly found. Common risk factors in the family domain were found to include familial history of substance abuse, parental attitudes, and modeling of deviant behavior. Within the peer domain, social expectancies and reinforcement by peer groups are common risk factors across addictions. Although some research has been undertaken to identify risk factors of problem adolescent gambling (7, 29, 73, 76–78), few studies have examined protective mechanisms, or more generally, resiliency for youth with respect to problem gambling. Dickson et al., after examining a wide number of variables, found that family cohesion and school connectedness served as protective factors for preventing gambling problems (73). Protective factors that have been examined across other youth risky behaviors and addictions generally fall into three categories: care and support, dispositional attributes such as positive and high expectations, and opportunities for participation (79).

In a number of recent studies Lussier and her colleagues (77–78) attempted to examine the role of resiliency and youth gambling behaviors. The construct of resiliency has changed over time to include not only social competence despite adversity, but to examine specific types of resiliency: educational resilience, emotional resilience, and behavioral resilience (33). Utilizing Jessor's (11) adolescent risk behavioral model, Lussier and her colleagues sought to explore the concept of resilience and its relationship to adolescent gambling problems (78). Of those identified as high risk in their sample, only 20% were deemed to be resilient. Though not finding overwhelming support for resilience as a predictor of gambling problems, both risk and protective factors did provide a unique contribution to the prediction model of gambling problems. In a follow-up study, Lussier reported that for adolescents from low-income immigrant homes, social bonding was associated with a decrease in severity for drug abuse, alcohol abuse, and gambling problems. Personal competence was similarly found to be associated with a decrease in substance abuse and deviant behaviors (77).

13.7 Current prevention programs

The past decade has witnessed an increased number of prevention programs attempting to reduce the incidence of problem gambling. Of those that are currently being implemented (although implementation is quite sporadic), most developed for youth have little or no science-based underlying principles and have failed to account for risk and protective factors. Few have been systematically evaluated (this has been gradually changing). The majority of these programs can be best described as primary and/or universal preventive efforts with the overall goal of reducing the incidence of problem gambling (a harm-minimization versus abstinence approach). Several programs have explicitly identified factors associated with the development of problem gambling, but these factors were not always defined as a risk or a protective factor, nor are there many programs that point to the scientific validity of such factors. A number of programs are based on increasing one's understanding of the mathematical laws of probability whereas others are focused on demystifying the myth that there is considerable skill involved in random activities (e.g., slots, roulette).

13.8 Commonalities and differences among programs

Prevention programs designed to reduce the incidence of gambling problems for youth have typically aimed at raising awareness concerning issues related to problem gambling. Most of these programs conceptualize gambling as an addiction and foster a harm-reduction framework. Some may try to advocate abstinence until one has the cognitive capacity necessary to set and maintain limits, but they typically emphasize responsible gambling. The distinction between responsible gambling and abstinence likely lies within the specific population targeted. Programs targeted toward populations where the prevalence of gambling and other addiction and/or mental health problems is high (e.g., First Nations) suggest prevention programs might encourage abstinence over harm-minimization, taking a tertiary approach in their prevention efforts.

Because the objective of the majority of current programs is to raise awareness, most provide information relevant to gambling and problem gambling, discuss motivations to gamble, warning signs, and consequences associated with excessive gambling, and detail how and where to get help for an individual with a gambling problem. Several curriculums go a little further than merely presenting factual information and dispelling erroneous cognitions, encouraging the development of interpersonal skills, fostering effective coping strategies, providing techniques and strategies to improve self-esteem, and offering ideas for resisting peer pressure. A number of current programs place greater emphasis on the mathematical/probabilistic aspects of gambling, including teaching students about the odds and probabilities associated with games of chance, whereas others emphasize issues related to erroneous cognitions and thoughts.

13.9 Gambling prevention programs

As previously noted, a growing number of gambling prevention programs has been developed. Some of these include Don't Bet on It in South Australia for children ages 6 to 9 years; Gambling Minimizing Health Risks in Queensland for children in levels 5 and 6; Facing the Odds in Louisiana for children in grades 5 to 8; Wanna Bet in Minnesota for children in grades 3 to 8; Gambling: A Stacked Deck in Alberta; and the Harvard/ Massachusetts Council Mathematics Curriculum for High School Students. Williams and his colleagues (16) introduced a high school program, Gambling: A Stacked Deck, in which they emphasized a general awareness of the nature of gambling and problem gambling, addressed erroneous cognitions, helped to foster generic decision-making and social problem-solving skills, and attempted to enhance youth's adaptive behaviors through a PowerPoint type workshop. Williams and his colleagues also introduced a module specifically focusing on probability theory in a statistics course as a way of modifying university students' gambling behavior. In this curriculum, they emphasized gambling-related odds, resistance to gambling fallacies, and gambling attitudes, with the ultimate goal of a reduction in gambling time and money expended.

For the past twenty years, the International Centre for Youth Gambling Problems and High-Risk Behaviors at McGill University has been examining the risk and protective factors associated with youth gambling and gambling problems. This research program has led to a better understanding of the factors necessary to include in our prevention initiatives. At the same time, we became aware of the importance of providing a variety of strategies for teachers and prevention specialists that they might adopt for classroom use. In spite of some evidence suggesting that single-trial inoculations are not necessarily effective for long-term gains in behavior changes, the Centre has adopted a multi-level approach, with some efforts directly student-based, others requiring minimal teacher intervention, and still others requiring greater teacher intervention. This buffet style approach is designed to appeal to teachers who are unfamiliar with the issue of teen gambling and/or gambling problems as well as those with limited time in which to administer a curriculum.

The prevention programs are also intended to address a number of different audiences: children and adolescents, teachers, parents, physicians, and attorneys/judges. All programs have been evaluated for their short-term gains (insufficient funding is available for long-term follow-up) and have generally been found beneficial in improving knowledge; increasing awareness of the warning signs for problem gambling; modifying inappropriate attitudes; correcting false cognitions, understandings, and erroneous beliefs (e.g., probabilities, skill vs. luck, strategies, superstitions, independence of events) with the intention of ultimately modifying and reducing gambling behavior and preventing excessive pathological gambling behavior disorders. Though it is not the intent to describe the specific goals for each of these prevention initiatives (see www.youthgambling.com), the more general goals are to enhance problem-solving skills, increase feelings of self-confidence, improve coping skills, resist peer pressure and social temptations, and facilitate good decision making. Many of these programs are currently being used in the United States, Canada, Europe, Australia, New Zealand, and Singapore. The following activities have been developed for use in primary and secondary schools.

13.9.1 The Amazing Chateau (grades 4–7) and Hooked City (grades 7–12)

These award-winning interactive educational software games are designed for youth to play individually. A teacher's manual accompanies these games. The games take approximately 60 minutes to complete and incorporate a problem-solving approach. The programs may be temporarily suspended, enabling the child to come back and continue at another time. The software allows the child to print valuable information, take a screening test for problem gambling, and maintain records of success while reinforcing a wide variety of concepts and misconceptions related to youth gambling issues.

13.9.2 Youth Awareness and Prevention Workshops (Levels I and II)

These PowerPoint workshops have been evaluated on over 7,000 school-age children and adolescents and have been shown to be successful in achieving a variety of prevention goals. Though intended to be completed in one sitting, they can and have been done over several days. An instructor manual accompanies each of these presentations, identifying the goals of each slide, background information, and questions to be raised.

13.9.3 Clean Break

This award-winning docudrama is approximately 25 minutes in length and was developed for high school students and delinquent youth. The production team, using MTV technology, follows a pathological gambler who attempted suicide and as a result is now a paraplegic. Interspersed throughout the DVD are scenes and examples of adolescent problem gambling behaviors based on the Centre's clinical experiences working with youth having gambling problems. This hard-hitting docudrama is accompanied by an examiner's manual and a PowerPoint presentation for follow-up discussions.

13.9.4 Know Limits

Issues around gambling, drug and alcohol use, tobacco use, and other high-risk behaviors are presented in a team game format. Incorporating elements of charades, Taboo, and word scramble, information is disseminated in a fun and enjoyable game format for high school students.

Other prevention programs are used to target individuals who frequently come into contact with adolescents and adolescent problem gamblers. For example, the Centre has developed two successful public service announcements (targeting Internet wagering and poker playing) that attempt to raise parental awareness that their children's gambling may in fact be becoming problematic. These 30-second PSAs have a clear message – "Talk with your children." Other programs designed for physicians (Youth Gambling Problems: Practical Information for Health Professionals), and those in the legal profession (Youth Gambling Problems: Practical Information for Professionals in the Criminal Justice System), provide DVDs with pertinent information on youth gambling problems and CD-ROMs with seminal papers, posters, and screening instruments, which can be downloaded and printed for the professional. Though other programs, in particular self-exclusion programs and the use of smart card technology for electronic gambling machines, have been implemented, these are not appropriate for adolescents given that their age prohibits them from these venues.

13.10 Mental health

Is problem gambling unique from other forms of addiction or are there commonalities? An examination of the commonalities of risk and protective factors for problem gambling and other addictions seems to provide evidence that gambling may be incorporated into more general addiction and adolescent risk behavior prevention programs. The current thinking is that gambling problems may be listed under a Behavioral Disorders in the upcoming revision of the American Psychiatric Association's Diagnostic and Statistical Manual-DSM-V. Everything being equal, we would suggest a more general mental health prevention program that addresses a diversity of adolescent risky behaviors (e.g., substance abuse, gambling, risky driving, eating disorders, truancy, and risky sexual activity). A number of science-based programs provide evidence that prevention programs for risky behaviors are indeed effective. Dickson et al. have suggested that there is strong support pointing to the need to examine similarities and differences among addictive behaviors, the need to analyze multiple risk and protective factors, and the importance of understanding the coping mechanisms of individuals engaging in risky behaviors (17).

13.11 New directions

There is little doubt that though our knowledge concerning youth with gambling problems has steadily increased during the past two decades, our need to incorporate such knowledge into a risk-protection-resilience prevention model needs further elaboration. Viewing risk and protective factors in light of the domains in which they operate provides a means to specify program goals (targeting specific factors), to establish outcome evaluation criteria, and to assess effectiveness of prevention programs. Though this research is still relatively new, we would suggest that the scientific standards expected from this field need to be no less rigorous.

Findings from the field of adolescent alcohol and substance abuse suggest that no one universal approach to prevention appears to be uniformly successful (32). As such, a combination of strategies seems to work best toward the goal of nurturing resilience. The Center for Substance Abuse Prevention has delineated a number of strategies that can be combined in the development of school, family, and community prevention programs that target each area impacting youth (80). Such strategies include information dissemination, prevention education, providing alternative activities in lieu of the particular addictive behavior, problem identification and referral, community-based processes (training community members and agencies in substance use and gambling education and prevention), and activities thought to reduce risk factors and enhance protective factors. In addition to adapting such programs for different cultural, ethnic and age groups, it is important to understand the venues in which such programs will occur. For example, if teachers remain reluctant to use one type of program then alternative approaches may be necessary. This is part of the underlying rationale for the Intentional Centre for Youth Gambling Problems and High-Risk Behavior's approach to developing alternative types of curriculum.

13.12 Prevention and social policy

Prevention programs in essence represent a form of social policy. This is particularly important within the context of the debate between harm-reduction versus abstinence (38). It has been argued that the strength of prevention programs that address problem gambling issues is highly dependent on clarity in the articulation of responsible social policies and assurance that they reflect research-based findings on resilience and effective program evaluations. Given the widespread increase in number of venues and normalization of gambling, current policies that reflect the predominant attitude that gambling has few negative consequences and is merely a form of entertainment leaves little credence to effective abstinence gambling prevention initiatives. Changing widespread attitudes about problem gambling in general, and youth gambling in particular, will be necessary before our prevention efforts will be successful in encouraging individuals to make wiser healthy decisions about gambling. To date, other potentially health-compromising behaviors – alcohol and substance use – have had significantly more visibility.

Our current social policies concerning problem gambling have generally been reactive to specific problems. For example, considerable attention has been focused on electronic gambling machines in certain jurisdictions. These machines, EGMs, Pokies, VLTs, often referred to as the crack cocaine of gambling, have resulted in a number of different policy initiatives, including limiting the number of machines per location, modifying hours of availability, or enforcement of smart card technology to help individuals preset limits and maintain those limits.

The lack of parental concern (8–9), and ineffective gambling law enforcement, in particular the selling of lottery and scratch tickets to youth (23, 52), remains a concern. Though there is preliminary research to suggest that perceptions of skill and luck can be modified for gambling activities (81), there is little evidence or empirical support that attitudes toward gambling can be modified and have long-lasting changes. Much basic and applied research funding is required to help identify common and unique risk and protective factors for gambling problems. In addition, longitudinal research to examine the natural history of pathological gambling from childhood to adolescence through later adulthood is required and will add substantially to our knowledge.

Only recently have health professionals, educators, and public policymakers acknowledged the need for prevention of problem gambling in light of the vast expansion of gambling. Nevertheless, state, provincial, or federal policies are virtually nonexistent. Though many existing programs are school-based targeting children and adolescents, this should not be misconstrued to suggest that only youth remain at high risk for the development of serious pathological gambling problems or that such behaviors cannot occur at any age. Other programs for adults have included self-exclusion programs, gambling education programs housed within casinos themselves, brochures, self-test assessment kiosks, and smart card technology.

In this chapter we have attempted to illustrate the importance of using a conceptual model as the foundation for prevention efforts and have argued that research, development of prevention programs, and their acceptability into school-based curriculum and community programs are important. There is a growing empirical base indicating that well-designed, appropriately implemented school-based prevention can positively impact multiple social, heath, and academic outcomes (37). Despite our limited knowledge of the role of protective factors in gambling problems, there is ample research to suggest that direct and moderator effects of protective factors can be used to guide the development of future prevention and intervention efforts to help minimize risk behaviors. Dickson et al.'s adaptation of the risk behavior model provides a promising framework from which to begin the much needed development of effective, science-based prevention initiatives for minimizing and ensuring a harm-reduction approach for problem gambling among youth as well as other selected groups (17).

There is a strong belief that competence and health-promotion programs are best initiated before youth are pressured to experiment with risky behaviors. Early intervention prevention programs that follow adolescents through high school will likely result in fewer youth with gambling problems. Sociocultural factors also remain crucial in developing effective programs. Prevention programming will need to account for the changing forms and opportunities for gambling. Ultimately, school-based initiatives may have to examine the commonalities among multiple risky behaviors before educators become inundated with the implementation of prevention programs for risky behaviors and have little time for the educational curriculum. Greater parental, teacher, and school administrator awareness of youth gambling problems will similarly be fundamental before real changes are realized.

References

1. National Research Council. Pathological gambling: A critical review. Washington, DC: National Academy Press; 1999.
2. Productivity Commission, Australia. Australia's Gambling Industries. Australian Government. Report number 10; 1999.
3. Volberg R, Gupta R, Griffiths MD, Ólason DT, Delfabbro P. An international perspective on youth gambling prevalence studies. In: Derevensky J, Shek DTL, Merrick J, eds. Youth gambling: The hidden addiction. Berlin: De Gruyter; 2011.
4. Derevensky J. Preface. In: Meyer G, Hayer T, Griffiths M, eds. Problem gambling in Europe. Challenges, prevention and interventions. New York. Springer; 2009.
5. Griffiths M, Parke J. Adolescent gambling on the internet: A review. Int J Adolesc Med Health 2010; 22:59–75.

6. McBride J, Derevensky J. Internet gambling behaviour in a sample of online gamblers. IJMA 2009;7:149–167.

7. Gupta R, Derevensky J. Adolescents with gambling problems: From research to treatment. J Gambl Stud 2000;16:315–342.

8. Ladouceur R, Jacques C, Ferland F, Giroux I. Parents' attitudes and knowledge regarding gambling among youths. J Gambl Stud 1998;14:83–90.

9. Campbell C, Derevensky J, Meerkamper E, Cutajar J. Parents' perceptions of adolescent gambling: A Canadian national study. J Gambl Stud, in press.

10 Bronfenbrenner U, McClelland P, Wethington E, Moen P, Ceci S. The state of Americans: This generation and the next. New York. Free Press; 1996.

11. Jessor R. New perspectives on adolescent risk behavior. In R. Jessor, ed. New perspectives on adolescent risk behavior. Cambridge, UK. Cambridge University Press; 1998.

12. Weissberg R, Walberg H, O'Brien M, Kuster C. Long-term trends in the well-being of children and youth. Washington, DC: Child Welfare League America Press; 2003.

13. Byrne A, Dickson L, Derevensky J, Gupta R, Lussier I. An examination of social marketing campaigns for the prevention of youth problem gambling. J Health Commun 2005;10:681–700.

14. Gaboury A, Ladouceur R. Evaluation of a prevention program for pathological gambling among adolescents. J Prim Prev 1993;14:21–28.

15. Williams R, Connolly D. Does learning about mathematics of gambling change gambling behavior? Psychol Addic Behav 2006;20:62–8.

16. Williams R, Connolly D, Wood R, Currie S, Meghan-Davis R. Program findings that inform curriculum development for the prevention of problem gambling. Gambling Research 2004;16:47–69.

17. Dickson L, Derevensky JL, Gupta R. The prevention of youth gambling problems: A conceptual model. J Gambl Stud 2002;18:161–84.

18. Evans R. Some theoretical models and constructs generic to substance abuse prevention programs for adolescents: Possible relevance and limitations for problem gambling. J Gambl Stud 2003;19(3):287–302.

19. Derevensky J, Gupta R, Dickson L, Deguire A-E. Prevention efforts toward reducing gambling problems. In: Derevensky J, Gupta R, eds. Gambling problems in youth: Theoretical and applied perspectives. New York. Kluwer Academic/Plenum; 2004:211–30.

20. Derevensky J, Gupta R. Youth gambling: A clinical and research perspective. Egambling 2000;2:1–10.

21. Derevensky JL, Gupta R, Winters K. Prevalence rates of youth gambling problems: Are the current rates inflated? J Gambl Stud 2003;19:405–25.

22. Jacobs D. Youth gambling in North America: Long term trends and future prospects. In: Derevensky J, Gupta R, eds. Gambling problems in youth: Theoretical and applied perspectives. New York. Kluwer Academic/Plenum; 2004:1–26.

23. Felsher J, Derevensky JL, Gupta R. Parental influences and social modeling of youth lottery participation. J Community Appl Soc Psychol 2003;13:361–77.

24. Ste-Marie C, Gupta R, Derevensky J. Anxiety and social stress related to adolescent gambling behavior. Int Gambl Stud 2002;2(1):123–41.

25. Gupta R, Derevensky J. Adolescent gambling behavior: A prevalence study and examination of the correlates associated with excessive gambling. J Gambl Stud 1998;14:319–45.

26. Jacobs DF. Juvenile gambling in North America: An analysis of long term trends and future prospects. J Gambl Stud 2000;16:119–52.

27. Shaffer HJ, Hall MN. Estimating the prevalence of adolescent gambling disorders: A quantitative synthesis and guide toward standard gambling nomenclature. J Gambl Stud 1996;12:193–214.

28. Shaffer HJ, Hall MN. Updating and refining prevalence estimates of disordered gambling behavior in the United States and Canada. Can J Public Health 2001;92:168–72.

29. Derevensky JL, Gupta R. Prevalence estimates of adolescent gambling: A comparison of SOGS-RA, DSM-IV-J, and the GA 20 Questions. J Gambl Stud 2000;16:227–52.
30. Svendsen R. Gambling among older Minnesotans. Prepared for the National Research Council Committee on the Social and Economic Impact of Pathological Gambling. Minnesota. Minnesota Institute of Public Health; 1998.
31. Shead, NW, Derevensky J, Gupta R. Youth problem gambling: Our current knowledge of risk and protective factors. In: Derevensky J, Shek DTL, Merrick J, eds. Youth gambling: The hidden addiction. Berlin: De Gruyter; 2011.
32. Baer J, MacLean M, Marlatt G. Linking etiology and treatment for adolescent substance abuse: Toward a better match. In: Jessor R, ed. New perspectives on adolescent risk behavior. Cambridge: Cambridge University Press; 1998.
33. Luthar S, Cicchetti D, Becker B. The construct of resilience: A critical evaluation and guidelines for future work. Child Dev 2000;71:543–62.
34. Wynne I IJ, Smith GJ, Jacobs DF. Adolescent gambling and problem gambling in Alberta. Alberta, Canada: Alberta Alcohol Drug Abuse Commission; 1996.
35. Nation M, Crusto C, Wandersman A, Kumpfer K L, Seybolt D, Morrissey-Kane E, et al. What works in prevention: Principles of effective prevention programs. Am Psychol 2003;58:449–56.
36. Coie J, Watt N, West S, Hawkins J, Asarnow J, Markman H, Ramey S, Shure M, Long B. The science of prevention. Am Psychol 1993;48:1013–22.
37. Greenberg MT, Weissberg RP, O'Brien MU, Zins JE, Fredericks L, Resnik H, et al. Enhancing school-based prevention and youth development through coordinated social, emotional, and academic learning. Am Psychol 2003;58:466–74.
38. Messerlian C, Derevensky JL, Gupta R. Youth gambling problems: A public health framework. Unpublished manuscript. Montreal: McGill University; 2003.
39. Beck J. 100 Years of "Just say no" versus "Just say know". Reevaluating drug education goals for the coming century. Eval Rev 1998;22:15–45.
40. Brown JH, D'Emidio-Caston M. On becoming 'at risk' through drug education: How symbolic policies and their practices affect students. Eval Rev 1995;19:451–92.
41. Gorman, DM. The irrelevance of evidence in the development of school-based drug prevention policy, 1986–1996. Eval Rev 1998;22:118–46.
42. Marlatt, GA. Basic principles and strategies of harm reduction. In: Marlatt GA, ed. Harm reduction: Pragmatic strategies for managing high-risk behaviors. New York. Guilford; 1998:49–66.
43. Poulin C, Elliott D. Alcohol, tobacco and cannabis use among Nova Scotia adolescents: Implications for prevention and harm reduction. Can Med Assoc J 1997;156:1387–93.
44. Thombs D, Briddick W. Readiness to change among at-risk Greek student drinkers. J Coll Student Dev 2000;41:313–22.
45. Dickson L, Derevensky J L, Gupta R. Harm reduction for the prevention of youth gambling problems: Lessons learned from adolescent high-risk prevention programs. J Adolesc Res 2004;19:233–63.
46. Battistich V, Schaps E, Watson M, Solomon D. Prevention effects of the Child Development Project: Early findings from an ongoing multisite demonstration trial. J Adolesc Res 1996;11:12–35.
47. Costello EJ, Erkanli A, Federman E, Angold A. Development of psychiatric comorbidity with substance abuse in adolescents: Effects of timing and sex. J Clin Child Psychol 1999;28:298–311.
48. Derevensky J, Gupta R. Adolescents with gambling problems: A review of our current knowledge. Egambling 2004;10:119–40.
49. Galambos, NL, Tilton-Weaver LC. Multiple risk behavior in adolescents and young adults. Health Rev 1998;10:9–20.
50. Loeber R, Farrington D, Stouthamer-Loeber M, Van Kammen W. Multiple risk factors for multi-problem boys: Co-occurrence of delinquency, substance use, attention deficit, conduct problems, physical aggression, covert behavior, depressed mood, and shy/withdrawn behavior. In:

Jessor R, ed. New perspectives on adolescent risk behavior. Cambridge: Cambridge University Press, 1998.

51. Gupta R, Derevensky J. An empirical examination of Jacobs' General Theory of Addictions: Do adolescent gamblers fit the theory? J Gambl Stud 1998;14:17–49.

52. St-Pierre R, Derevensky, J, Gupta R, Martin I. Preventing lottery ticket sales to minors: Factors influencing retailers' compliance behaviour. Unpublished manuscript, 2011.

53. Meghan C. Harm reduction or reducing harm? Can Med Assoc J 2001;164:173.

54. Riley D, Sawka E, Conley P, Hewit, D, Mitic W, Poulin C, Room R, Single E, Topp J. Harm reduction: Concepts and practice – a policy discussion paper. Subst Use Misuse 1999;34: 9–24.

55. Cohen J. Achieving a reduction in drug-related harm through education. In: Heather N, Wodak A, Nadelmann E, O'Hare P, eds. Psychoactive drugs and harm reduction: From faith to science. London: Whurr; 1993.

56. DiClemente, C. Prevention and harm reduction for chemical dependency: A process perspective. Clin Psychol Rev 1999;19:173–86.

57. Denning P, Little J. Harm reduction in mental health: The emerging work of harm reduction psychotherapy. Harm Reduct Comm 2001;11:7–10.

58. Heather N, Wodak A, Nadelmann E, O'Hare P. Psychoactive drugs and harm reduction: From faith to science. London: Whurr; 1993.

59. Messerlian C, Gillespie M, Derevensky J. Beyond drugs and alcohol: Including gambling in our high-risk behavior framework. Paediatr Child Health 2007;12(3):199–204.

60. Stinchfield R. Demographic, psychosocial and behavioral factors associated with youth gambling and problem gambling. In: Derevensky J, Gupta R, eds. Gambling problems in youth: Theoretical and applied perspectives. New York. Kluwer Academic/Plenum; 2004:27–40.

61. Felsher J, Derevensky J, Gupta R. Lottery playing amongst youth: Implications for prevention and social policy. J Gambl Stud 2004;20(2):127–53.

62. Fleming AM. Something for nothing: A history of gambling. New York: Delacorte Press; 1978.

63. Schwartz D. Roll the bones: The history of gambling. New York: Gotham Books; 2007.

64. Boys A, Marsden J, Griffiths P, Fountain J, Stillwell G, Strang J. Substance use among young people: the relationship between perceived functions and intentions. Addiction 1999;94:1043–50.

65. Kandel DB. On processes of peer influences in adolescent drug use: A developmental perspective. Adv Alcohol Subst Abuse 1985;4139–63.

66. Cheung, YW, Erickson PG, Landau T. Experience of crack use: Findings from a community-based sample in Toronto. J Drug Issues 1991;21:121–40.

67. Erikson EH. The life cycle completed: A review. New York: Norton; 1982.

68. Murphy SB, Reinarman C, Waldorf D. An 11-year follow-up of a network of cocaine users. Br J Addict 1989;84:427–36.

69. Gillespie M, Derevensky J, Gupta R. The utility of outcome expectancies in the prediction of adolescent gambling behaviour. J Gambl Issues 2007;19:69–85.

70. Brown JH, D'Emidio-Caston M, Benard B. Resilience education. Thousand Oaks, CA: Corwin Press; 2001.

71. Masten A, Best K, Garmezy N. Resilience and development: Contributions from the study of children who overcome adversity. Dev Psychopathol 1990;2:425–44.

72. Derevensky J, Gupta R, Dickson L, Deguire AE. Prevention efforts toward minimizing gambling problems. Paper prepared for the National Council on Problem Gambling, Center for Mental Health Services (CMS) and the Substance Abuse and Mental Health Services Administration (SAMHSA). Washington, DC; 2001.

73. Dickson L, Derevensky JL, Gupta R. Youth gambling problems: The identification of risk and protective factors. Report prepared for the Ontario Problem Gambling Research Centre, Guelph, Ontario; 2003.

74. Bournstein PJ, Zweig JM, Gardner SE. Understanding substance abuse prevention-toward the 21st century: A primer on effective programs. Rockville: U.S. Department of Health and Human Services, Substance Abuse and Mental Health Services Administration, Center for Substance Abuse Prevention, Division of Knowledge Development and Evaluation; 1999.

75. Jessor R, Van Den Bos J, Vanderryn J, Costa FM, Turbin MS. Protective factors in adolescent problem behavior: Moderator effects and developmental change. Dev Psychol 1995;31:923–33.

76. Griffiths MD, Wood RT. Risk factors in adolescence: The case of gambling, videogame playing, and the internet. J Gambl Stud 2000;16:199–226.

77. Lussier I. Risk, compensatory, protective and vulnerability processes influencing youth gambling problems and other high risk behaviors. Unpublished doctoral dissertation, McGill University; 2009.

78. Lussier I, Derevensky J, Gupta R, Bergevin T, Ellenbogen S. Youth gambling behaviors: An examination of the role of resilience. Psychol Addict Behav 2007;21:165–73.

79. Werner E. High risk children in young adulthood: A longitudinal study from birth to 32 years. Am J Orthopsychiatr 1989;59:72–81.

80. Center for Substance Abuse Prevention. Principles of substance abuse prevention (DHHS Publication No. SMA 01–3507). Rockville, MD: National Clearinghouse for Alcohol and Drug Information; 2001.

81. Baboushkin H, Derevensky JL, Gupta R. Modifying children's perception of the amount of skill and luck involved in gambling activities. Paper presented at the annual meeting of the National Council on Problem Gambling, Detroit; June 1999.

14 Prevention of gambling problems in adolescents: The role of problem gambling assessment instruments and positive youth development programs

Daniel T. L. Shek and Rachel C. F. Sun

Although adolescent gambling behavior is a growing problem, there are unfortunately few adolescent gambling prevention programs, and the existing programs are seldom guided by well-articulated theories and systematic research. In the design of universal gambling prevention programs for adolescents, it is argued that the programs should be developed with reference to the risk factors for problem gambling, including cognitive, coping, emotional, behavioral, and interpersonal antecedents. It is argued that programs incorporating positive youth development constructs would help adolescents to develop competencies incompatible with the above-mentioned characteristics of problem gambling, hence reducing the likelihood of problem gambling. The issues related to the application of positive youth development constructs to adolescent problem gambling prevention are discussed.

14.1 Introduction

A survey of the Western literature showed that adolescent gambling behavior is a growing problem. Shaffer and Hall (1) reported that 10 to 14% of the young respondents were at-risk for problem gambling. Griffiths and Wood (2) revealed that high levels of adolescent gambling were found in Europe, the United States, Canada, and Australia. Gupta and Derevensky (3) showed that 63% of underage adolescents in grades 7 to 12 were found gambling and that out of the total population, 2.7% were found to be probable pathological gamblers, 6.6% were gamblers at-risk, and 54% were social gamblers. Dickson, Derevensky, and Gupta (4) reported that 4 to 8% of the adolescents were problem gamblers, which was as high as two to four times the adult population. Hardoon, Gupta, and Derevensky (5) suggested that 4.9% of the respondents were pathological gamblers whereas 8.0% of them were at-risk. In Hong Kong, there are very few studies examining problem gambling in adolescents. The Chinese Young Men Christian Association of Hong Kong (6) found that 3.5% of the young respondents were pathological gamblers and 0.8% of them were probable pathological gamblers. Although the reported prevalence rates of problem gambling in adolescents in different countries and/or cities may not be directly comparable because of different operational definitions of problem gambling, these figures do give us some idea about the seriousness of the problems in adolescents. All governments should work to find means to tackle the problem.

This chapter attempts to examine the issue of how adolescent problem gambling programs could possibly be constructed. The first approach that we can adopt is to examine the risk factors associated with adolescent problem gambling and develop prevention programs attempting to reduce the influence of the risk factors. Within this context, prevention programs based on problem gambling assessment tools such as the Maroondah Assessment Profile for Problem Gambling (G-MAP) will help to develop the related programs and identify adolescent problem gamblers. The second approach we can consider is to make use of the positive youth development (PYD) approach to develop positive youth development programs by applying PYD constructs. The basic logic of this approach is that with the strengthening of adolescent development, adolescent developmental problems would be reduced.

14.2 Prevention of problem gambling in adolescents

In view of the growth of problem gambling in adolescents, one obvious question is how problem gambling in adolescents can be prevented (7, 8). From the prevention science perspective, two approaches dominate the development of preventive strategies. The first approach adopts the "traditional" conception (9), which includes three levels of dealing with the problem: (a) primary prevention (elimination of the occurrence of problems), (b) secondary prevention (early identification of high-risk groups and early intervention), and (c) tertiary prevention (prevention of further deterioration of the problem). The second approach adopts the "changing" conception (10), which includes three target groups: (a) universal prevention (targeting all adolescents regardless of their risk status), (b) selective prevention (targeting adolescents who have above-average risk of behaviors but with no indication that their participation in risky behaviors is a problem), and (c) indicated prevention (targeting adolescents with noticeable signs and markers of a behavioral problem even if they are not diagnosable). The focus on primary prevention and universal prevention initiatives has been commonly used to prevent adolescents' risky behaviors such as substance abuse.

It is noteworthy that prevention programs regarding problem gambling are underdeveloped. As pointed out by Dickson, Derevensky, and Gupta (4), "despite increased awareness of the need to begin educating young children about the potential dangers of gambling, empirical knowledge of the prevention of adolescent gambling and its translation into science-based prevention initiatives is scarce" (p. 97). They argued that "the field of prevention of youth gambling problems can draw upon the substantial research on adolescent alcohol and substance abuse prevention which has a rich history of research, program development and implementation, and evaluation" (p. 99).

Currently, a majority of intervention programs are developed by applying the risk-factor concept. For example, the common strategy used in adolescents' substance abuse prevention programs is to identify the risk and protective factors in substance abusers in order to minimize the risk factors and maximize the protective factors in young people (2, 11). Use of this strategy in problem gambling prevention is critical because it helps identify the risk factors involved in problem gambling and reduce them while strengthening the protective factors at the same time.

Gupta and Derevensky (12) have done an excellent job in summarizing some of the major risk factors for young people with serious gambling problems, as follows:

1. problem gambling is more popular among males
2. risk-takers have greater risk for problem gambling
3. prevalence rates of adolescents' problem gambling are 2 to 4 times those of adults
4. problem gamblers have relatively lower self-esteem
5. problem gamblers have higher rates of depression
6. dissociation during gambling frequently occurs in problem gambling
7. high risk of suicidal ideation and suicidal attempts exists in problem gamblers
8. loss of quality friendships and relationships are common in problem gamblers, and they have more gambling associates than do the nonproblem gamblers
9. problem gamblers have increased risk for multiple addictions
10. problem gamblers have higher excitability than nonproblem gamblers
11. problem gamblers have poorer general coping skills
12. relative to nonproblem gamblers, problem gamblers display increased delinquency and crime

Another excellent review of risk and protective factors in adolescent problem gambling can be seen in another chapter in this book.

14.2.1 Relevance of problem gambling assessment frameworks to adolescent problem gambling prevention

It is argued that understanding of the risk factors involved in adolescent problem gambling would help to develop adolescent problem gambling prevention programs. A survey of the literature shows that researchers have developed different assessment tools to identify risk factors in problem gambling. The G-MAP developed by Loughnan, Pierce, and Sagris-Desmond (13) is one such example. According to the G-MAP, the common risk factors identified in problem gambling are as follows:

1. **Problematic beliefs about winning** (i.e., faulty cognitive problems): faulty belief in the efficacy of one's cognitive system (control factor), use of intuition and ideas about luck to achieve successful outcomes (prophecy factor), and belief that gambling is a reasonable way to make money (uninformed factor).
2. **Emotional and coping problems**: use of gambling to lift mood (good feelings factor), use of gambling to control stress (relaxation factor), use of gambling to alleviate boredom (boredom factor), and dissociation as well as disconnection from emotional responses when engaging in gambling (numbness).
3. **Problem situations**: using gambling behavior as an "escape" from the perceived demands in life (oasis), and gambling as a result of the desire to be "naughty" or rebellious (mischief factor).
4. **Attitudes to self** (cognitive/psychological problem): belief that others see them as "losers" and wish that gambling can help them to be "winners" (low self-image factor), gambling as a result of the desire to maintain self-image of being a "winner" (winner factor), belief that gambling is a disease or affliction that can only be solved by life-long abstinence (entrenchment), and conscious use of gambling to punish or hurt oneself (harm to self factor).

5. **Social problem**: social factors that may contribute to gambling (systems factor) and use of gambling to satisfy the desire to be around people but minimize the pressure to interact with them (shyness factor).

To help to assess and develop intervention programs in the Chinese context, Shek and Chan (14) translated and validated the G-MAP in Hong Kong. Based on the responses of 8 problem gamblers and 125 pathological gamblers seeking help from a problem gambling treatment center, reliability analyses showed that the G-MAP and its related domains and scales were generally internally consistent. There are also several lines of evidence suggesting that the Chinese G-MAP and the various domains are valid.

As the original G-MAP developed in Australia may not be suitable for people in Asian countries due to cultural differences, Shek, Sun, Lee, and Chan (15) developed the modified Chinese version of the G-MAP (Chinese G-MAP) for the assessment of problem gambling. This modified Chinese G-MAP has 10 domains and 23 scales resembling eight groups of factors related to pathological gambling, as follows:

1. Beliefs about Winning Domain (Cognitive Problems)
    1. Control: belief in the efficacy of one's system in winning money
    2. Prophecy: use of intuition and ideas about luck to achieve successful outcomes
2. Feelings Domain (Emotional Problems)
    1. Boredom: use of gambling to alleviate boredom
    2. Good Feelings: use of gambling to lift one's mood
    3. Numbness: dissociation and disconnection from emotional responses when engaging in gambling
    4. Relaxation: use of gambling to cope with stress
3. Situations Domain (Life Situations Related to Pathological Gambling)
    1. Desperation: gambling as a result of desperation
    2. Rebellion: gambling as a result of the desire to be rebellious
    3. Oasis: use of gambling to reward oneself
    4. Transition: relationship between gambling and transitional events in lives
4. Attitudes to Self Domain (Self-Concept and Psychological Problem)
    1. Low Self-Image: belief that one is a "loser" and wish that gambling can help one to be a "winner"
    2. Winner: gambling as a result of the desire to maintain self-image of being a "winner"
    3. Low Self-Efficacy: belief that one is able to control his/her gambling behavior
5. Social Domain (Social Influences)
    1. Friendship: use of gambling to increase social encounter
    2. Shyness: use of gambling to satisfy the desire to be around by people but minimize the pressure to interact with them
6. Behavior Domain (Behavioral Influences)
    1. Habit: gambling in familiar environment or with familiar people
    2. Leisure: gambling as a hobby or an interest
7. Spirituality Domain (Spiritual Influences)
    1. Lack of Life Goal: belief that gambling and winning money are meaningful in one's life
    2. Self-Worth: gambling as a way to search for one's value
8. Family Domain (Family Influences)

1. Reinforcements: gambling for the sake of one's family
2. Escape: gambling as a way to escape from family problems
9. Attitudes to Financial Management Domain (Attitudinal Influences)
   1. Attitudes to Financial Management: gambling as a way to deal with one's debts
10. Culture Domain (Cultural Influences)
    1. Chinese Beliefs about Gambling: beliefs in the Chinese proverbs about gambling

Shek, Sun, Lee, and Chan (15) reported findings supporting the reliability and validity of the modified Chinese G-MAP. The findings suggest that the Chinese G-MAP and the various domains and scales are internally consistent in both the nonproblem gambling group and the problem gambling group. The findings suggest that the Chinese G-MAP and the various domains and scales are valid: The various G-MAP domain and scale measures were significantly correlated among themselves; the G-MAP measures were significantly correlated with pathological gambling behavior assessed by the DSM-IV; the G-MAP total scale and domain measures were able to discriminate problem gamblers and nonproblem gamblers. Obviously, the modified G-MAP dimensions can be used to develop adolescent prevention programs in the Chinese culture. For example, it would be helpful to train adolescents to deal with Chinese beliefs about gambling. Furthermore, the modified Chinese G-MAP can be used to identify Chinese adolescent problem gamblers who may need early intervention.

14.2.2 An alternative but complementary approach: Positive youth development

Although the prevention science approach focusing on risk and protective factors of high-risk adolescent behaviors has generated much research and produced many prevention programs in the past few decades, it has been criticized as taking a negative view about adolescent development. Based on the belief that adolescents are assets to be developed rather than problems to be solved, an alternative approach to tackle adolescent gambling problem is in order.

Some researchers (16) look on positive youth development (PYD) to accomplish this goal. Damon (17) stated that the field of PYD focuses on adolescents' talents, strengths, interests, and future potentials. This focus is in sharp contrast to prevention science's focus on adolescents' personal disadvantages, disabilities, and behavioral problems, such as learning disabilities and substance abuse. Many researchers and intervention program developers believe that the effort to identify and promote young people's talents and strengths will raise their self-esteem, self-image, and life goals. As a result, PYD constructs should be used to promote development of adolescents.

There are many PYD programs in the West. Catalano, Berglund, Ryan, Lonczak, and Hawkins (18, 19), based on their revision of 77 PYD programs, have concluded that there are 25 successful programs involving 15 identified PYD constructs. These 15 constructs are useful in developing adolescent problem gambling prevention programs. The meaning of these PYD constructs and the rationales for including them in problem gambling prevention programs are explained below.

1. *Promotion of Bonding:* Promotion of bonding means developing strong affective relationships with and commitment to people (healthy adults and positive peers) and

institutions (school, community, and culture). It is believed that strong linkages with healthy adults and significant others are important to prevent problem gambling in adolescents. Researchers found that many adolescent gamblers are negatively impacted by the following situations: (a) many parents and friends of adolescent gamblers are gamblers; (b) perceived family support in adolescent problem gamblers is poor (5); and (c) quality friendships and relationships are lost and replaced by gambling associates among problem gamblers (12). According to family theories, adolescents' developmental problems are regarded as outcomes of their problematic family processes. In a longitudinal study examining the linkage between parental behavioral and psychological control and adolescents' adjustment, Shek (20–22) showed that parental psychological and behavioral control are related to the children's psychological well-being (such as life satisfaction, mastery, life satisfaction, and hopelessness). This construct is intimately linked to adolescents' gambling behavior.

2. *Promotion of Social Competence*: Social competence refers to interpersonal skills (such as communication, assertiveness, conflict resolution, and interpersonal negotiation), ability to build up positive human relationships and provision of opportunities to practice such skills. There are several rationales for developing social competence as a means to prevent problem gambling: (a) the social competence in adolescent gamblers is poor (e.g., outcomes of the G-MAP assessment), (b) many friends and peers of adolescents with gambling problems are gamblers, and (c) there is poorly perceived peer support among adolescent problem gamblers (5).

3. *Promotion of Emotional Competence*: Emotional competence includes awareness of one's own emotions, ability to understand others' emotions, ability to use the vocabulary of emotion, capacity for empathy, ability to differentiate internal subjective emotional-experience from external emotional-expression, capacity to control emotional distress, awareness of emotional messages within relationships, and capacity for emotional management. The justification for including this PYD construct is that there are greater emotional problems (such as depression and suicidal ideation) in adolescent gamblers (3) and in problem gamblers.

4. *Promotion of Cognitive Competence*: Cognitive competence includes cognitive abilities, processes, or outcomes (such as logical thinking, problem solving, and goal setting), and critical thinking (such as making inferences, self-reflection, and coordination of multiple views). The cultivation of cognitive competence as a preventive strategy is important because researchers have found that there are illusions of control and unrealistic perceptions of luck in adolescent problem gamblers (23). The control factor (belief in the efficacy of their system), prophecy factor (use of intuition and ideas about luck to achieve successful outcomes), and uninformed factor (belief that gambling is a reasonable way to make money) in the G-MAP also suggest that cognitive dysfunction is a source of concern in problem gamblers. According to cognitive theories of problem gambling, cognitive dysfunction and irrational thoughts about gambling are basic factors conducive to problem gambling.

5. *Promotion of Behavioral Competence*: This PYD construct includes the ability to use nonverbal and verbal strategies to perform socially acceptable and normative behavior in social interactions and to make effective behavior choices. The basic justification for including this construct in the prevention toolbox is that peer pressure plays an important role in adolescent problem gambling (24). A significant proportion of adolescent gambling activities take place in friends' homes. How to

help adolescents resist negative peer influence has become a central focus in many of the current programs on the prevention of adolescents' high-risk behaviors.

6. *Promotion of Moral Competence*: Moral competence refers to the orientation to perform altruistic behavior, ability to judge moral issues, as well as to promote the development of justice and altruistic behaviors in adolescents. It is argued that the promotion of this PYD construct is important because problem gamblers are unable to judge the negative consequences of pathological gambling. Adolescent problem gamblers have weak moral constraint as reflected by the findings that they usually have a history of delinquency such as stealing money to fund their gambling (2).

7. *Development of Self-Efficacy*: Self-efficacy refers to belief in one's ability to organize and execute the courses of action required to produce given attainments as well as techniques to change negative self-defeating cognitions to positive ones. There are two reasons to support the inclusion of this PYD construct in problem gambling prevention programs. First, problem gamblers may either have very low self-efficacy (so that they wish to attain control via gambling) or overestimate their ability to control the outcomes of gambling. Second, as there is increasing research evidence showing that self-efficacy is negatively related to substance abuse, development of self-efficacy is hypothesized to reduce the likelihood of problem gambling.

8. *Fostering Prosocial Norms*: Prosocial norms are clear and healthy standards, beliefs, and behavior guidelines that promote socially desirable behavior. Prosocial norms often include altruism, solidarity, and volunteerism leading to prosocial behaviors, such as cooperation and sharing. As pointed out by Hardoon, Gupta, and Derevensky (5), adolescent gambling is closely related to delinquency and conduct problems. Because prosocial norms and behaviors can be viewed as incompatible with aggressive or deviant behaviors, it is expected that the promotion of prosocial behaviors (i.e., the PYD construct), will be conducive to the reduction of high-risk behaviors.

9. *Cultivation of Resilience*: Resilience can be conceived as a capacity (the ability of an individual for adapting to changes in a healthy way), a process (a reintegration process for an individual to recover), or a result (positive outcomes after going through stressful events). Cultivation of resilience means fostering adolescents' capacity against unconstructive developmental changes and life stresses in order to "bounce back" from stressful life experience and achieve healthy outcomes. The inclusion of resilience as a PYD construct is important for two reasons. First, research studies have shown that coping behaviors in adolescent gamblers are poor (3) and that problem gambling may occur after negative life events (G-MAP). Second, studies show that resilience is negatively related to adolescent high-risk behaviors.

10. *Cultivation of Self-Determination*: Self-determination refers to an adolescent's ability to set goals and make choices according to his/her own thinking. Regarding skills and strategies that promote self-determination, they include self-awareness of strengths and limitations, goal setting and action planning, problem solving, choice-making, and self-evaluation. There are two justifications for promoting self-determination as a strategy to prevent problem gambling. First, problem gambling represents poor choice-making in adolescent behaviors. Second, as impulsivity is involved in adolescent problem gamblers, cultivation of self-determination is important (24).

11. *Cultivation of Spirituality*: Cultivation of spirituality refers to promotion of the development of beliefs in a higher power or a sense of spiritual identity, meaning, or practice. There are two arguments supporting the use of this PYD construct in the prevention of adolescent problem gambling. First, research shows that purpose in life is negatively related to adolescents' high-risk behavior and positively related to psychological well-being (25). Second, according to the existential theory of Victor Frankl, psychopathological behavior such as problem gambling is a result of an existential vacuum that is created by a lack of meaning in an individual.

12. *Promotion of Beliefs in the Future*: Beliefs in the future refers to hope and optimism, including valued and attainable goals, positive appraisal of one's capability and effort (a sense of confidence), and positive expectancies of the future. As problem gamblers have heightened risk for suicidal ideation and attempts (4), it is assumed that such negative views about the future are antecedents of problem gambling and promotion of beliefs in the future will reduce the likelihood of problem gambling.

13. *Development of a Clear and Positive Identity*: This PYD construct refers to the building of self-esteem and facilitation of exploration and commitments in self-definition. As many studies have shown that the self-esteem of adolescent problem gamblers is lower than that of the control participants (4), it can be argued that promotion of self-esteem in adolescents will prevent the development of problem gambling in adolescents.

14. *Opportunity for Prosocial Involvement*: This PYD construct refers to events and activities that promote adolescents' participation in prosocial behaviors and maintenance of prosocial norms. As prosocial involvement is negatively related to delinquency and psychological problems (26, 27), it can be argued that providing opportunities for prosocial involvement would prevent the development of problem gambling.

15. *Recognition for Positive Behavior*: This construct refers to the development of systems for rewarding or recognizing participants' positive behaviors such as prosocial behaviors or positive changes in behaviors. This PYD construct is important because adolescent problem gamblers may attempt to derive achievement from excessive gambling and many adolescent problem behaviors occur as a result of the lack of proper recognition for their positive behaviors.

14.2.3 The development of positive youth development programs in Hong Kong

The development of positive youth development programs is in its infancy in Hong Kong. To promote the holistic development among adolescents in Hong Kong, The Hong Kong Jockey Club Charities Trust in 2004 approved HK$400 million (note: the official exchange rate between US$ and HK$ is 1:7.8) to launch a project entitled "P.A.T.H.S. to Adulthood: A Jockey Club Youth Enhancement Scheme". "P.A.T.H.S." denotes Positive Adolescent Training through Holistic Social Programmes. The Trust invited academics of five universities in Hong Kong to form a research team to develop a multi-year universal PYD program to promote holistic adolescent development in Hong Kong, with Daniel Shek as the principal investigator and The Hong Kong Polytechnic University as the lead institution. Besides developing the program, the research team also provides training for teachers and social workers who implement the program, and carries out longitudinal evaluation of the project. There are two tiers of programs (Tier 1 and Tier 2) in this project. The Tier 1 Program is a universal PYD program in which students in Secondary 1 to Secondary 3 participate, normally with 20 hours of training in the school year at each grade. Because research findings suggest that roughly one-fifth of adolescents will need help of a deeper nature, the Tier 2 Program will generally be provided for at least one-fifth of the students who have greater psychosocial needs at each grade (i.e., selective program). Because of the overwhelming success of the project, the Trust earmarked another HK$350 million to implement the project for another cycle and to revamp the curriculum.

The overall objective of the Tier 1 Program is to promote holistic development among junior secondary school students in Hong Kong. To achieve this objective, program elements related to PYD constructs are included in the Tier 1 Program (28). These include promotion of bonding, cultivation of resilience, promotion of social competence, promotion of emotional competence, promotion of cognitive competence, promotion of behavioral competence, promotion of moral competence, cultivation of self-determination, promotion of spirituality, development of self-efficacy, development of a clear and positive identity, promotion of beliefs in the future, provision of recognition for positive behavior, provision of opportunities for prosocial involvement, and fostering prosocial norms (28, 29). Both Chinese and English curriculum manuals have been produced with reference to all PYD constructs except the recognition for positive behavior. For recognition for positive behavior, it is argued that it should be implemented as a regular principle inside and outside classrooms. As such, no specific curricula are needed.

For the evaluation of the program, objective outcome evaluation, subjective outcome evaluation, secondary data analyses, process evaluation, interim evaluation, qualitative evaluation based on focus groups, student weekly diaries, and case studies have been used. Based on these strategies, existing research findings generally revealed that different stakeholders have positive perceptions of the program, workers, and benefits of the program, and that the program is effective in promoting holistic PYD among Chinese adolescents in Hong Kong (28–33).

14.3 Discussion

Although the utilization of PYD programs represents a reasonable approach to prevent adolescent problem gambling, there are several issues that should be considered for developing adolescent prevention programs in Hong Kong.

First, it is important to examine the two possible goals of problem gambling prevention programs: abstinence of gambling vs. harm-minimization or harm-reduction of problem gambling (7, 8). With specific reference to the Chinese culture of Hong Kong, parents basically do not tolerate gambling in adolescents. As such, abstinence of gambling is regarded as the legitimate objective of gambling prevention programs. This goal is clearly exemplified by the anti-gambling program initiated by the Hong Kong Education City. On the other hand, gambling prevention programs in the West are commonly designed within the context of harm-reduction or minimization.

The second issue is whether specific gambling prevention programs or generic PYD programs should be designed. Though the former has the advantage of having a specific focus on problem gambling as well as spending less manpower and financial resources, the stigmatizing effect of such programs should not be underestimated. For example, most schools admitting "better" students tend to deny any gambling problems exist among their students. They will not join such prevention programs as a defense mechanism. As "generic" PYD programs targeting the total youth population are non-stigmatizing in nature, school administrators, teachers, and parents will accept these prevention programs more readily. Nevertheless, the basic question that should be asked is whether PYD program should be a panacea to all adolescents with high-risk behaviors.

Third, though it is reasonable to propose that researchers can apply the elements and principles of substance abuse prevention programs to problem gambling prevention programs, one query that should be raised is whether there are any meaningful similarities between substance abuse prevention programs and problem gambling prevention programs. Basically, one has to identify the lowest common multiples of both types of prevention programs. Although there are many common risk factors involved in substance abuse and problem gambling (e.g., sensation seeking and higher predisposition in males), there are some differences involved. For example, though parents generally do not tolerate problem gambling behavior in adolescents, their tolerance for substance abuse in their children is even less.

Fourth, to ensure that problem gambling prevention programs are effective, one should ask what theoretical mechanisms intrinsic to those programs can contribute to the effectiveness of the programs (34). It is noted that the theory of reasoned action, self-concept theories, and cognitive theories have been applied to many existing gambling prevention programs. Hardoon and Derevensky (35) also pointed out that there are different theories of gambling behaviors, including personality, cognitive, learning/behavioral, general addiction, and social learning. With reference to the ecological approach, there can be different personal and environmental risk and protective factors that may contribute to the success of problem gambling prevention programs. Hence, it is important to argue for the use of theoretical mechanisms in problem gambling prevention programs because these theories will serve as the backbone in designing the programs.

The fifth issue concerns the universality of problem gambling prevention programs. A survey of the literature shows that most of the existing gambling prevention programs are designed in Western countries. If one assumes that knowledge transcends culture and prevention theories are universally applicable, one can simply translate the English version of such programs and apply them in different cultures. Nevertheless, as the meaning of gambling is different under different cultures, there are researchers arguing for the design of indigenous gambling prevention programs utilizing the "emic" approach rather than the "etic" approach.

Sixth, although it is conceptually desirable to have problem gambling prevention programs, whether such programs are really effective in reducing problem gambling behavior in adolescents is an empirical question to be considered. Evaluation of the effectiveness of the gambling prevention program is an important issue yet to be addressed. Unfortunately, program evaluation is not a simple and straightforward task and there are many types and approaches of evaluation (36). In his discussion of the major strategies of evaluation, Patton (37) outlined three basic types of evaluation: quantitative evaluation, qualitative evaluation, and utilization-focused evaluation. Ginsberg (38) summarized the major forms of evaluation, including quantitative and qualitative approaches, cost-benefit analyses, satisfaction studies, needs assessment, single-subjects designs, experimental approaches and models, utilization focused evaluation, empowerment evaluations, fraud and abuse detection, client satisfaction and journalistic evaluation. Using starting alphabets as the bases of classification, Patton (37) suggested that there are more than 100 types of evaluation. Because of the complexity of the nature of evaluation and the different paradigms involved, researchers are confronted with the task of developing appropriate evaluation approaches and strategies in the field of gambling prevention. Ideally speaking, different evaluation strategies should be used to examine program effectiveness (39–41).

Finally, it would be exciting if the key elements of prevention approach and positive youth development approach can be integrated. According to Catalano et al. (18), there are several attributes of the prevention science perspective. These include (a) identification of risk and protective factors, (b) adoption of a developmental perspective, (c) assertion that problem behaviors share many common antecedents, and (d) assertion that risk and protective factors change youth outcomes. Characteristics associated with the positive youth development approach were also identified, as (a) emphasis on integrated youth development (i.e., focusing on a range of youth developmental possibilities and problems) rather than dealing with a single youth problem; (b) upholding of the belief that "problem-free is not fully prepared"; (c) emphasis of person-in-environment perspective; and (d) focus on developmental models on how young people grow, learn, and change. In their discussion of the positive youth development approach, Catalano et al. (19) noted that the attributes of positive youth development and characteristics of the prevention science approach are compatible, and that both approaches could be cooperative rather than competitive. It will be theoretically and practically interesting to see how we can design an integrated program for Chinese adolescents based on the dimensions of G-MAP and the PYD constructs.

In summary, with the growing severity of adolescent problem gambling, prevention of such problem is an urgent issue that should be addressed by researchers, professional workers, prevention program developers, and policymakers (42). It is argued that the utilization of the G-MAP findings as well as the application of PYD constructs is a promising approach for the problem gambling prevention field in the West as well as in Hong Kong.

Acknowledgements

The preparation of this work was financially supported by The Hong Kong Jockey Club Charities Trust.

References

1. Shaffer HJ, Hall MN. Estimating prevalence of adolescent gambling disorders: A quantitative synthesis and guide toward standard gambling nomenclature. J Gambl Stud 1996;12:193–214.
2. Griffiths M, Wood RTA. Risk factors in adolescence: The case of gambling, videogame playing, and the Internet. J Gambl Stud 2000;16:199–225.

3. Gupta R, Derevensky JL. An examination of the differential coping style of adolescents with gambling problems. Montreal, Quebec: Int Centre Youth Gambl Problems High-Risk Behav; 2001.
4. Dickson LM, Derevensky JL, Gupta R. The prevention of gambling problems in youth: A conceptual framework. J Gambl Stud 2002;18:97–159.
5. Hardoon KK, Gupta R, Derevensky JL. Psychosocial variables associated with adolescent gambling. Psychol Addict Behav 2004;18:170–79.
6. Chinese Young Men Christian Association of Hong Kong. A research report on adolescent gambling in Hong Kong. Hong Kong: Chinese Young Men Christian Assoc Hong Kong; 2004.
7. Dickson LM, Derevensky JL, Gupta R. Harm reduction for the prevention of youth gambling problems: Lessons learned from adolescent high-risk behavior prevention programs. J Adolesc Res 2004;19:233–63.
8. Dickson L, Derevensky JL, Gupta R. Youth gambling problems: A harm reduction prevention model. Addict Res Theory 2004;12:305–16.
9. Caplan G. Principles of preventive psychiatry. New York: Basic; 1964.
10. Levine M, Perkins DV, eds. Principles of community psychology: Perspectives and applications. New York: Oxford Univ Press; 1997.
11. Elias MJ, Gager P, Leon S. Spreading a warm blanket of prevention over all children: Guidelines for selecting substance abuse and related prevention curricula for use in the schools. J Prim Prev 1997;18:41–69.
12. Gupta R, Derevensky JL. Adolescents with gambling problems: From research to treatment. J Gambl Stud 2000;16:315–42.
13. Loughnan T, Pierce M, Sagris-Desmond A. Maroondah Assessment Profile for Problem Gambling: Administrator's Manual. Melbourne: Aust Council Educ Res; 1999.
14. Shek DTL, Chan EML. Assessment of problem gambling in a Chinese context: The Chinese G-MAP. ScientificWorldJournal 2009;9:548–56.
15. Shek DTL, Sun RCF, Lee JJ, Chan EML. Development and validation of an indigenous Chinese measure of problem gambling. Hong Kong: Even Centre, Tung Wah Group Hospitals, Dept Appl Soc Sci, Hong Kong Polytech Univ; 2009.
16. Benson PL, Saito RN. The scientific foundation of youth development. Youth Development: Issues, Challenges, and Directions 2000;125–48. http://www.ppv.org/indexfiles/yd-index.html. Accessed November 17, 2004.
17. Damon W. What is positive youth development? Ann Am Acad of Polit Soc Sci 2004;591:13–24.
18. Catalano RF, Berglund ML, Ryan JAM, Lonczak HS, Hawkins JD. Positive youth development in the United States: Research findings on evaluations of positive youth development programs. Prev Treatment 5, Article 15. 2002 Jun 22. http://www.journals.apa.org/prevention/volume5/pre0050015a.html. Accessed November 17, 2004.
19. Catalano RF, Berglund ML, Ryan JAM, Lonczak HS, Hawkins JD. Positive youth development in the United States: Research findings on evaluations of positive youth development programs. Ann Am Acad of Polit Soc Sci 2004;591:98–124.
20. Shek DTL. Perceived parental control and parent-child relational qualities in Chinese Adolescents in Hong Kong. Sex Roles 2005;53(9–10):635–46.
21. Shek DTL. Conceptual framework underlying the development of a positive youth development program in Hong Kong. Int J Adoles Med Health 2006;18(3):303–14.
22. Shek DTL. Perceived parental behavioral control and psychological control in Chinese adolescents in Hong Kong. Am J Fam Ther 2006;34(2):163–76.
23. Gupta R, Derevensky JL. Adolescent gambling behavior: A prevalence study and examination of the correlates associated with problem gambling. J Gamb Stud 1998;14:319–45.
24. Langhinrichsen-Rohling J, Rohde P, Seeley JR, Rohling ML. Individual, family, peer correlates of adolescent gambling. J Gambl Stud 2004;20:23–46.
25. Shek DTL. Meaning in life and psychological well-being: An empirical study using the Chinese version of the Purpose in Life Questionnaire. J Genet Psychol 1992;153:185–200.

26. Ma HK, Shek DTL, Cheung PC. The relation of social influences and social relationships to prosocial and antisocial behavior in Hong Kong Chinese adolescents. In: Shohov SP, ed. Advances in psychology research. New York: Nova Science; 2002:177–201.

27. Shek DTL, Ma HK, Cheung PC. A longitudinal study of adolescent antisocial and prosocial behavior. Psychologia 2000;43:229–42.

28. Shek DTL, Ma HK, Sun RCF. Interim evaluation of the Tier 1 Program (Secondary 1 Curriculum) of the Project P.A.T.H.S.: First year of the Full Implementation Phase. ScientificWorldJournal 2008;8:47–60.

29. Shek DTL, Sun RCF, Siu AMH. Interim evaluation of the Secondary 2 Program of Project P.A.T.H.S.: Insights based on the Experimental Implementation Phase. ScientificWorldJournal 2008;8:61–72.

30. Shek DTL. Evaluation of Project P.A.T.H.S. in Hong Kong: Triangulation of findings based on different evaluation strategies. ScientificWorldJournal 2008;8:1–3.

31. Shek DTL, Siu AMH, Lee TY, Cheung CK, Chung R. Effectiveness of the Tier 1 Program of Project P.A.T.H.S.: Objective outcome evaluation based on a randomized group trial. ScientificWorldJournal 2008;8:4–12.

32. Shek DTL, Sun RCF, Lam CM, Lung DWM, Lo SC. Evaluation of Project P.A.T.H.S. in Hong Kong: Utilization of student weekly dairy. ScientificWorldJournal 2008;8:13–21.

33. Shek DTL, Ma HK. Design of a positive youth development program in Hong Kong. Int J Adolesc Med Health 2006;18(3):315–27.

34. Evans RI. Some theoretical models and constructs generic to substance abuse prevention programs for adolescents: Possible relevance and limitations for problem gambling. J Gambl Stud 2003;19:287–302.

35. Hardoon KK, Derevensky JL. Child and adolescent gambling behavior: Current knowledge. Clin Child Psychol Psychiatry 2002;2:263–81.

36. Chelimsky E, Shadish WR. Evaluation for the 21st century: A handbook. Thousand Oaks, Calif.: Sage; 1997.

37. Patton MQ. Utilization-focused evaluation: The new century text. Thousand Oaks, CA: Sage; 1997.

38. Ginsberg LH. Social work evaluation: Principles and methods. Boston: Allyn and Bacon; 2001.

39. Shek DTL, Sun RCF. Effectiveness of the Tier 1 Program of Project P.A.T.H.S.: Findings based on three years of program implementation. ScientificWorldJournal 2010;10:1509–19.

40. Shek DTL, Ma CMS, Sun RCF. Evaluation of a positive youth development program for adolescents with greater psychosocial needs: Integrated views of program implementers. ScientificWorldJournal 2010;10:1890–1900.

41. Shek DTL, Ma CMS. Longitudinal data analyses using linear mixed models in SPSS: Concepts, procedures, and illustrations. ScientificWorldJournal 2011;11:42–76.

42. Derevensky JL, Shek DTL, Merrick J. Adolescent gambling. Int J Adolesc Med Health 2010;22:1–2.

Acknowledgements

15 About the editors

Jeffrey L. Derevensky, PhD, is Professor and Director of Clinical Training in the School of Applied Child Psychology, Department of Educational and Counselling Psychology and Professor, Department of Psychiatry at McGill University, Canada. He is a clinical consultant to numerous hospitals, school boards, government agencies, and corporations. At McGill, he has developed a comprehensive research program investigating many facets of youth gambling, is actively involved in treating youth with severe gambling problems, helps coordinate multiple prevention initiatives, and is the Co-Director of the McGill University Youth Gambling Research and Treatment Clinic and the International Centre for Youth Gambling Problems and High-Risk Behaviors. He is on the editorial board of several journals, is a member of multiple international scientific committees, and has been the recipient of numerous research and training grants. Much of his work has focused on furthering our understanding of youth gambling problems and high-risk behaviors. He has provided expert testimony before international governmental commissions, and has over 200 published refereed journal articles, book chapters, and research reports. He was the recipient of the Connecticut Council on Problem Gambling Award for his "International leadership in addressing youth problem gambling through research, training and advocacy" and the International Centre for Youth Gambling Problems and High-Risk Behaviors was the recipient of the U.S. National Council on Problem Gambling Outstanding Program Award.

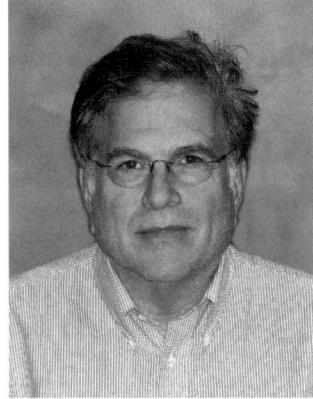

Professor Daniel T. L. Shek, PhD, FHKPS, BBS, JP, is Chair Professor of Applied Social Sciences, Department of Applied Social Sciences, The Hong Kong Polytechnic University, Hunghom, Hong Kong, PRC, Advisory Professor of East China Normal University, Honorary Professor of Kiang Wu Nursing College of Macau, PRC and Adjunct Professor, University of Kentucky College of Medicine, Lexington, United States. He is Chief Editor of *Journal of Youth Studies*, past Consulting Editor of *Journal of Clinical Psychology*, past international consultant of *American Journal of Family Therapy*, and editorial board member of *Social Indicators Research, International Journal of Adolescent Medicine and*

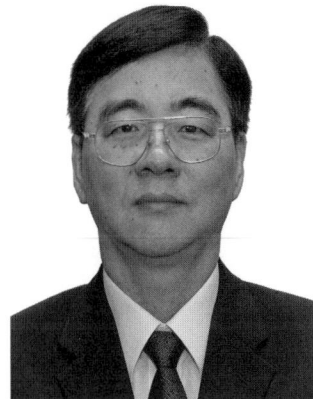

Health, The Scientific World Journal (Child Health and Human Development and Holistic Health and Medicine domains*), Asian Journal of Counseling, International Journal on Disability and Human Development,* and *Bentham Open Family Studies Journal.* He has served on many government advisory bodies, including the Action Committee against Narcotics, Commission on Youth, Fight Crime Committee, and Family Council. He has published numerous books, book chapters, and more than 300 scientific articles in international refereed journals.

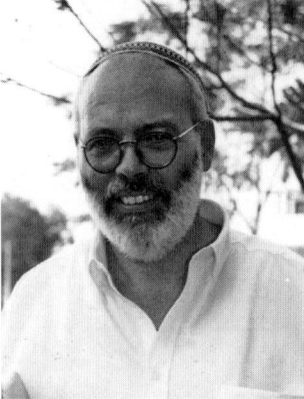

Joav Merrick, MD, MMedSci, DMSc, is professor of pediatrics, child health and human development affiliated with Kentucky Children's Hospital, University of Kentucky, Lexington, United States and the Division of Pediatrics, Hadassah Hebrew University Medical Centers, Jerusalem, Israel, the medical director of the Health Service, Division for Intellectual and Developmental Disabilities, Ministry of Social Affairs, Jerusalem, the founder and director of the National Institute of Child Health and Human Development in Israel. His credits include numerous publications in the field of pediatrics, child health and human development, rehabilitation, intellectual disability, disability, health, welfare, abuse, advocacy, quality of life, and prevention. He received the Peter Sabroe Child Award for outstanding work on behalf of Danish children in 1985 and the International LEGO-Prize ("The Children's Nobel Prize") for an extraordinary contribution toward improvement in child welfare and well-being in 1987.

16 The International Centre for Youth Gambling Problems and High-Risk Behaviors (Centre International d'étude sur le jeu et les comportements à risque chez les jeunes)

Jeffrey L. Derevensky and Rina Gupta

16.1 Background

There remains indisputable evidence that a relatively large percentage of children and adolescents are engaging in gambling activities in spite of legal and to some extent parental restrictions. Prevalence studies conducted over the past decade suggest that gambling has become particularly attractive to today's youth (see the review by Volberg et al. in Chapter 2). Volberg and her colleagues' review, summarizing studies in the United States, Canada, Europe, Nordic countries, Australia, and New Zealand, confirms high prevalence rates of gambling among youth. They concluded that although adolescent and young adult gambling is widespread, there remains significant variability in both prevalence of gambling and the incidence of problem and pathological gambling among adolescents. Much of this discrepancy is likely a result of methodological and sampling differences, availability of gambling venues and opportunities, and cultural, gender, and age differences. Issues such as instrumentation, method of data collection (i.e., classroom data collection, telephone sampling, data collected via Internet surveys), sampling procedures (i.e., sampling size, gender distribution), age differences (e.g., the required legal age in order to gamble varies considerably between jurisdictions), and ease of accessibility all impact the prevalence rates.

Independent of this variability, there is little doubt that gambling remains a highly popular activity among adolescents and that the prevalence rates for problem and pathological gambling typically exceed those found for adults. The conclusions of the earlier National Research Council (NRC) (1) review of adolescent studies were that the estimates of youth gambling ranged from 52 to 89%, with the median estimate being 73%. Their conclusion was that "most adolescents not only gamble, but also have gambled fairly recently." Recognizing differences in methodologies used, the results of the NRC task force concluded that in the 1990s, nine out of ten studies reported problem gambling among adolescents to be 20% (median), with serious past year gambling problems to be 6.1% (median). Volberg and her colleagues and Stinchfield in this volume all highlight some of the methodological issues and concerns associated with assessing adolescent prevalence rates of pathological gamblers. Nevertheless, there is ample evidence to suggest that youth gambling is a common activity and that rates of problem gambling among adolescents, as currently measured, exceed those of adults.

An emerging concern is the recent explosion of Internet and mobile gambling and its impact on young people (see the chapter by Griffiths and Parke). Volberg and her colleagues and Griffiths and Parke suggest strong links between online gambling, role-playing games, and "gambling" on Internet gambling free/practice sites. Adolescents and young adults appear to be migrating between free sites and actual gambling sites. In spite of our growing body of knowledge in the area, there remains much to do to better understand the risk factors and determinants placing certain youth at risk for developing a gambling problem (2).

Problematic gambling among adolescents is part of a larger problem centered on youth risky behaviors (3). Adolescent gambling has been repeatedly shown to be related to other substance use, and precedes engaging in any other potentially addictive behaviors (e.g. smoking, alcohol, and drug consumption). Adolescents with gambling problems have been shown to experience increased delinquency, antisocial behavior, criminal activity, and the disruption of relationships that negatively affect overall school performance and work activities. These behaviors lead to serious psychosocial and economic costs to the individual, his/her family, and society (4).

Derevensky (2), in summarizing the existing research, concluded that despite some conflicting findings there appears to be an overall consensus that (a) gambling is more popular among males than females, (b) probable pathological gamblers are greater risk takers, (c) adolescent prevalence rates of pathological gambling are 2 to 4 times that of adults, (d) adolescent problem/pathological gamblers have lower self-esteem, (e) adolescent problem gamblers have higher rates of depression, (f) youth problem gamblers dissociate more frequently when gambling, and (g) adolescents remain at increased risk for the development of an addiction or multiple addictions. Still further, personality correlates reveal specific at-risk traits, with adolescent pathological gamblers higher on excitability, extroversion, and anxiety, and lower on conformity and self-discipline. These personality traits have also been found to be positively correlated with risk-taking behaviors in general (5). Age of onset has also been shown to be a risk factor, with pathological gamblers reporting starting serious gambling at early ages, usually around the age of 10 or 11 (4). Still further, results indicate that children start gambling with family members, especially parents and grandparents. In fact, of those children reporting gambling, 81% report gambling with family members (6). Contrary to involvement with alcohol, drug, and cigarette use, most children do not feel the need to hide their gambling behavior from their families. An early "big win" has also been reported to be a contributing factor underlying problem gambling behavior. It should be noted that an early big win for an adolescent may be considerably more reinforcing than for an adult.

16.2 The context for the development of the International Centre for Youth Gambling Problems and High-Risk Behaviors

The concern among educators, clinicians, treatment providers, and the industry with respect to underage gambling has continuously grown in recent years. Spurred by the 1995 North American Think Tank on Youth Gambling Issues held at Harvard University, a Think Tank held in 2001 at McGill University (the second Think Tank was a collaborative effort between Harvard Medical School and McGill University), the attention given to problem gambling by the National Research Council (Washington, DC), the National Gaming Impact Commission (Washington, DC), local legislative concerns (Commission des Finances Publiques-Consultations sur le project de loi no. 84), government commissions throughout the world (e.g., British Gambling Commission, Australian Productivity

Commission), and the importance placed on restricting youth from specific gambling activities by regulators, considerable research attention began to focus on underage gambling.

Since 1992, Drs. Derevensky and Gupta and their graduate students at McGill University have been attempting to identify and understand the underlying determinants and critical factors related to youth gambling problems. With research support and funding from multiple governmental, industry, and foundation grants, their on-going research efforts have been crucial in helping to identify the determinants placing youth at-risk for gambling problems, and in the development of effective treatment strategies and prevention programs.

The McGill Youth Gambling Research and Treatment Clinic and the International Centre for Youth Gambling Problems and High-Risk Behaviors have served as focal points for research, treatment of youth with gambling-related problems, and outreach and training programs for graduate students, clinicians, and researchers. Collaborative work with national and international researchers has significantly advanced understanding of youth problem gambling behavior, and this book is a testament to our current knowledge. Nevertheless, the changing landscape of gambling continues to evolve, with new technological forms of gambling (e.g., Internet and mobile wagering) revolutionizing the industry and bringing easier accessibility to youth.

The change in perception of gambling from an association with a host of negative associations to a socially acceptable form of entertainment (e.g., "gaming") has had an impact not only on adults but adolescents as well. This changing environmental framework, along with the normalization of gambling (movement away from sin and vice to gaming as a form of entertainment) has presented new challenges. The McGill Youth Gambling Research and Treatment Clinic and the International Centre for Youth Gambling Problems and High-Risk Behaviors have served as central points for the dissemination of information within Quebec, Canada, and internationally. Of critical importance has been their role in impacting public health and social policy. Drs. Derevensky and Gupta, the co-directors of the Centre, have provided expert testimony before government commissions, legislative committees, and regulators in the United States, Canada, South America, Europe, Southeast Asia, and Australasia. They have worked as research consultants for numerous public and private commissions, foundations, and governmental agencies in an effort to reduce and minimize the harms associated with excessive, problematic gambling.

16.3 An international center

We have witnessed unprecedented growth worldwide in the expansion of gambling opportunities and venues. The need for basic and applied research meeting the highest scientific standards, and the development of scientifically validated youth prevention programs, treatment programs, training, and governmental consultations has never been greater. McGill's International Centre has become the central focal point for our continued efforts to help understand, inform, and prevent youth gambling problems.

The Centre is housed on McGill University's main campus in Montréal, Canada, and has maintained a prominent presence in the development and coordination of a number of national and international research projects. The Centre works in close collaboration with other international research centers and researchers. Collaborative research, training, and policy development is realized through specific projects, interchange of staff, seminars, and jointly sponsored conferences with other institutions of higher learning and research centers. The Centre augments the training of applied child psychologists, clinical psychologists, social workers, psychiatrists, prevention specialists, and educators through its collaborative memberships. It remains instrumental in the articulation and development of responsible social policies related to youth gambling and risk-taking.

The International Centre for Youth Gambling Problems and High-Risk Behaviors mandate can be best understood in the areas of research, training and service, treatment, prevention and public awareness, the dissemination of information, and policy development.

16.4 Research

The primary role for the Centre is the advancement of knowledge concerning youth gambling and risk-taking behaviors through the development of empirically based basic and applied research. Though the field of youth gambling and our knowledge in this area is increasing, there still remains much work needed to further our understanding of youth problem gambling. Members of the Centre, along with our international collaborators, have been actively engaged in multiple funded and non-funded research projects directly addressing youth gambling problems and co-occurring disorders. This research has been published in peer-reviewed scientific journals, multiple book chapters, several books, presented at national and international conferences, and has been instrumental in the development of effective prevention programs (see the Centre's Web site for publications and prevention initiatives – www.youthgambling.com).

The Centre continues to provide an ideal forum for enhanced collaborative efforts and has incorporated a psychological, psychiatric, biological, neurological, sociological, social policy, and socioeconomic program of research. The Centre and its members have fostered the development and coordination of a national and international research agenda addressing youth gambling issues.

16.5 Training and service

A significant effort has been made to help build research capacity in the field. This includes the training of post-doctoral, doctoral, and master's level graduate students from McGill University. A seminar series concerning research and clinical issues dealing with youth risk-taking has been ongoing, with some sessions incorporating visiting faculty. The Centre is frequently visited by international faculty, graduate students, clinicians, and prevention specialists, as well as legislators and members of the industry. Members of the Centre frequently provide lectures in courses, teach in graduate training programs, provide research expertise for funding and governmental agencies, and engage in Grand Rounds and hold staff positions at various teaching hospitals.

Workshops aimed at enhancing knowledge and awareness of youth gambling issues have been held for teachers, clinicians, treatment providers, community agencies, and parents. As well, the Centre provides expert knowledge for media consultations, has hosted a number of symposia, conferences and international visitors, and has provided expert testimony for legislative committees in multiple countries.

16.6 Treatment

For the past 15 years the Centre has provided therapeutic services for youth problem gamblers and their families. This is deemed an essential component within the Centre's mandate and has been instrumental in the development of innovative treatment modalities. The Centre offers expertise in the evaluation of effective treatment models aimed at establishing *best practices* (additional details about the Centre's treatment philosophy are found in this book).

16.7 Prevention and public awareness

The Centre remains actively engaged in the development of empirically based prevention programs and coordination of prevention efforts on an international level. Whether using school-based products such as the Centre's award-winning CD-Rom interactive games (*The Amazing Chateau* or *Hooked City*), a docudrama entitled *Clean Break*, workshop-based PowerPoint presentations (*Youth Gambling: An Awareness and Prevention Workshop, Levels I & II*), a paper-pencil curriculum program entitled *Count Me Out*, or a group game, *Know Limits*, these innovative prevention initiatives have been translated into several languages and are currently being used worldwide. As well, the Centre has developed two public service announcements (Teen Poker, Teen Internet Gambling) targeting parents, and most recently developed a set of multimedia Tool Kits for physicians and medical professionals (*Youth Gambling Problems: Practical Information for Health Professionals*) and attorneys/judges (*Youth Gambling Problems: Practical Information for Professionals in the Criminal Justice System*). Additional programs include an annual holiday media campaign in collaboration with the U.S. National Council on Problem Gambling and lottery corporations in Canada, United States, Mexico, Austria, Portugal, and Sweden urging parents not to purchase lottery tickets for underage minors as holiday gifts. All prevention activities and examples of the prevention materials can be found at www.youthgambling.com. Other awareness activities include holding poster contests and multimedia projects for youth in high school.

The Centre is playing a prominent role in a national and international effort toward developing responsible social policy guidelines. This also includes guidelines for advertising and prevention efforts.

16.8 Information dissemination

The Centre maintains an online database and central depository of research articles concerning youth gambling, co-occurring addictive disorders, and youth risk-taking behaviors through its Web site. The Centre also provides spokespersons and experts for

meetings and conference presentations and publishes a free, quarterly online newsletter, *Youth Gambling International (YGI),* which has a wide international distribution
network.

16.9 Policy development

The Centre's staff provides valuable information and is influential in the development
and articulation of responsible social policy recommendations, funding advice at a
policy and research level, and law enforcement recommendations. The Centre has
worked with the World Health Organization in trying to develop a global response to
the issues of gambling problems.

The Centre has become an attractive site where visiting academics, graduate students,
industry representatives, and social policy experts spend time. Seminars, workshops,
and research projects take advantage of visiting expertise. Emphasis continues on the
multidisciplinary nature and complexity associated with youth risk-taking behaviors.

Finally, the Centre's staff has provided expert testimony before legislators and legislative hearings in Canada, United States, Europe, Norway, Australia, New Zealand, and
South Korea in an effort to develop responsible gambling policies.

Our knowledge of youth gambling has significantly increased during the past 15 years
yet new challenges continue to emerge. The gambling industry is not static and has
quickly adapted to technological advances and changing governmental perspectives.
As the worldwide recession escalated, so too has government's desire to provide additional gambling opportunities to help increase revenues. More and more governments
around the world have relied on the expansion of gambling venues and opportunities
to increase needed revenues. This new availability and accessibility for both adults and
youth remains potentially problematic and will represent new challenges in helping
formulate responsible gambling practices. Our knowledge in this field is just beginning
and the need for responsible public policies remains strong. The Centre continues to
play an important role in meeting these objectives.

References

1. National Research Council. Pathological gambling: A critical review. Washington, DC: National Academy Press; 1999.
2. Derevensky J. Gambling behaviors and adolescent substance use disorders. In: Kaminer Y,
Buckstein OG, eds. Adolescent substance abuse: Psychiatric comorbidity and high risk behaviors. New York: Haworth Press; 2008:403–33.
3. Dickson L, Derevensky J, Gupta, R. Youth gambling problems: A harm reduction prevention
model. Addict Res Theory 2004;12(4):305–16.
4. Gupta R, Derevensky J. Adolescent gambling behavior: A prevalence study and examination of
the correlates associated with excessive gambling. J Gambl Stud 1998;14:319–45.
5. Gupta R, Derevensky J, Ellenbogen S. Personality characteristics and risk-taking tendencies
among adolescent gamblers. Can J Behav Sci 2006;38(2):201–13.
6. Gupta, R, Derevensky, J. Familial and social influences on juvenile gambling behavior.
J Gambl Stud 1997;13(3):179–92.

17 About the Department of Applied Social Sciences, The Hong Kong Polytechnic University

The Department of Applied Social Sciences (APSS) of The Hong Kong Polytechnic University is one of the largest and most vibrant centers in the region dedicated to the education and training of professional social workers, social policy and welfare administrators, psychologists, and counselors in Hong Kong.

The Department started as the Institute of Social Work Training in 1973. It joined the Hong Kong Polytechnic in 1977 and became its School of Social Work. The School was eventually renamed the Department of Applied Social Sciences. APSS celebrated its 35th anniversary in the academic year of 2007/08. Currently there are 93 full-time academics, over 80 research/project staff, 20 fieldwork supervisors, and 34 colleagues in other categories, including administrative and supporting personnel.

The Department has six thriving research centers: Centre for Social Policy Studies, China Research and Development Network, Network for Health and Welfare Studies, Professional Practice and Assessment Centre, Centre for Third Sector Studies, and the Manulife Centre for Children with Specific Learning Disabilities, providing platforms for collaborative research and practice projects with government departments and NGOs.

The Department of Applied Social Sciences offers taught programs in the fields of social work, social policy and administration, counseling, and applied psychology, as well as research degrees at MPhil and PhD levels. In 2008/09, APSS offered some 20 programs for higher diploma, degree, postgraduate, MPhil and PhD students. There are currently about 1,500 students enrolled in the various APSS programs and we have graduated more than 14,000 students over the years.

In the past decade, the Department has successfully expanded into the Chinese mainland. The Department currently offers a MSW(China) Program in collaboration with Peking University and a Joint PolyU-PekingU Social Work Research Centre has been established to foster research in Social Work and Social Policy.

Contact:

Professor Daniel T. L. Shek, PhD, FHKPS, BBS, JP
Chair Professor of Applied Social Sciences
Department of Applied Social Sciences
The Hong Kong Polytechnic University
Hunghom, Hong Kong
E-mail: daniel.shek@polyu.edu.hk

18 About the National Institute of Child Health and Human Development in Israel

The National Institute of Child Health and Human Development (NICHD) in Israel was established in 1998 as a virtual institute under the auspices of the Medical Director, Ministry of Social Affairs and Social Services, in order to function as the research arm for the Office of the Medical Director. In 1998 the National Council for Child Health and Pediatrics, Ministry of Health, and in 1999 the Director General and Deputy Director General of the Ministry of Health endorsed the establishment of the NICHD that since 2011 is affiliated with the Division of Pediatrics, Hadassah Hebrew University Medical Centers, Jerusalem, Israel.

18.1 Mission

The mission of a National Institute for Child Health and Human Development in Israel is to provide an academic focal point for the scholarly interdisciplinary study of child life, health, public health, welfare, disability, rehabilitation, intellectual disability, and related aspects of human development. This mission includes research, teaching, clinical work, information, and public service activities in the field of child health and human development.

18.2 Service and academic activities

Over the years many activities became focused in the south of Israel due to collaboration with various professionals at the Faculty of Health Sciences (FOHS) at the Ben Gurion University of the Negev (BGU). Since 2000 an affiliation with the Zusman Child Development Center at the Pediatric Division of Soroka University Medical Center has resulted in collaboration around the establishment of the Down Syndrome Clinic at that center. In 2002 a full course on "Disability" was established at the Recanati School for Allied Professions in the Community, FOHS, BGU, and in 2005 collaboration was started with the Primary Care Unit of the faculty and disability became part of the master of public health course on "Children and society." In the academic year 2005–2006 a one-semester course on "Aging with disability" was started as part of the master of science program in gerontology in our collaboration with the Center for Multidisciplinary Research in Aging. In 2010 collaborations began with the Division of Pediatrics, Hadassah Hebrew University Medical Centers, Jerusalem, Israel.

18.3 Research activities

The affiliated staff have over the years published work from projects and research activities in this national and international collaboration. The International Journal of

Adolescent Medicine and Health (in 2000), the International Journal on Disability and Human Development of De Gruyter Publishing House (in 2005, Berlin and New York), the TSW-Child Health and Human Development and the TSW-Holistic Health and Medicine of the Scientific World Journal (in 2006, New York and Kirkkonummi, Finland), all peer-reviewed international journals, were affiliated with the National Institute of Child Health and Human Development. In 2008 the International Journal of Child Health and Human Development (Nova Science, New York), the International Journal of Child and Adolescent Health (Nova Science), and the Journal of Pain Management (Nova Science) affiliated, and the International Public Health Journal (Nova Science) and Journal of Alternative Medicine Research (Nova Science) joined in 2009.

18.4 National collaborations

Nationally the NICHD works in collaboration with the Faculty of Health Sciences, Ben Gurion University of the Negev; Department of Physical Therapy, Sackler School of Medicine, Tel Aviv University; Autism Center, Assaf HaRofeh Medical Center; National Rett and PKU Centers at Chaim Sheba Medical Center, Tel HaShomer; Department of Physiotherapy, Haifa University; Department of Education, Bar Ilan University, Ramat Gan, Faculty of Social Sciences and Health Sciences; College of Judea and Samaria in Ariel, and recent collaborations have been established with the Center for Pediatric Chronic Diseases, Division of Pediatrics, Hadassah Hebrew University Medical Centers, Mt Scopus Campus in Jerusalem.

18.5 International collaborations

International affiliations include with the Department of Disability and Human Development, College of Applied Health Sciences, University of Illinois at Chicago; Strong Center for Developmental Disabilities, Golisano Children's Hospital at Strong, University of Rochester School of Medicine and Dentistry, New York; Centre on Intellectual Disabilities, University of Albany, New York; Centre for Chronic Disease Prevention and Control, Health Canada, Ottawa; Chandler Medical Center and Children's Hospital, Kentucky Children's Hospital, Section of Adolescent Medicine, University of Kentucky, Lexington; Chronic Disease Prevention and Control Research Center, Baylor College of Medicine, Houston, Texas; Division of Neuroscience, Department of Psychiatry, Columbia University, New York; Institute for the Study of Disadvantage and Disability, Atlanta; Center for Autism and Related Disorders, Department Psychiatry, Children's Hospital Boston, Boston; Department of Paediatrics, Child Health and Adolescent Medicine, Children's Hospital at Westmead, Westmead, Australia; International Centre for the Study of Occupational and Mental Health, Düsseldorf, Germany; Centre for Advanced Studies in Nursing, Department of General Practice and Primary Care, University of Aberdeen, Aberdeen, United Kingdom; Quality of Life Research Center, Copenhagen, Denmark; Nordic School of Public Health, Gottenburg, Sweden; Scandinavian Institute of Quality of Working Life, Oslo, Norway; Centre for Quality of Life of the Hong Kong Institute of Asia-Pacific Studies and School of Social Work, Chinese University, Hong Kong.

18.6 Targets

Our focus is on research, international collaborations, clinical work, teaching, and policy in health, disability, and human development and establishment of the NICHD as a permanent institute at one of the residential care centers for persons with intellectual disability in Israel in order to conduct model research and together with the four university schools of public health/medicine in Israel establish a national master and doctoral program in disability and human development at the institute to secure the next generation of professionals working in this often nonprestigious/low-status field of work.

Contact:

Joav Merrick, MD, DMSc
Professor of Pediatrics, Child Health and Human Development
Medical Director, Health Services, Division for Intellectual and Developmental Disabilities,
    Ministry of Social Affairs and Social Services,
    POB 1260, IL-91012 Jerusalem, Israel.
E-mail: jmerrick@inter.net.il

Index

abstinence from gambling 170–4, 216–18, 221, 239–40
academic achievement of gamblers 65–6
accessibility of gambling opportunities 10, 69
Addiction Foundation of Manitoba 35
addictions, general theory of 11–12, 61, 64
Adolescent Risk Communication Institute 33
advertisements for gambling 10, 70
African Americans 33
age of onset of gambling activity 7–8, 100, 217
age restrictions on gambling and age verification procedures 126–7, 138–9, 217
alcohol consumption *see* binge drinking; drink problems
Alcohol Use Disorders Identification Test (AUDIT) 84
American Psychiatric Association 4
analysis of gambling episodes 176–7
Anderson, S. 45
Anjoul, F. 168
anticipated regret about gambling 92
antidepressants 203–5
antisocial behavior 67, 69
assessment instruments for gambling 91, 147–62, 233–5; classification accuracy of 153; reliability of 148; validity of 153
attention deficit hyperactivity disorder (ADHD) 65
attitudes towards gambling 10, 71, 74, 225; *see also* social acceptability of gambling
atypical antipsychotics 206–7
Australia 43–5, 69
awareness-raising 60, 253

Baiocco, R. 39
Bandura, A. 82
baselines for gambling behaviour 177
Bebo 134–5
Becoña, E. 39

behavioral competence 237
behaviorally-conditioned gamblers 13
Belgium 38
belief in the future, promotion of 238
Best, K. 219
Biganzoli, A. 38
binge drinking 79, 82, 90, 92–3, 193
binge gambling 79–80, 97, 261; definition of 91; prevalence of 90
biologically-vulnerable gamblers 13–14
Blaszczynski, A. 12, 67, 81–3, 92
bonding 236
Boudreau, B. 157
Bournstein, P.J. 219
brain function 201
Brunelle, N. 127–8, 138
bupropion 205
Byrne, A. 131

Cada, Joe 70
Campbell, C. 138
Canada 33–6, 45, 48, 131–2
Canadian Adolescent Gambling Inventory (CAGI) 147–8, 152, 160–1
Capitanucci, D. 38
Catalano, R.F. 100, 114, 120, 235, 241
Center for Substance Abuse Prevention 224–5
childhood maltreatment 9, 64, 68
China 99–108, 113–21
Chinese communities 71
Chinese G-MAP 234–5
Chinese PYD Scale 101, 115–16
Cicchetti, D.V. 153
Clean Break (docudrama) 223
clomipramine 203–4
cognitive-behavioral therapy 169
cognitive competence 236–7
cognitive therapy 177–8
community influences 69–70
competencies for healthy development 121, 231, 236–7
conditioning of gamblers 13